Haematology in Critical Care

A Practical Handbook

EDITED BY

Jecko Thachil, MRCP, FRCPath
Consultant Haematologist
Department of Haematology
Central Manchester University Hospitals NHS Foundation Trust
Manchester, UK

Quentin A. Hill, MRCP, FRCPath
Consultant Haematologist
Department of Haematology
Leeds Teaching Hospitals NHS Trust
Leeds, UK

WILEY Blackwell

This edition first published 2014
© 2014 by John Wiley & Sons, Ltd.

Registered Office
John Wiley & Sons, Ltd, The Atrium, Southern Gate, Chichester, West Sussex, PO19 8SQ, UK

Editorial Offices
9600 Garsington Road, Oxford, OX4 2DQ, UK
The Atrium, Southern Gate, Chichester, West Sussex, PO19 8SQ, UK
111 River Street, Hoboken, NJ 07030–5774, USA

For details of our global editorial offices, for customer services and for information about how to
apply for permission to reuse the copyright material in this book please see our website at
www.wiley.com/wiley-blackwell

Library of Congress Cataloging-in-Publication Data

Haematology in critical care : a practical handbook / edited by Jecko Thachil, Quentin A. Hill.
    p. ; cm.
  Includes bibliographical references and index.
  ISBN 978-1-118-27424-8 (cloth)
I. Thachil, Jecko, editor.   II. Hill, Quentin A., editor.
[DNLM: 1. Hematologic Diseases–diagnosis–Handbooks.   2. Hematologic Diseases–therapy–
Handbooks.   3. Critical Care–methods–Handbooks.   4. Hematology–methods–Handbooks. WH 39]
  RC633
  616.1'5–dc23
                                                        2014005978

A catalogue record for this book is available from the British Library.

Wiley also publishes its books in a variety of electronic formats. Some content that appears in print may not
be available in electronic books.

Cover images: blood film images – courtesy of Quentin A. Hill; ICU monitor – iStockphoto/© flubydust;
blood bag – iStockphoto/© pictorico; respiratory mask – iStockphoto/© Juanmonino
Cover design by Andy Meaden

Set in 9/12pt Minion by SPi Publisher Services, Pondicherry, India
Printed and bound in Malaysia by Vivar Printing Sdn Bhd

1   2014

Contents

iii

List of Contributors

Shubha Allard, MD, FRCP, FRCPath
Consultant Haematologist and Honorary Clinical
Senior Lecturer
Clinical Haematology
Barts and the London NHS Trust
NHS Blood and Transplant
London, UK

Arvind Arumainathan, MBChB (Hons),
MRCP, FRCPath
Consultant Haematologist
Department of Haematology
Royal Liverpool University Hospital
Liverpool, UK

Roopen Arya, MA, PhD,
FRCP, FRCPath
Professor of Thrombosis and Haemostasis
King's Thrombosis Centre
Department of Haematological Medicine
King's College Hospital NHS Foundation Trust
London, UK

Jon Bailey
Academic Clinical Fellow in Emergency Medicine
Oxford University Hospitals
John Radcliffe Hospital
Oxford, UK

Sarah A. Bennett, MRCP
Clinical Research Fellow in Coagulation
King's Thrombosis Centre
Department of Haematological Medicine
King's College Hospital NHS Foundation Trust
London, UK

Andrew Breen, MBChB, FRCA, FFICM
Consultant in Critical Care Medicine
Adult Critical Care
St James's University Hospital
Leeds, UK

Therese A. Callaghan, BSc (Hons),
MB ChB, FRCP, FRCPath
Consultant Haematologist
NHS Blood and Transplant
Liverpool, UK

Medical Department
Royal Liverpool University Hospital
Liverpool, UK

Joydeep Chakrabartty, MBBS,
MRCP, FRCPath
Consultant Haematologist
MIOT Hospital
Chennai, India

Leon Cloherty, MB ChB,
FRCA, FFICM
Consultant in Anaesthesia and Intensive Care Medicine
Department of Critical Care
Royal Liverpool University Hospital
Liverpool, UK

Daniel Collins, BPharm (Hons),
PGDipClinPharm, MRPharmS, IP
Haematology Pharmacist
Department of Pharmacy
Royal Liverpool University Hospital
Liverpool, UK

Tim Collyns, MA, MB, BChir,
FRCPath
Consultant Microbiologist
Leeds Teaching Hospitals Trust
St James's University Hospital
Leeds, UK

Nicola S. Curry, MA, MRCP, FRCPath
Consultant Haematologist
Oxford Haemophilia and Thrombosis Centre
Oxford University Hospitals
Oxford, UK

Department of Haematology
Oxford University Hospitals
Oxford University
Oxford, UK

Khaled El-Ghariani, MA, FRCP, FRCPath
Consultant in Haematology and Transfusion Medicine &
Clinical Director
Department of Stem Cells and Therapeutic Apheresis Services
NHS Blood and Transplant and Sheffield Teaching Hospitals
NHS Trust
Sheffield, UK

Honorary Senior Lecturer
University of Sheffield
Sheffield, UK

Peter A. Hampshire, FRCA, FFICM
Consultant in Intensive Care and Anaesthesia
Department of Critical Care
Royal Liverpool and Broadgreen University Hospitals
NHS Trust
Liverpool, UK

Fran Hartley, RGN, BSc,
PG Cert (Clinical Education)
Transfusion Practitioner
Hospital Transfusion Team
Leeds Teaching Hospitals NHS Trust
Leeds, UK

Catharina Hartman, MB ChB, MCEM
Specialty Registrar
Intensive Care Unit
Aberdeen Royal Infirmary
Aberdeen, UK

Stephen F. Hawkins, MB ChB (Hons),
MRCP, FRCPath, PhD
Consultant Haematologist
Department of Haematology
Royal Liverpool University Hospital
Liverpool, UK

Quentin A. Hill, MRCP, FRCPath
Consultant Haematologist
Department of Haematology
Leeds Teaching Hospitals NHS Trust
Leeds, UK

Jo Howard, MB BChir, MRCP, FRCPath
Consultant Haematologist
Department of Haematology
Guy's and St Thomas' NHS Foundation Trust
London, UK

Charlotte Kallmeyer, MD, MRCP, FRCPath
Consultant Haemotologist
Department of Haematology
St James's University Hospital
Leeds Teaching Hospitals NHS Trust
Leeds, UK

Anne Kelly, MA, MB, Bchir, MRCPCH
Clinical Research Fellow
Department of Haematology
Division of Transfusion Medicine
University of Cambridge/NHS Blood and Transplant
Cambridge
Cambridge, UK

Suzanne Kite, MA, FRCP
Consultant in Palliative Medicine
Palliative Care Team
St James's University Hospital
Leeds, UK

Jerrold H. Levy, MD, FAHA, FCCM
Professor of Anesthesiology
Department of Anesthesiology and Critical Care
Duke University School of Medicine
Durham, NC, USA

Vanessa Martlew, MA, MB ChB, FRCP,
FRCPath, FRCPEdin
Consultant Haematologist
Department of Haematology
Royal Liverpool Hospital
Liverpool, UK

Helen V. New, PhD, FRCP, FRCPath
Honorary Senior Lecturer
Consultant in Paediatric Haematology and Transfusion Medicine
Department of Paediatrics
Imperial College Healthcare NHS Trust/NHS Blood and
Transplant
London, UK

Derek R. Norfolk, MB, BS, FRCP, FRCPath
Consultant in Haematology and Transfusion Medicine
NHS Blood and Transplant
Leeds Teaching Hospitals NHS Trust
Leeds, UK

Elankumaran Paramasivam, MBBS,
MD, MRCP, EDICM, FICM
Consultant in Respiratory and Intensive Care Medicine
St James's University Hospital
Leeds, UK

Amrana Qureshi, MB BChir, MRCPCH,
FRCPath
Consultant Paediatric Haematologist
Paediatric Haematology and Oncology Children's Hospital
John Radcliffe Hospital
Oxford, UK

Amin Rahemtulla, PhD, FRCP
Consultant Haematologist
Department of Haematology
Imperial College Healthcare NHS Trust
Hammersmith Hospital
London, UK

Andrew Retter, MBBS, BSc, MRCP, DICM
Haematology Registrar
Department of Haematology
Guy's and St Thomas' NHS Foundation Trust
London, UK

Intensive Care Department
Guy's and St Thomas' NHS Foundation Trust
London, UK

Michael Richards, MA, BM, BCh, DM,
MRCP, FRCPath
Department of Paediatric Haematology
Consultant Paediatric Haematologist
Leeds Children's Hospital
Leeds, UK

Marie Scully, BSc (Hons), MD, MRCP,
FRCPath
Consultant Haematologist
Department of Haematology
University College Hospital London
London, UK

John Snowden, BSc (Hons), MB ChB,
MD, FRCP, FRCPath
Consultant Haematologist and Director of BMT
Department of Haematology
Sheffield Teaching Hospitals NHS Foundation Trust
South Yorkshire, UK

Honorary Professor
Department of Oncology
University of Sheffield
Sheffield, UK

Simon J. Stanworth,
FRCP, FRCPath, DPhil
Consultant Haematologist
NHS Blood and Transplant/Oxford University
Hospitals NHS Trust
John Radcliffe Hospital
Oxford, UK

Honorary Senior Clinical Lecturer
Department of Haematology
University of Oxford
Oxford, UK

Jecko Thachil, MRCP, FRCPath
Consultant Haematologist
Department of Haematology
Central Manchester University Hospitals NHS
Foundation Trust
Manchester, UK

Mari Thomas, MA (Cantab),
MRCP, FRCPath
Clinical Research Fellow
Haemostasis Research Unit
University College London
London, UK

Joost J. van Veen,
FRCP, FRCPath, MD
Consultant Haematologist
Department of Haematology
Sheffield Haemophilia and Thrombosis Centre
Sheffield Teaching Hospitals NHS Foundation Trust
Sheffield, UK

Jonathan Wallis,
BA, MB BS, FRCP, FRCPath
Consultant Haematologist
Department of Haematology
Newcastle upon Tyne NHS Acute Hospitals Trust
Newcastle upon Tyne, UK

Stephen Webber, MBChB, FRCA, FFICM
Critical Care Consultant
Department of Anaesthesia and Critical Care
Sheffield Teaching Hospitals NHS Foundation Trust
South Yorkshire, UK

Nigel Webster, MBChB, PhD, FRCA,
FRCP, FRCS, FFICM
Professor of Anaesthesia and Intensive Care
Anaesthesia and Intensive Care
Institute of Medical Sciences
University of Aberdeen
Aberdeen, UK

Richard Wenstone, MBChB,
FRCA, FFICM
Consultant Intensivist
Department of Critical Care
Royal Liverpool University Hospital
Liverpool, UK

Anne M. Winkler, MD
Assistant Professor
Department of Pathology and Laboratory Medicine
Emory University School of Medicine
Atlanta, GA, USA

Medical Director
Grady Health System Transfusion Service
Atlanta, GA, USA

Assistant Medical Directory
Emory Special Coagulation Laboratory
Atlanta, GA, USA

Stephen Wright, MRCP, FRCA, FFICM
Consultant in Intensive Care and Anaesthesia
Department of Perioperative and Critical Care
Freeman Hospital
Newcastle upon Tyne, UK

Preface

Patients with a primary haematological disorder account for 1–2% of admissions to intensive care units. In the UK, patients are usually managed on a mixed medical and surgical unit where low patient numbers may limit the degree of expertise that can be developed. In contrast, almost all critically ill patients require a full blood count and coagulation screen. These tests are frequently abnormal and require interpretation. Issues of thrombosis, bleeding, and transfusion are also extremely common in critically ill patients.

This book is a practical guide to the investigation and management of these common problems as well as the acute aspects of care in patients with a primary haematological disorder. We are full-time clinical haematologists, and both regularly attend on intensive care. We have started with an approach to abnormal laboratory tests and then taken a disease-orientated approach to topics such as coagulation and haematological malignancy. Other key topics include paediatric and neonatal care, transfusion, point-of-care testing and the emergency presentation of haematological disease.

Quentin A. Hill
Jecko Thachil

Acknowledgements

I would like to thank a number of individuals for kindly reviewing and commenting on specific areas of the text, including Dr Andy Breen, Dr Sharon English, Dr Mike Bosomworth, Dr Mervyn Davies and Professor David Bowen.

I would also like to thank my family for their support: my parents who have led by example, to Anita for her patience and to Lila and Reuben, stars twinkling at ground level.

QAH

I would like to thank my parents for their continued blessings, my wife Gail for her patience and support and my children Nimue, Neah and Izahak for the tremendous bliss.

JT

SECTION 1

Approach to Abnormal Blood Tests

CHAPTER 1

Diagnostic Approach to Anaemia in Critical Care

Stephen F. Hawkins[1] and Quentin A. Hill[2]

[1]Department of Haematology, Royal Liverpool University Hospital, Liverpool, UK
[2]Department of Haematology, Leeds Teaching Hospitals NHS Trust, Leeds, UK

Anaemia was defined by the World Health Organization as a haemoglobin (Hb) concentration less than 120 g/L (Hb < 36%) in females and less than 130 g/L (Hb < 39%) in males, but the lower level of the reference range for Hb may vary between laboratories. It is common in critically ill patients, occurring in up to 80% of those in intensive care units (ICUs) [1] with 50–70% having a Hb less than 90 g/L during their admission. By reducing oxygen delivery to the tissues, this may be tolerated poorly in those with cardiorespiratory compromise. In critical care, anaemia is commonly due to multiple factors such as inflammation, blood loss, renal impairment and nutritional deficiencies [2, 3] (see Table 17.1), but it is important to consider treatable causes and identify when more detailed investigation is needed. The role of transfusional support is considered in Chapter 17.

Tissue hypoxia exerts physiological control of Hb by triggering the release of erythropoietin (EPO) by the kidneys, which stimulates bone marrow (BM) erythropoiesis. Hb will increase so long as there are no underlying BM disorders (e.g. myelodysplasia) and there are adequate supplies of iron, vitamin B12 and folic acid. When a rapid marrow response occurs (e.g. following haemorrhage or replacement of a deficient vitamin), reticulocytes (young erythrocytes) enter the blood in large numbers and can be identified on the blood film (polychromasia) or by an elevated reticulocyte count. The normal lifespan for erythrocytes is 120 days, before being removed by the reticuloendothelial system (predominantly in the spleen and liver), but their lifespan may be shortened by inflammation, haemorrhage or haemolysis.

Diagnostic approach to anaemia in critical care

In the history, note pre-existing co-morbidities including renal and cardiac impairment. Also note medications, diet and symptoms suggestive of blood loss. Examine for jaundice, lymphadenopathy or organomegaly.

- If there is a sudden unexpected drop in Hb, this may be a sampling error; consider repeating the full blood count (FBC).
- Is the anaemia acute or chronic? This may inform the diagnosis, likely tolerance of anaemia and treatment strategy. Only 10–15% of ICU patients have chronic anaemia prior to admission [4].
- Is the anaemia isolated or are there other cytopenias? Thrombocytopenia (Chapter 3) is also a common finding (~40% of ICU patients) and will therefore often coexist with anaemia in critically ill patients. Common causes of both include sepsis, organ failure and acute blood loss, but important differentials include disseminated intravascular coagulation (DIC) (Chapter 9) and thrombotic microangiopathies (TMAs) (Chapter 11). Review the

Haematology in Critical Care: A Practical Handbook, First Edition. Edited by Jecko Thachil and Quentin A. Hill.

clotting and blood film. Haemophagocytic lymphohistiocytosis (HLH) is an important cause of fever and cytopenias that can present with single or multiple organ failure (see succeeding text under extrinsic causes of extravascular haemolysis).

• Pancytopenia may be an artefact (i.e. dilution during sampling) or result from BM failure or infiltration, infection, HLH, hypersplenism, drugs, autoimmune disease or megaloblastic anaemia. If pancytopenia is present, examine for splenomegaly and request a blood film and haematinics. If the cause remains unclear, the advice of a haematologist should be sought as a BM examination may be required.

If the cause of an *isolated* anaemia remains unclear, it is worth classifying on the basis of the mean cell volume (MCV) as this helps to direct further investigation (Figure 1.1).

Normocytic anaemia (MCV within the normal range)

Anaemia is most commonly normocytic in critically ill patients and usually multifactorial [4]. Iatrogenic reasons include frequent blood sampling and haemodilution (intravenous fluid administration). Occult blood loss can occur as a result of gastrointestinal mucosal inflammation and contributed to by coagulation defects, thrombocytopenia and uraemia. Another important reason is secondary anaemia, also termed *anaemia of chronic disease* (AoCD) or *anaemia of inflammation*. This is the most common cause of anaemia in hospitalized patients and can be caused by infection, cancer, autoimmune disease or chronic kidney disease [5]. This results in a *functional* iron deficiency, whereby adequate iron stores are present but the availability of iron for erythropoiesis is reduced. Hepcidin, a peptide produced by the liver in

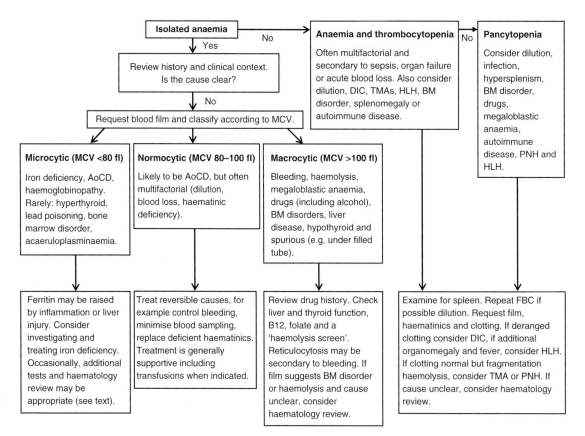

Figure 1.1 Investigation of anaemia in critical care. MCV, mean cell volume; DIC, disseminated intravascular coagulation; TMAs, thrombotic microangiopathies; HLH, haemophagocytic lymphohistiocytosis; BM, bone marrow; AoCD, anaemia of chronic disease; PNH, paroxysmal nocturnal haemoglobinuria.

response to inflammatory cytokines, may be at least in part responsible for this phenomenon. Typically, ferritin is elevated and serum iron and transferrin saturation are low. Iron supplementation usually produces no improvement (in contrast to true iron deficiency). In addition to functional iron deficiency, inflammation results in reduced EPO production, reduced marrow sensitivity to EPO and shortened red cell survival.

Check haematinics as combined deficiencies can result in a normal MCV. Additionally, due to the acute phase response, a normal ferritin does not exclude iron deficiency. Consideration should be given to the possibility of occult or recent bleeding. The anaemia is likely to resolve with improvement of the underlying conditions. Meanwhile, supportive management (including transfusion when required; see Chapter 17) is the mainstay of therapy, and blood sampling should be kept to a minimum.

Microcytic anaemia (MCV below the normal range)

This is often a result of iron deficiency (blood loss, malabsorption or dietary deficiency). It can also occur during prolonged and severe illness as an extreme form of AoCD. Less commonly, microcytosis can be due to a haemoglobinopathy (e.g. thalassaemia trait), acaeruloplasminaemia, myelodysplasia, hyperthyroidism, lead poisoning and some rare congenital conditions (e.g. congenital sideroblastic anaemia).

Iron deficiency can be associated with a thrombocytosis, especially with bleeding. Less frequently, severe iron deficiency may also result in a leukopenia and thrombocytopenia. The blood film may show hypochromic, microcytic red cells, polychromasia and pencil cell poikilocytes. The usual tests of iron status (ferritin and iron studies) are less likely to be informative in the critically ill patient. A reliable measure of iron storage is specially stained BM aspirate slides, but this may not identify acute blood loss and is not usually justifiable solely for this purpose. Instead, if the clinical picture and blood film are compatible, consider a trial of iron replacement and appropriate investigations to identify a cause.

Consider additional testing:
• Lead level if prominent basophilic stippling on film or clinical suspicion
• Thyroid function if relevant clinical symptoms/signs
• BM if dysplastic blood film (haematology referral)

• Hb electrophoresis if target cells, long-standing microcytosis, iron replete or not of northern European ethnicity

Macrocytic anaemia (MCV above the normal range)

The leading causes of macrocytic anaemia are alcohol abuse, megaloblastic anaemia (deficiency of vitamin B12 and/or folic acid) and accelerated erythropoiesis (e.g. in response to bleeding or haemolysis).

Other causes include medications (e.g. some chemotherapy agents, hydroxycarbamide, methotrexate, azathioprine, zidovudine, phenytoin), liver dysfunction, hypothyroidism, aplastic anaemia and myelodysplasia. Macrocytosis can occur in pregnancy, in Down syndrome and in smokers.

Spurious causes of macrocytosis include cold agglutinins (red cells agglutinate due to an autoantibody; this will correct by warming a repeat FBC sample), high white cell counts (e.g. acute leukaemia), severe hyperglycaemia (in patient or by sampling close to an intravenous dextrose infusion causing osmotic swelling) or an underfilled tube at venepuncture (increased concentration of EDTA anticoagulant).
• Initial Investigations would include liver and thyroid function, B12/folate levels and screening tests for haemolysis (lactate dehydrogenase [LDH], reticulocyte count, haptoglobin, direct Coombs' test [DCT], bilirubin and blood film examination).

Alcohol excess may be suggested by the history, examination or other blood results (e.g. raised gamma glutamyl transferase). The resulting anaemia and macrocytosis are usually mild, in contrast to megaloblastic anaemia where the MCV may be as high as 120 fl. The blood film may show typical megaloblastic features such as oval macrocytosis and neutrophil hypersegmentation. Folic acid replacement should not be given unless the vitamin B12 level is known as by stimulating erythropoiesis, folic acid may aggravate B12 deficiency thereby precipitating subacute combined degeneration of the cord. In B12 deficiency, heart failure may arise through overenthusiastic blood transfusion, and B12 replacement is usually sufficient. If transfusion is judged essential, transfuse one unit slowly, consider diuretic cover, and then reassess.

Myelodysplasia is a clonal BM disorder characterized by ineffective erythropoiesis. There may be dysplastic changes on blood film or additional cytopenias. Although onset is usually insidious, patients may present acutely with infection or transformation to acute myeloid leukaemia and, if suspected, require a haematology referral.

Haemolysis causes anaemia when increased red cell destruction exceeds the marrow's capacity to compensate. Typical findings include a reduced haptoglobin, raised LDH and raised unconjugated bilirubin, but these are not fully sensitive or specific. For example, haptoglobin rises as an acute phase response and may fall in liver disease and megaloblastic anaemia and can be congenitally low. The reticulocyte count will only rise if the marrow is healthy. A positive DCT suggests autoimmune haemolysis but can also be positive in other circumstances such as following therapeutic immunoglobulin infusion, recent stem cell or organ transplantation or alloimmunization following recent blood transfusion. Results must therefore be taken in clinical context before diagnosing haemolysis.

Haemolysis can be intravascular or extravascular. Acute intravascular haemolysis can be life-threatening and may require renal or cardiovascular support. Patients may develop chills, fevers, rigors, flank or back pain, dyspnoea, dizziness, tachycardia, hypotension, dark urine, oliguria and shock. Red cell fragments may be present on the blood film; LDH is more markedly elevated compared with extravascular haemolysis. Urine and plasma may become red or brown due to the presence of free Hb. Some Hb is taken up by renal cells and iron stored as haemosiderin is subsequently shed into the urine where it can be detected 1–2 weeks after the onset of haemolysis.

In patients where severe intravascular haemolysis is a major presenting feature, consider:
• Was there recent blood transfusion? Most immediate haemolytic transfusion reactions are due to ABO mismatch. Bacterial contamination can present with a similar picture. Investigation and management of transfusion reactions are discussed in Chapter 14.
• Is there a history of fever and foreign travel or splenectomy? Investigate for falciparum malaria with thin and thick films (also antigen testing if available). Bartonellosis and babesiosis can also invade the red cell, cause haemolysis and be visible on the blood film (see Chapter 6). Severe babesiosis often occurs in patients with a history of prior splenectomy.
• Always consider *Clostridium perfringens* sepsis. Massive intravascular haemolysis due to alpha-toxin occurs in approximately 10% of cases and is associated

with shock and mortality of up to 80%, usually within hours of presentation. Risk factors include diabetes, malignancy or following abdominal surgery. The primary focus is usually hepatobiliary, intestinal or uterine. Infection of a traumatic injury (gas gangrene) can also lead to sepsis. Spherocytes and ghost cells (depigmented red cells) feature on the blood film. Tissue or blood cultures confirm diagnosis. Treatment involves early high-dose antibiotics (e.g. penicillin and clindamycin) and surgical debridement of devitalized tissue.
• Review medications (including peri-operative antibiotics and over-the-counter medication). An important differential is drug (or drug metabolite)-induced immune haemolytic anaemia (e.g. second- or third-generation cephalosporins or diclofenac). The DCT may be negative if haemolysis is massive. Further exposure to the causative drug can be fatal.
• Has there been accidental (or intentional) ingestion/inhalation of toxic substances? Haemolysis is caused by oxidative damage with the formation of physiologically useless methaemoglobin and denatured Hb, which precipitates (Heinz bodies), damaging the red cell membrane and leading to extravascular and, if severe, intravascular haemolysis. Symptoms of methaemoglobinaemia may also be prominent including cyanosis, headache and fatigue, leading to arrhythmias, seizures and coma in severe cases. Blood is characteristically a chocolate brown colour.
  ○ Nitrates. Present in fertilizer and can result in methaemoglobinaemia in infants exposed to well water or vegetable juice. Inhaled amyl nitrite (poppers, liquid gold) used *recreationally* can cause fatal oxidant injury.
  ○ Copper sulphate poisoning. Rare in the UK but in some countries is sold over the counter for pesticide and home-made glue and is burnt in houses for religious purposes by Buddhists and Hindus. Hydrated crystals are marine blue and attractive to children. Ingestion is also associated with erosive gastropathy, hepatitis, acute renal failure and rhabdomyolysis.
  ○ Sodium chlorate (a weed killer). Not authorized in the European Union member states after May 2010 (decision 2008/865/EC).
  ○ Arsine gas. Produced in industrial processes.
• Are symptoms associated with cold exposure? In paroxysmal cold haemoglobinuria (PCH), haemolysis is provoked by the cold, resulting in haematuria, back or abdominal pain and fever. It usually follows a viral

infection in children and, although often transient, can be severe. The DCT is positive and PCH is confirmed by the Donath–Landsteiner test.

• Also consider glucose-6-phosphate dehydrogenase (G6PD) deficiency. There may be a personal or family history and a recent trigger for haemolysis. It is an inherited, X-linked red cell enzyme defect resulting in susceptibility to oxidative damage. It affects an estimated 400 million people worldwide and is most prevalent in sub-Saharan African countries. As well as a variably severe chronic extravascular haemolysis, oxidative stress such as infection, ingestion of fava (broad) beans and various medications (e.g. dapsone, primaquine, nitrofurantoin) leads to acute intravascular haemolysis and bite cells on the blood film. Blood tests are readily available but false-negative results can occur in the presence of a reticulocytosis (higher G6PD levels).

• Are there additional cytopenias or a history of venous thrombosis? Paroxysmal nocturnal haemoglobinuria (PNH) is an acquired stem cell disorder that renders blood cells susceptible to complement-mediated injury. It is readily diagnosed with peripheral blood flow cytometry. See Chapter 32 for further details.

Intravascular haemolysis may not be the major clinical feature of a disorder and is not always fulminant. Examples are listed:

• Renal failure – red cell fragments may be present due to uraemia, complications of haemodialysis or the underlying cause of renal failure (e.g. lupus nephritis).

• Other extracorporeal circuits (e.g. ventricular assist devices, cardiopulmonary bypass circuits) or following placement of an indwelling transjugular intrahepatic portosystemic shunt (TIPS).

• Severe burns.

• Drowning.

• TMAs. Associations include HIV, autoimmune disease, malignancy, pregnancy, diarrhoeal illness, hypertension and certain drugs (e.g. ciclosporin).

• DIC.

• Cardiac periprosthetic or perivalvular leaks.

• Cold agglutinin disease (CAD). Autoimmune haemolytic anaemia (AIHA) is caused by a cold reactive IgM antibody. The DCT is usually positive to complement only and agglutination is seen on the blood film. The patient and blood products for transfusion should be kept warm

• March haemoglobinuria. Caused by intensive exercise, e.g. long-distance running.

• Oxidant drugs (e.g. dapsone, salazopyrin) and inherited unstable haemoglobins can give rise to chronic intravascular haemolysis.

• Zieve's syndrome. Rarely, intravascular haemolysis has been described associated with cirrhosis and alcohol excess.

• Wilson's disease. Usually presents with liver or neurological disease, or through family screening, but can occasionally present with acute intravascular haemolysis.

Haemolysis that is mainly extravascular can be caused by intrinsic red cell defects or extrinsic factors.

Intrinsic defects: inherited conditions give rise to a long-term haemolytic state, but decompensated anaemia can occur with additional stress such as haematinic deficiency, pregnancy or infection. Aplastic crisis, classically by parvovirus B19, results in transient interruption of red cell production and reticulocytopenia, which can cause a life-threatening anaemia. Intrinsic defects are reviewed in more depth in Chapter 32.

• Disorders of Hb. In thalassaemia, an imbalance of globin chains leads to their precipitation and reduced red cell survival. Structural Hb variants can give rise to sickle cell disease (see Chapter 18).

• Red cell membrane defects (e.g. hereditary spherocytosis). May be suspected from blood film appearance. Variable severity and age of presentation. Sometimes require splenectomy.

• Red cell enzyme deficiencies (e.g. pyruvate kinase or pyrimidine 5′ nucleotidase deficiency). These rare inherited conditions usually give rise to a chronic non-spherocytic haemolytic anaemia.

Extrinsic factors:

• Liver disease. Mild effect due to alteration of the red cell membrane (e.g. acanthocytes, stomatocytes).

• Splenomegaly. Results in increased red cell sequestration and destruction.

• Delayed haemolytic transfusion reaction – typically seen 1–2 weeks after transfusion, caused by an anamnestic immune response due to an antibody undetectable during routine pre-transfusion testing.

• Warm AIHA. Spherocytes are seen on the blood film. DCT is positive.

• Immune haemolysis can also be drug induced or follow solid organ and BM transplantation.

• HLH. May be primary or secondary to infection or malignancy. Phagocytosis in the marrow, liver, spleen or lymph nodes leads to cytopenias, organomegaly, fever, deranged liver function and coagulopathy. There may also be neurological symptoms and lymphadenopathy. Fibrinogen may be low and fasting triglycerides and ferritin high.

In conclusion, anaemia is common and usually multi-factorial. The cause may be clear from the clinical context, but, if not, classification according to the MCV is helpful in directing investigations. Anaemia is most often normo-cytic and contributed to by blood loss, haemodilution, impaired EPO release and functional iron deficiency. Consider a haematology referral: where anaemia is promi-nent and the cause unclear despite investigation and where haemolysis, haemoglobinopathy, TMA or myelodysplasia are suspected or in cases of an unexplained pancytopenia.

References

1 Walsh TS, Saleh EE. Anaemia during critical illness. Br J Anaesth 2006;97:278–91.
2 Fink MP. Pathophysiology of intensive care unit-acquired anemia. Crit Care 2004;8(Suppl. 2):S9–10.
3 Hayden SJ, Albert TJ, Watkins TR et al. Anemia in critical illness: Insights into etiology, consequences and management. Am J Respir Crit Care Med 2012;185(10):1049–57.
4 Walsh TS, Wyncoll DLA, Stanworth SJ. Managing anaemia in critically ill adults. BMJ 2010;341:547–51.
5 Davis SL, Littlewood TJ. The investigation and treatment of secondary anaemia. Blood Rev 2012;26(2):65–71.

CHAPTER 2
Leukopenia

Stephen F. Hawkins[1], Jecko Thachil[2] and Quentin A. Hill[3]

[1]Department of Haematology, Royal Liverpool University Hospital, Liverpool, UK
[2]Department of Haematology, Central Manchester University Hospitals NHS Foundation Trust, Manchester, UK
[3]Department of Haematology, Leeds Teaching Hospitals NHS Trust, Leeds, UK

Leukopenia is defined as a total white blood count (WBC) or leukocyte count below the lower limit of the reference range for the laboratory in question (e.g. $<3.5 \times 10^9/L$). Leukopenia on admission to intensive care occurs in approximately 7% of admissions and is associated with increased mortality [1]. It can be a result of a reduction in any of the major subtypes of WBC (neutrophils, lymphocytes, monocytes, eosinophils or basophils), but most frequently neutrophils and/or lymphocytes, which contribute most to the total WBC count. The differential diagnosis of neutropenia and lymphopenia can be seen in Table 2.1.

Neutropenia

The severity of neutropenia may be divided into mild ($1.5 - 2 \times 10^9/L$), moderate ($0.6 - 1.4 \times 10^9/L$) or severe ($\leq 0.5 \times 10^9/L$). Persistent and severe neutropenia is more likely to be clinically significant and lead to complications. The pathogenesis of neutropenia can include decreased production from the bone marrow, increased destruction in the blood circulation, increased margination to the vascular endothelium, neutrophil aggregation and splenic pooling.

In the ICU setting, neutropenia is usually secondary, most commonly to drugs or infection. A primary haematological cause such as leukaemia or another malignancy will rarely develop in a patient who arrived in the ICU with a normal neutrophil count. A drug-induced cause for neutropenia can easily be overlooked due to the multiple agents the patients may receive. A temporal relationship between the commencement of any drug and the development of neutropenia is usually the only clue and may not be considered. A sudden drop in the count can also suggest drug-induced neutropenia, and often, the neutropenia resolves soon after the discontinuation of the drug.

Any infection can lead to neutropenia, most often viral infections such as influenza, cytomegalovirus (CMV) and respiratory syncytial virus. The most likely bacterial cause for neutropenia is a chronic infection like tuberculosis, brucellosis or typhoid rather than streptococcal or staphylococcal infections. The pathogenesis for this neutropenia includes margination and sequestration in the spleen and in the lungs. HIV infection can frequently cause neutropenia, with over two-thirds of patients being neutropenic sometime during their illness. The mechanisms for this include antibody formation, bone marrow suppression and cytokine-mediated neutrophil destruction, while certain antiretroviral agents may decrease neutrophil counts.

Immunological causes like vasculitis and systemic lupus erythematosus can lead to neutropenia through antibody-mediated destruction. Disease control often leads to resolution of the neutropenia. Haemophagocytic

Haematology in Critical Care: A Practical Handbook, First Edition. Edited by Jecko Thachil and Quentin A. Hill.
© 2014 John Wiley & Sons, Ltd. Published 2014 by John Wiley & Sons, Ltd.

Table 2.1 Differential diagnosis of leukopenia.

Sepsis
Infection
    Viral (e.g. HIV)
    Bacterial (e.g. TB)
Post-infective
Drug-induced (e.g. phenytoin, cotrimoxazole)
B12 and/or folate deficiency
Immunological (e.g. SLE)
Bone marrow failure (e.g. haematological malignancies)

syndrome can cause cytopenias due to macrophage overactivity, consuming blood cells and their precursors. This is can be primary or associated with rheumatological diseases, malignancy and viral infections. Presenting features are discussed in Chapter 1.

Vitamin B12 or folate deficiency can present with neutropenia, with folic acid deficiency developing relatively quickly in patients not supplemented. Associated macrocytic anaemia may provide a clue to this diagnosis and can easily be treated with replacement. Copper deficiency may also be associated with neutropenia due to maturation arrest in the bone marrow or antibody formation. This can occur in patients receiving total parenteral nutrition without adequate copper supplementation, typically with a normocytic anaemia and a normal platelet count. Bone marrow examination can support the diagnosis. Some rarer causes of neutropenia include patients with ketoacidosis and hyperglycaemia, haemodialysis (activation of complement by dialyser membranes, which causes neutrophil aggregation) and cardiopulmonary bypass surgery.

When neutropenia is identified, determine whether it is isolated or associated with other cytopenias. Pancytopenia usually suggests the presence of bone marrow failure (from any cause including drugs) or hypersplenism, usually merits a haematology referral and is discussed in more detail in Chapter 1. The risk of severe, potentially life-threatening infection increases as the neutrophil count drops and is highest for those with severe neutropenia ($<0.5 \times 10^9$/L) [2], especially when the mechanism is marrow failure since there is no reserve capacity to produce neutrophils. Also review the trend in the WBC count to ascertain whether the problem is new or potentially long standing and to correlate its development with any changes in medication. Neutropenia developing in a septic patient is most likely to be a result

of the sepsis, and little specific testing is required other than examination of the blood film which may show characteristic features in the remaining neutrophils (e.g. toxic granulation and left shift). The count should improve as the sepsis resolves, but if not, alternative diagnoses should be considered. If the cause remains unclear, or if the neutropenia is severe, a haematology opinion should be requested as a bone marrow aspirate and trephine biopsy may be required.

Lymphopenia

Lymphopenia can be a pre-existing problem or can develop during the course of an illness. The approach is similar to neutropenia in terms of reviewing the history and previous results. Long-standing lymphopenia is most likely a result of chronic viral infection (such as HIV) but can occur due to generalized marrow failure diseases or (rarely) congenital immunodeficiency syndromes. A sudden-onset lymphopenia may be a result of an acute viral infection (including HIV, EBV and CMV) or due to marrow suppression by drugs (again numerous causes).

Management

In addition to identifying and treating the root cause of leukopenia where possible, it is important to recognize that patients are susceptible to infection and that infections can progress more rapidly than in those with normal WBC counts. Consequently, patients with leukopenia should ideally be managed in a side room (i.e. protective isolation), and if infection is suspected (due to fever or other clinical features such as hypotension), urgent treatment is required. Cultures should be taken and antibiotics started without delay (approach to neutropenic fever in haematology patients is discussed in Chapter 20). The choice of antibiotics should take into account local policy. In some centres, initial empirical therapy for neutropenic sepsis is with intravenous piperacillin–tazobactam, but in others, this is combined with an aminoglycoside (most commonly gentamicin) if renal function has previously been satisfactory. In patients who are allergic to penicillin, options may include meropenem or aztreonam with gentamicin. This will depend on the severity of the penicillin allergy and on local policy, which is influenced by

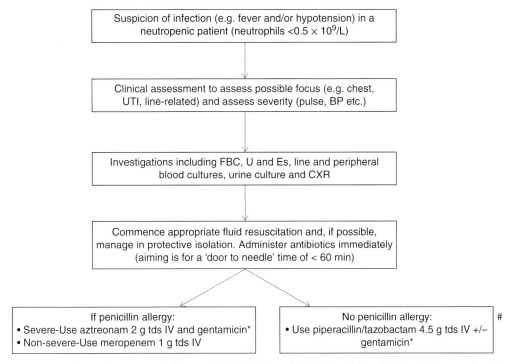

Figure 2.1 A suggested approach to neutropenic fever. *, Initial dosing is determined by body weight and eGFR and subsequent doses should be guided by plasma gentamicin levels. #, Antibiotic choices will differ according to local resistance patterns and local policy should be consulted.

regional variations in microbiological data. Figure 2.1 shows a suggested pathway for neutropenic fever though it is advisable to consult local guidelines.

In some cases, granulocyte colony-stimulating factor (G-CSF) may be given to facilitate neutrophil recovery, but this can make bone marrow interpretation difficult. Studies looking at G-CSF in the setting of chemotherapy-induced febrile neutropenia have shown that its use reduces the duration of neutropenia and shortens hospital stays but does not improve overall survival [3]. As a result, its use is generally limited to selected groups of patients such as those with severe neutropenia (<0.1 × 10⁹/L) expected to last for more than 10 days and patients with severe hypotensive sepsis. The use of G-CSF remains controversial in the setting of intensive care, and discussion with a haematologist is advisable.

In summary, leukopenia is not uncommon in critical care and is usually due to neutropenia. In the setting of critical illness, infection and sepsis are the predominant causes of leukopenia, though drug-induced reductions are also common. Laboratory investigations should include a blood film and assays of B12 and folate. A haematology referral may be appropriate when the leukopenia is severe or persistent and if advice is needed regarding the management.

References

1 Waheed U, Williams P, Brett S, Baldock G, Soni N. White cell count and intensive care outcome. Anaesthesia 2003;58(2):180–2.
2 Munshi HG, Montgomery RB. Evidence-based case review: severe neutropenia, a diagnostic approach. West J Med 2000;172(4):248–52.
3 Clark OA, Lyman GH, Castro AA, Clark LG, Djulbegovic B. Colony-stimulating factors for chemotherapy-induced febrile neutropenia: a meta-analysis of randomized controlled trials. J Clin Oncol 2005;23:4198–214.

CHAPTER 3

Thrombocytopenia in the Intensive Care Unit

Jecko Thachil

Department of Haematology, Central Manchester University Hospitals NHS Foundation Trust, Manchester, UK

Introduction

Thrombocytopenia is the most common haemostatic abnormality seen in the intensive care unit (ICU). The reported incidence of thrombocytopenia in this setting ranges from 15% to 60% and is more frequently seen in surgical and trauma patients (35–41%) compared to medical patients (20–25%). Approximately half of the patients with thrombocytopenia already have this on arrival at the ICU, while the remainder usually develops it in the first 4 days of being in the ICU.

Prognostic significance

The degree of thrombocytopenia has been regarded as a marker of illness severity in critically ill patients. A lower platelet count on admission to ICU correlates with higher Simplified Acute Physiology Scores (SAPS), Multiple Organ Dysfunction Scores (MODS) and Acute Physiology and Chronic Health Evaluation (APACHE) scores than those with normal platelet counts. It is also an independent predictor of mortality in ICU with the severity of thrombocytopenia being inversely related to survival. A four- to sixfold increase in mortality has been reported if the platelet count is reduced by more than 50% during ICU admission or if the thrombocytopenia is sustained for more than 4 days. Thrombocytopenia has also been associated with longer hospital and ICU stays.

Clinical presentation

Although the well-recognized clinical manifestations of thrombocytopenia are purpura, petechiae and bleeding, it is more common for these symptoms to be absent when the low platelet count is detected. Although the classical definition of thrombocytopenia is a platelet count less than 150×10^9/L, significant or spontaneous bleeding rarely occurs with a platelet count above 50×10^9/L (unless there are coexistent reasons for platelet dysfunction). Diffuse bleeding and haemorrhage from venepuncture sites may accompany thrombocytopenia and often due to increased vascular permeability and poor vasoconstriction rather than the low platelet count per se. At the same time, the risk of bleeding increases four- to fivefold with a count less than 50×10^9/L. Spontaneous intracerebral haemorrhage is rare in ICU patients with low platelet count (frequency of 0.3–0.5%) and is most commonly seen when the platelet count is less than 10×10^9/L.

In contrast to bleeding, thrombocytopenia in ICU may be the result of increased platelet aggregation in the different vasculature. Often, thrombocytopenia is an accompaniment of organ failure, especially renal impairment and respiratory distress syndrome. Platelet aggregation in the organs has been described as a contributory factor in these clinical states. In this regard, a dropping platelet count may be considered as a predictor of impending organ failure, and the aetiological causes may be sought

Haematology in Critical Care: A Practical Handbook, First Edition. Edited by Jecko Thachil and Quentin A. Hill.
© 2014 John Wiley & Sons, Ltd. Published 2014 by John Wiley & Sons, Ltd.

and treated early. In addition to microvascular thrombosis, low platelet count can also be associated with an increased risk of thrombosis in disorders such as microangiopathic haemolytic anaemia or heparin-induced thrombocytopenia, where once again platelet aggregation is the underlying pathophysiological mechanism.

Another consequence of thrombocytopenia is the increased vascular permeability, which occurs with the very low platelet count. Platelets are integral constituents of the mechanisms necessary for the maintenance of the vascular integrity. Hence, in cases of thrombocytopenia, there are increased capillary leakage and consequent vascular oedema, clinically evident as generalized oedema, and adult respiratory distress syndrome.

Specific characteristics of thrombocytopenia in the ICU

• The cause of thrombocytopenia in ICU patients is usually multifactorial.
• Although an easily recognizable cause of drop in platelet count may be identified, several other reasons may coexist.
• Different reasons for thrombocytopenia may develop over the course of time – for example, drug-induced thrombocytopenia may not *improve* since sepsis has set in, causing thrombocytopenia due to a different mechanism.
• Unsuccessful management of thrombocytopenia may mean all the underlying reasons have not been adequately managed.
• As discussed earlier, low platelet count can present as organ failure, thrombosis and, less often, bleeding.

Causes of thrombocytopenia in the ICU

For practical purposes, five different mechanisms for thrombocytopenia may be considered:
• Decreased platelet production
• Increased destruction
• Increased aggregation
• Dilution
• Sequestration

Decreased platelet production

Bone marrow suppression leading to thrombocytopenia can occur in response to drugs, infections and nutritional deficiencies (vitamin B_{12}, folate, copper) and as a consequence of bone marrow infiltration with metastases and haematological disorders such as leukaemia.

Drug-induced thrombocytopenia is extremely common in ICU and can be due to myelosuppression, e.g. chemotherapy agents, or via immune-mediated mechanisms, e.g. heparin. Many antibiotics like teicoplanin, penicillin derivatives and meropenem can cause low platelet count and are often overlooked. Proton pump inhibitors and diuretics are the other common, but not often considered, culprits. Temporal relationship with the commencement of the drug and the drop in platelet count is the only way to suspect drug-induced thrombocytopenia, while confirmation requires their discontinuation and recovery of the platelet count over the next few days. Definitive laboratory investigations to confirm the implicated drug are often difficult.

Acute viral infections such as rubella, mumps, varicella, cytomegalovirus (CMV) and Epstein–Barr virus (EBV) can cause thrombocytopenia as well as more chronic infections such as hepatitis C and human immunodeficiency virus (HIV). Bacterial infections and fungal diseases often cause thrombocytosis initially and then cause thrombocytopenia due to platelet aggregation rather than a problem of platelet production. In this context, it is useful to note that platelets actively participate in the immune effector function of the body by secreting granules, which are microbicidal. It also works alongside the different white cells including neutrophils and monocytes to destroy the invading microorganisms. In the case of viral infections, thrombocytopenia is often a consequence of the phenomenon *molecular mimicry* where the virus resides inside a protective barrier created by the platelets, which then become immunogenic and are destroyed by the body's defence system.

Excessive alcohol intake can also have a direct toxic effect on megakaryocytes, resulting in decreased platelet production. This can be exacerbated further by coexisting nutritional deficiencies such as vitamin B_{12} or folate deficiency. In addition to the effect on bone marrow, alcohol excess affects the platelets through the development of liver cirrhosis. The liver produces the platelet hormone thrombopoietin, which becomes deficient in liver cirrhosis, leading to low platelet count.

Portal hypertension, which can accompany liver cirrhosis, can also cause thrombocytopenia.

Bone marrow disorders like leukaemia and lymphoma are not common presentations in the ICU. It may be argued for this reason that bone marrow examination may not be an ideal test in the ICU patient for the diagnosis of cause for thrombocytopenia, although one reason for performing this procedure is to obtain specimens for microbiological culture in some chronic infections like tuberculosis.

Increased platelet destruction

Thrombocytopenia due to increased platelet destruction occurs via immune- or nonimmune-mediated mechanisms. Immune-mediated thrombocytopenia results from the production of antibodies against platelets, which can occur in response to viral infections (EBV, CMV), drugs (heparin-induced thrombocytopenia) or following transfusion of blood products (post-transfusion purpura (PTP)). Nonimmune thrombocytopenia arises from the physical destruction of platelets by extracorporeal circuits used in cardiopulmonary bypass and haemofiltration machines and by intravascular devices such as intra-aortic balloon pumps. Increased platelet destruction can also occur in vasculitides, where immune-mediated destruction is the cause.

Increased platelet aggregation

Increased platelet aggregation is probably the main cause of thrombocytopenia in bacterial sepsis. Platelets can aggregate with each other and also with other cells including monocytes and neutrophils, decreasing the number of total circulating individual platelets. In addition, there is also an increased binding of platelets to activated endothelium, which leads to platelet sequestration and destruction in micro-vessels. Bacterial lipopolysaccharide and inflammatory cytokines also induce platelet aggregation.

Increased platelet consumption also occurs in acute and chronic disseminated intravascular coagulation (DIC) and in the thrombotic microangiopathic disorders, thrombotic thrombocytopenic purpura (TTP), haemolytic uremic syndrome (HUS) and HELLP syndrome in pregnant women (characterized by haemolysis, elevated liver enzymes and low platelets). Platelet aggregation can also be a manifestation of massive pulmonary embolism. Recently, acute drop in platelet count has been described as a phenomenon in thrombotic storm where widespread thrombosis occurs in different organs and leads to thrombocytopenia due to increased consumption.

Dilution

Patients with massive blood loss develop thrombocytopenia via the direct loss of platelets in the blood from the site of bleeding and through the consumption of platelets utilized in clot formation in response to the haemorrhage. Dilutional thrombocytopenia may also arise in this setting if large volumes of crystalloid or colloid solutions are infused into the patient or if inadequate replacement of platelets occurs in relation to the transfusion of red cells and plasma blood products.

Sequestration

Platelet sequestration secondary to splenomegaly can occur in cirrhosis, congestive heart failure, portal hypertension, infection and myeloproliferative disorders. Approximately one-third of the total platelet mass is sequestered in the spleen normally, and this can increase to 90% in massive splenomegaly. These patients are less likely to bleed from their thrombocytopenia as the platelets are able to enter the circulation in response to bleeding and have a normal lifespan.

Diagnostic approach to thrombocytopenia in the ICU setting

- In order to establish the cause of thrombocytopenia in critically ill patients, it is important to obtain an accurate history of their current illness and past medical history.
- Drug history is one of the most important checks in a thrombocytopenic ITU patient. A review of all the medications which the patient has recently received (including non-prescription and recreational drugs) should be done. The timing of onset of each medication in relation to the development of thrombocytopenia should be considered.
- Exposure to heparin in the ICU setting as a result of central catheter flushes or haemofiltration/dialysis should also be excluded as a potential cause of thrombocytopenia.
- A review of the timing of all transfusions of blood products received by the patient should also occur in order to consider PTP as a possible diagnosis.
- Clinical examination should focus on any evidence of bleeding or microthrombosis. Splenomegaly may be a relevant finding in this context.

Investigations

1 Previous laboratory results can be used to determine the rate of thrombocytopenia development and if the thrombocytopenia is an acute or a chronic problem. A gradual decrease in platelet count over 5–7 days is more in keeping with decreased platelet production or a consumptive cause of thrombocytopenia, while a more abrupt drop in platelet count occurring within 2 weeks of transfusion or commencement of a new drug points towards an immunological cause such as drug-induced thrombocytopenia or PTP.

2 Valuable diagnostic information can be gained from examining a blood film, and this should be requested in all patients with thrombocytopenia:

   a. The presence of platelet clumping on the blood film indicates that the thrombocytopenia maybe spurious and that the full blood count should be repeated in a heparin- or citrate-containing blood collection tube.

   b. The presence of schistocytes (red blood cell fragments) indicates a microangiopathic process.

   c. A leukoerythroblastic blood film with teardrop cells, nucleated red blood cells and immature granulocyte precursors present is suggestive of an underlying bone marrow abnormality.

   d. Macrocytosis of red cells is seen in patients with folate or vitamin B12 deficiency, hypothyroidism or alcohol toxicity.

   e. For those with history of foreign travel, the blood film can also be examined for the presence of parasites such as malaria.

3 Clotting screen abnormalities may suggest sepsis or DIC.

4 Liver function tests.

5 Haemolysis screen to include lactate dehydrogenase (LDH) and reticulocyte count, bilirubin and haptoglobin.

6 HIT screen if appropriate.

7 Vasculitic screen.

8 Nutritional deficiencies – serum vitamin B12 and folate levels.

9 Blood cultures.

10 Viral screen including HIV, EBV, CMV and hepatitis C.

Although the aforementioned is a rough guide to the investigations which may be considered for an ITU patient with thrombocytopenia, all these tests may not be required in every patient.

Management

In general, the management of thrombocytopenia is to treat the underlying cause. However, platelet transfusions may be considered if there is active bleeding or if a procedure with bleeding risk is required. The following guidance may be followed for practical purposes:

• If platelet count is below 10×10^9/L, one adult dose of platelets may be transfused.

• If the platelet count is below 20×10^9/L and patient is septic or very ill, one adult dose of platelets may be transfused (in these clinical situations, increased platelet consumption can occur).

• If the platelet count is below 30×10^9/L and the patient is bleeding, one adult dose of platelets may be transfused.

• If the platelet count is over 30×10^9/L, platelet transfusion is avoided unless:

   ○ Patient requires an interventional procedure (threshold is most often 50×10^9/L).

   ○ Patient requires anti-platelet agent (threshold is 50×10^9/L).

In certain conditions like TTP and heparin-induced thrombocytopenia, platelet transfusions are best avoided unless active and life-threatening bleeding occurs.

Further reading

Crowther MA, Cook DJ, Meade MO et al. Thrombocytopenia in medical-surgical critically ill patients: Prevalence, incidence, and risk factors. J Crit Care 2005;20(4):348–53.

Greinacher A, Selleng K. Thrombocytopenia in the intensive care unit patient. Hematol Am Soc Hematol Educ Program 2010;2010:135–43.

Rice TW, Wheeler AP. Coagulopathy in critically ill patients: Part 1: platelet disorders. Chest 2009;136(6):1622–30.

Wang HL, Aguilera C, Knopf KB, Chen TM, Maslove DM, Kuschner WG. Thrombocytopenia in the intensive care unit. J Intensive Care Med 2013;28(5):268–80.

CHAPTER 4

High Blood Counts

Quentin A. Hill

Department of Haematology, Leeds Teaching Hospitals NHS Trust, Leeds, UK

Thrombocytosis

Thrombocytosis, defined as a platelet count greater than $450 \times 10^9/L$, has been reported in 1–2% of patients attending hospital. It is a common finding in the intensive care unit (ICU), present in approximately 20% of patients at some stage during the admission [1–3]. The differential diagnosis of thrombocytosis can be seen in Table 4.1. As with unselected patients attending hospital [4], the vast majority of thrombocytosis cases are reactive in a critical care setting.

Secondary (reactive) thrombocytosis

Circulating platelets are derived from bone marrow megakaryocytes. Thrombopoietin is the main regulator of platelet count, driving megakaryocyte maturation and proliferation. However, reactive thrombocytosis appears to be secondary to pro-inflammatory cytokines such as interleukins (especially IL-6) and TNF which are also known to affect thrombocytopoiesis. Patients may also have raised inflammatory markers and a leukocytosis. Severe illness can cause a *left shift* on blood film where myeloid stem cell precursors not normally seen in peripheral blood are visible. These include band forms, metamyelocytes, myelocytes and, less frequently the more immature forms, promyelocytes and myeloblasts. The blood film may reveal other features of inflammation such as rouleaux formation and *reactive* neutrophilia (see neutrophilia in the following text). If hyposplenism is the cause of thrombocytosis, additional supportive features may be found in the film (Howell–Jolly bodies, target cells, lymphocytosis and acanthocytes).

In patients attending hospital, the most common causes are tissue damage, infection, iron deficiency, malignancy (most commonly gastrointestinal, lymphoma and lung) and chronic inflammatory disorders (most commonly inflammatory bowel disease, rheumatoid arthritis, chronic pancreatitis and systemic lupus erythematosus (SLE)) [4, 5]. Most critically ill trauma patients with thrombocytosis have additional predisposing conditions such as nosocomial infection, acute lung injury, bleeding and catecholamines [3], while in one study, independent risk factors for thrombocytosis included obesity, laparotomy, injury severity and mechanical ventilation [2].

The main concern with thrombocytosis is thrombosis. However, in the general hospital population, thrombosis only occurs in approximately 1% of patients with a reactive thrombocytosis, generally when additional risk factors (e.g. post-operative patient or underlying malignancy) are also present [4, 5]. Even at very high platelet counts, the risk appears low, and in a study of 231 patients with a reactive platelet count greater than $1000 \times 10^9/L$ (sometimes labelled as *extreme* thrombocytosis), only 3 (1%) had vaso-occlusive symptoms/events [6]. Venous thromboembolic events (VTE) also appear infrequent in trauma patients with thrombocytosis admitted to the ICU (1/34 (2.9%) [3] and 28/614 (4.6%) [2]). In the series of Salim et al. [2], those with thrombocytosis had a significantly higher rate of pulmonary embolus compared to patients with normal platelet counts, but the overall rate of thrombosis was not significantly different. Thrombosis was no more likely in the 41 patients with a platelet count greater than $1000 \times 10^9/L$ than those with platelets counts of $450–1000 \times 10^9/L$.

Haematology in Critical Care: A Practical Handbook, First Edition. Edited by Jecko Thachil and Quentin A. Hill.
© 2014 John Wiley & Sons, Ltd. Published 2014 by John Wiley & Sons, Ltd.

Table 4.1 Causes of thrombocytosis.

Primary
Inherited
Hereditary (e.g. mutations in gene for TPO or c-Mpl)
Acquired
Polycythaemia vera (PV)
Essential thrombocythaemia
Primary myelofibrosis (PMF)
Chronic myeloid leukaemia (CML)
Myelodysplastic syndrome (MDS)
Chronic myelomonocytic leukaemia (CMML)
Secondary
Infection (acute/chronic)
Inflammatory disorders
Tissue injury (including surgery)
Hyposplenism (surgical or functional)
Severe exercise
Severe haemolysis
Haemorrhage or iron deficiency
Malignancy
Drugs (steroids, adrenaline, vincristine, thrombomimetics)
Rebound post chemotherapy or alcohol withdrawal
Pseudo-thrombocytosis
Schistocytes (red cell fragments)
Microspherocytes (e.g. severe burns)
Cytoplasmic fragments (e.g. chronic lymphocytic leukaemia (CLL))
Bacteria
Haemoglobin H disease
Cryoglobulinaemia

Critically ill patients with thrombocytosis surprisingly have lower mortality compared to patients with normal counts [1–3], and individuals with a blunted platelet response (low rate of change following ICU admission), on the contrary, have higher mortality. The reason for this is not understood, but reactive thrombocytosis may be a marker of the host's ability to successfully initiate a response to injury [2]. The onset of thrombocytosis is typically 7–14 days after ICU admission [1–3]. In one study, all patients' platelet counts normalized with resolution of the acute illness at a mean of 35 days after admission [3].

Primary thrombocytosis
Most primary thrombocytosis is caused by myeloproliferative neoplasms (MPNs) such as essential thrombocytosis (ET), polycythaemia vera (PV), primary myelofibrosis (PMF) and chronic myeloid leukaemia (CML). Thrombocytosis can also be due to myelodysplastic syndrome (MDS)/MPN overlap syndromes,

e.g. chronic myelomonocytic leukaemia (CMML) and MDS with isolated del(5q-). Vasomotor symptoms such as headache, transient visual disturbance, chest pain, syncope and erythromelalgia (burning pain in hands or feet with erythema and warmth) occur in up to 40% of ET patients but are rare in reactive thrombocytosis [7]. Patients may also have splenomegaly, weight loss, night sweats, fatigue and loss of appetite. Other potential blood count abnormalities include a raised white count (e.g. CMML, CML), raised haematocrit (PV) or anaemia (PMF, MDS). Pseudohyperkalaemia can occur due to *in vitro* leakage of intracellular potassium during clotting. Thrombotic complications (mostly arterial) develop in 10–40% of those with ET and PV. Venous thrombosis usually occurs in the lower limbs but also in the abdominal veins (hepatic, portal or mesenteric) or the cerebral sinuses. Bleeding risk is also increased, especially when the platelet count is greater than $1000–2000 \times 10^9$/L. This has been attributed to platelet dysfunction and an acquired von Willebrand disease caused by large von Willebrand factor multimers being absorbed onto platelets. Definitive diagnosis usually requires a bone marrow aspiration and biopsy with cytogenetics. Peripheral blood testing for the $JAK2^{V617F}$ mutation is positive in approximately 50% of ET and PMF patients and over 90% of those with PV but is not found in reactive thrombocytosis. Treatment will depend on the exact diagnosis. ET patients typically receive aspirin, but platelets greater than 1000×10^9/L is a relative contraindication, requiring initial cytoreduction. Those at high risk of thrombosis (age > 60, prior ET-related thrombotic event) or haemorrhage (prior ET-related haemorrhage, platelet count $>1500 \times 10^9$/L) will also receive cytoreductive therapy such as hydroxycarbamide, interferon or anagrelide.

Approach to thrombocytosis in critical care
A blood film should be requested in all cases as this will exclude a pseudo-thrombocytosis (Table 4.1) and may detect features suggestive of a primary disorder such as macrocytosis, basophilic stippling, teardrop poikilocytes or a leukoerythroblastic picture. Other features suggesting a primary disorder include B symptoms, splenomegaly, vasomotor symptoms, and additional full blood count (FBC) abnormalities. Check inflammatory markers, but if there is an obvious secondary cause (e.g. acute blood loss, recent surgery/trauma, active

infection or splenectomy scar), extensive investigation is not required. If no secondary cause can be found or the thrombocytosis preceded or persists despite resolution of the acute illness, haematology advice should be sought.

• An anti-platelet agent such as aspirin is not generally required for secondary thrombocytosis, even if the count is greater than $1000 \times 10^9/L$. However, VTE prophylaxis with low-molecular-weight heparin should be considered for patients with a reactive thrombocytosis, if no contraindication exists. The platelet count should be monitored to ensure resolution.

• If thrombosis occurs (especially at an atypical site), even if a reactive condition is present, consider haematology review to exclude a primary disorder. In rare cases acutely presenting with life-threatening bleeding or critical thrombosis, platelet apheresis may be appropriate to rapidly reduce extreme thrombocytosis while diagnostic assessment is being undertaken [7].

• Patients with bleeding and an MPN should be investigated with platelet function and von Willebrand factor studies. Anti-platelet agents should be discontinued and the patient considered for cytoreductive therapy. Other treatments including platelet transfusion, desmopressin, von Willebrand factor containing concentrate and recombinant activated factor VII may also be considered on an individual basis but benefit balanced against the potential to increase thrombotic risk [8, 9].

Leukocytosis

Leukocytosis is defined as an elevation of the total white blood count (WBC) greater than two standard deviations above the mean (or a WBC > $11 \times 10^9/L$ in adults). Leukocytosis is a common finding in critical care and is a marker of poor outcome in commonly used prognostic scoring systems. In most cases, the reason for leukocytosis is readily apparent, and treatment is of the underlying disorder. Instances when a more careful assessment is required are highlighted in the following text as well as the approach to, and differential diagnosis of, elevation in leukocyte subsets.

Leukemoid reaction

Leukemoid reaction has been used to describe a marked reactive leukocytosis (sometimes defined as >$50 \times 10^9/L$) with associated left shift. Common causes include severe

bacterial infection, severe haemorrhage, tuberculosis, growth factors (e.g. granulocyte colony-stimulating factor (G-CSF)) and a paraneoplastic reaction to solid organ malignancy (the latter usually associated with large tumour burden and poor prognosis). Most importantly, leukemoid reaction must be distinguished from leukaemia. In leukemoid reaction, leukocytes are predominantly more mature cells, neutrophils typically have reactive changes (see neutrophilia in the following text), and there may be a reactive thrombocytosis. By contrast, in CML, the presenting WBC may be as high as 500 × $10^9/L$ with prominence of myelocytes and basophils, while splenomegaly can be massive (Figure 4.1). Hypogranular neutrophils, a predominance of blast cells and presence of Auer rods in blast cells favour leukaemia [10]. If leukaemia is suspected, send peripheral blood for immunophenotyping, but bone marrow examination with cytogenetics may be required.

Hyperleukocytosis and leukostasis

• Hyperleukocytosis describes a very high WBC in patients with leukaemia. This has arbitrarily been defined as a WBC greater than $100 \times 10^9/L$, but the level at which clinical complications arise depends on the type of leukaemia. It occurs in 5–13% of patients with acute myeloid leukaemia (AML) and 10–30% of patients with acute lymphoblastic leukaemia (ALL) [11]. Hyperleukocytosis is a poor prognostic factor in AML and ALL and is associated with a high rate of early mortality (up to 40% in AML and around 5% in ALL) [12] due to leukostasis, disseminated intravascular coagulopathy (DIC) and tumour lysis syndrome (TLS).

• Leukostasis is the term used to describe tissue injury from vascular obstruction by a high level of circulating blasts and is a medical emergency. Stasis arises from obstruction of the microvasculature by large-sized and non-deformable blasts. Blast cytokine secretion and interaction with endothelium may contribute to vessel wall injury and tissue hypoxia. Leukostasis is most commonly seen in AML and blast crisis of CML. Symptoms typically occur in AML patients with a WBC greater than $100 \times 10^9/L$ but can occur at lower counts. Leukostasis is less prevalent in ALL when the WBC is less than 400 × $10^9/L$ and is very rare in chronic lymphocytic leukaemia (CLL). Symptoms most commonly arise from the central nervous system (CNS) and lungs. Early death is often caused by intracranial haemorrhage. Leukostasis can

(a)

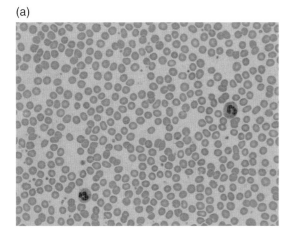

(b)

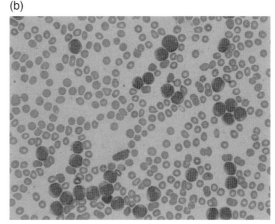

(c)

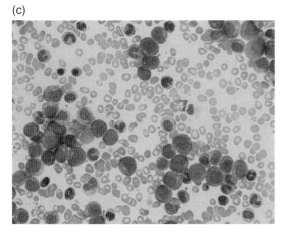

Figure 4.1 Leukocytosis. All are peripheral blood films at × 50 magnification. (a) Normal blood film. White blood count (WBC) 9 × 10^9/L. (b) Patient with acute myeloid leukaemia. Presenting WBC 197 × 10^9/L. (c) Patient with chronic myeloid leukaemia (CML). Presenting WBC 376 × 10^9/L (presented with blurred vision, retinal haemorrhage and massive splenomegaly).

occur even after cytoreduction has been initiated with leukapheresis or chemotherapy. Patients may develop:

- Blurred vision, dizziness, ataxia, headache, confusion or coma. There may be papilloedema, retinal haemorrhage, cranial nerve defects and intracranial haemorrhage on CT/MRI.
- Dyspnoea, tachypnoea and diffuse pulmonary infiltrates on chest X-ray/CT chest. PaO$_2$ may be spuriously low due to oxygen consumption by metabolically active blast cells.
- High fever is common.
- DIC (20–40% of patients with acute leukaemia and leukostasis).
- TLS.
- Other manifestations include right ventricular overload, priapism, renal vein thrombosis, bowel infarction and limb ischaemia.

- Management of hyperleukocytosis and leukostasis:
  - Urgent peripheral blood immunophenotyping, polymerase chain reaction (PCR) for BCR-ABL (if CML is suspected) and bone marrow with cytogenetics to secure the diagnosis of leukaemia.
  - ECG, CXR or CT head if relevant symptoms.
  - If pyrexia, blood cultures and consider empirical antibiotics.
  - Screen for DIC with FBC (automated platelet count may be falsely elevated by blast fragments), blood film, clotting and fibrinogen. In the absence of bleeding, maintain platelets greater than 20 × 10^9/L. If DIC, especially if evidence of haemorrhage, consider correction of coagulopathy (see also Chapter 9).
  - Screen for TLS with U&E, uric acid, phosphate and calcium (pseudohyperkalaemia can occur due to leakage of intracellular potassium during blood clotting

in vitro; a lithium-heparin/plasma sample will be more accurate). Ensure adequate hydration and pre-scribe allopurinol or rasburicase (dependent on TLS risk; see also Chapter 35) prior to cytoreduction. Recheck electrolytes 4–6 h after initiation of cytore-ductive therapy.

○ Generally avoid transfusion of packed cells and diu-retics, which will increase blood viscosity and can worsen or precipitate leukostasis.

○ Urgent cytoreductive therapy is required along with the general measures outlined earlier. Therapeutic options are chemotherapy and leukapheresis:

▪ Emergency induction chemotherapy is the treat-ment of choice and can significantly reduce the WBC within 24 h. Patients with hyperleukocytosis without leukostasis awaiting definitive chemother-apy may receive hydroxycarbamide which has been shown to reduce WBC by 50–80% within 24–48 h without worsening DIC. A typical oral dose would be 50–100 mg/kg/day, sometimes divided into a 12 or 6 h regimen.

▪ Leukapheresis: there is a lack of prospective randomized studies to demonstrate benefit. Retrospective data shows it to be effective at reducing the WBC (by 20–50% per procedure), but it does not influence long-term outcome. Some but not all studies suggest a reduction in early mortality. Leukapheresis is indicated for patients with leukostasis without immediate access to induction chemotherapy. Side effects include citrate-induced hypocalcaemia and thrombocy-topenia. The WBC may recover rapidly requiring repeat procedures and hydroxycarbamide can be started concomitantly. Avoid leukapheresis in acute promyelocytic leukaemia (APL).

Acute promyelocytic leukaemia (APL)

A rare but important cause of leukocytosis, this subtype of AML is characterized by abnormal hypergranular pro-myelocytes in the bone marrow and the production of a PML-RARA oncoprotein, usually due to a balanced translocation (t15:17). Its importance lies in its excellent outcome (cure rate approaching 80%) combined with its high rate of early death from a complex coagulopathy and secondary haemorrhage (most often brain and lungs), making it a medical emergency. It commonly presents with pancytopenia, but its hypogranular variant presents

with leukocytosis and circulating blasts. The risk of thrombosis is also increased. A WBC greater than $10–20 \times 10^9$/L is a risk factor for haemorrhage.

If APL is suspected:

• Test for coagulopathy and transfuse platelets to keep greater than $30–50 \times 10^9$/L and cryoprecipitate (or fibrinogen concentrate) to keep fibrinogen greater than 1.5 g/L [13].

• All-*trans*-retinoic acid (ATRA) should be commenced urgently based on morphology and clinical suspicion. ATRA induces differentiation of the leukaemic cells that are then able to undergo apoptosis. This leads to resolu-tion of the coagulopathy in 1–2 weeks.

• If WBC greater than 10×10^9/L, commence induction chemotherapy on an urgent basis (higher risk of differen-tiation syndrome; see succeeding text).

• Rapid genetic confirmation from bone marrow aspirate, either by PCR, fluorescent in situ hybridization (FISH), conventional karyotyping or an anti-promyelocytic leu-kaemia (PML) monoclonal antibody assay.

Patients treated with ATRA (or arsenic trioxide) can develop a potentially life-threatening differentiation syndrome:

• Fever, weight gain, dyspnoea, hypotension, pulmonary infiltrates, renal impairment, pleural and pericardial effusions.

• If suspected, treat with dexamethasone 10 mg intrave-nously twice daily. Ensure good fluid balance. Consider interruption of ATRA or arsenic therapy if severe.

Neutrophilia

Mild persistent neutrophilia in asymptomatic individuals may sometimes represent a normal variant. Neutrophilia and left shift can occur in normal pregnancy and the postpartum period. Possible causes of neutrophilia are listed in Table 4.2. Epinephrine, exercise and pain are thought to cause a rapid-onset neutrophilia due to the movement of cells into the circulating pool that were previously marginated against the vessel walls. Corticosteroids act by increasing output from marrow stores. Cigarette smoking usually only causes a mild neu-trophilia (dependent on the degree of tobacco intake), but this can persist for several years after cessation. Neutrophilia can occur in chronic conditions such as inflammatory bowel disease, rheumatoid arthritis or gout, especially with active disease. In cases of hyperther-mia (e.g. heat stroke), in addition to neutrophilia, there are a variable number of *botryoid* neutrophils with nuclei resembling a bunch of grapes (also seen following severe burn injuries).

Neutrophilia in the critically ill patient will often be due to infection or inflammation and may be multifactorial. *Reactive* changes occur in neutrophils in response to acute infection/inflammation including the appearance of Döhle bodies, cytoplasmic vacuoles and toxic granulation. Inflammation results in the bone marrow releasing less mature myeloid cells resulting in *left shift* in the blood film. A mild normocytic anaemia and thrombocytosis may also be present. Leukoerythroblastic changes (presence of immature white and red cells) reported on blood film are a *stressed* marrow response to severe bleeding, inflammation, hypoxia or trauma but can also occur in bone marrow infiltration or haematological malignancy.

History will focus on the differentials listed in Table 4.2 and the cause will often be readily apparent. Examine for signs of an infective focus, skin or joint abnormalities, surgical scars, lymphadenopathy or organomegaly. Assess with inflammatory markers and blood film to determine if further investigation is needed. Bone marrow examination will not usually be required for an isolated neutrophilia, but additional abnormalities such as raised haematocrit, a (unexpected) leukoerythroblastic blood film or splenomegaly may prompt investigation for a primary haematological disorder. Otherwise, treatment is of the underlying disorder.

Table 4.2 Causes of leukocytosis.

Neutrophilia	Lymphocytosis	Eosinophilia	Monocytosis
Primary			
AML	CLL, ALL	Leukaemia	AML, CML, CMML
MPDs, e.g. CML	Lymphoma	Lymphoma	MDS
CMML	Other LPDs	Mastocytosis	Hodgkin's lymphoma
Secondary			
Infection	Viral infection	Allergic disorders	Malignancy
Tissue damage	MMR, Hep A	Atopic eczema	Chronic infection
Trauma, surgery	Infectious mononucleosis	Asthma, allergic rhinitis	Tuberculosis
SCD crisis	Influenza, CMV	Drug reactions	Brucellosis
Burns	Rickettsial infection	NSAIDs	Protozoa
Inflammation	Chronic infection	Antibiotics	Chronic inflammation
Drugs	Tuberculosis	Parasitic infections	Crohn's disease
Steroids	Syphilis	Fungal infections	Rheumatoid arthritis
Epinephrine	Brucellosis	HIV	SLE
G-CSF	Whooping cough	Skin disorders	
ATRA	Stress related, e.g. MI, trauma, surgery	Connective tissue disorders	
Lithium	Endocrine disorders	Vasculitis	
Acute pain, bleeding or hypoxia	Drug allergy	Adrenal insufficiency	
Acute stress, heat stroke	Cytokines, e.g. G-CSF	Hypereosinophilic syndrome (HES)	
Smoking	Smoking	Malignancy	
Splenectomy	Splenectomy	Bowel disorders	
Malignancy	Epinephrine	Crohn's disease	
Diabetic ketoacidosis	Status epilepticus (muscle contraction)	Eosinophilic enteritis	
Venom (snake, bee, scorpion)	Thymoma	Cholesterol embolization	

AML, acute myeloid leukaemia; CLL, chronic lymphocytic leukaemia; ALL, acute lymphoblastic leukaemia; CML, chronic myeloid leukaemia; CMML, chronic myelomonocytic leukaemia; MPD, myeloproliferative disorders; MDS, myelodysplastic syndromes; LPDs, lymphoproliferative disorders; MMR, measles, mumps, rubella; Hep A, hepatitis A; SCD, sickle cell disease; HIV, human immunodeficiency virus; SLE, systemic lupus erythematosus; ATRA, all-trans-retinoic acid; MI, myocardial infarction; G-CSF, granulocyte colony-stimulating factor.

Lymphocytosis

The normal range for lymphocytes is higher in neonates and young children. Some causes of lymphocytosis are shown in Table 4.2. Blood film examination will usually detect lymphocyte abnormalities in primary disorders, and if these are suspected, peripheral blood immunophenotyping can often confirm the diagnosis. Cytology may appear normal, for example, in lymphoma-associated reactive lymphocytosis. Therefore, if a primary cause is suspected (e.g. B symptoms, additional cytopenias, organomegaly), then bone marrow or lymph node biopsy may be required.

Acute infective lymphocytosis due to infectious mononucleosis (positive heterophil agglutination test, e.g. Monospot®) or other viral agents (e.g. Coxsackie) can elevate the lymphocyte count to above 50×10^9/L. Large *atypical* lymphocytes are present on blood film. Infectious mononucleosis can additionally be complicated by thrombocytopenia, haemolytic anaemia, splenomegaly, hepatitis and rarely aplastic anaemia.

Epinephrine- and stress-induced lymphocytosis is due to redistribution of lymphocytes and may resolve within hours.

Eosinophilia

Common and important causes of eosinophilia are listed in Table 4.2. Eosinophilia can also occur in the recovery phase following infection. Marked eosinophilia ($>5 \times 10^9$/L) requires assessment for end-organ damage and may be seen in parasitic infection (e.g. toxocariasis, strongyloides and filariae), drug reactions (e.g. cephalosporins, carbamazepine, phenytoin, allopurinol and dapsone), Churg–Strauss syndrome, eosinophilic leukaemia and hypereosinophilic syndrome (HES) [10].

Hypereosinophilic syndrome has been defined as a count greater than 1.5×10^9/L for at least 6 weeks, lack of evidence of parasitic, allergic or other known cause and evidence of end-organ damage secondary to eosinophilic infiltration (most commonly the heart, skin, lungs and nervous system). Correct diagnosis is important because mortality can be high, especially with cardiac involvement and because those patients expressing the fusion protein FIP1L1-PDGFRA can achieve durable remission with the tyrosine kinase inhibitor imatinib.

Two studies have tested critically ill patients with relative eosinophilia (defined as >3%) by a corticotrophin stimulation test. A quarter of patients (23–25%) [14, 15]

were found to have relative adrenal insufficiency, and the majority of these responded to hydrocortisone with haemodynamic improvement.

- History should include medications, known atopic conditions or food allergy and detailed travel history including exposure to animals, raw food and untreated water.
- Examine for skin lesions, nail beds for splinter haemorrhages, lymphadenopathy, organomegaly, arthropathy and respiratory or cardiac signs.
- Investigation would include blood film, clotting, liver and renal function, inflammatory markers, immunoglobulins with immunofixation for a monoclonal protein and autoantibody screen. Dependent on symptoms, geographic exposure and suspected parasite, serological testing as well as repeated stool analysis may be required. Additional tests for parasites may include duodenal aspirate (e.g. strongyloides, ascariasis), blood film (filariasis), urine (schistosomiasis, filariasis), sputum (e.g. strongyloides, ascariasis, schistosomiasis) or tissue biopsy (bladder, liver or muscle) [16]. Consider lymph node biopsy or bone marrow examination with cytogenetics if haematological malignancy is suspected, biopsy of suspect skin lesions, human immunodeficiency virus (HIV) serology, chest X-ray and echocardiogram. Also consider testing for adrenocortical deficiency, especially if other evidence of hypoadrenalism (fever, weakness, fatigue, delirium, nausea, vomiting, hyponatraemia or vasopressor-dependent refractory hypotension).

The causes of monocytosis are listed in Table 4.2. Basophilia can be due to myeloproliferative and leukaemic disorders such as CML and systemic mastocytosis. Secondary causes include myxoedema, ulcerative colitis, urticaria and post-splenectomy.

Polycythaemia

Polycythaemia is suspected when the haematocrit is raised (>0.48 women, >0.52 men). However, haematocrit is influenced by plasma volume as well as red cell mass (RCM). An absolute polycythaemia (erythrocytosis) can be proven when blood volume studies (calculated using autologous red cells labelled with a radioactive isotope) indicate a RCM greater than 25% above the mean predicted value. Blood volume analysis is time consuming and not always available, especially in acute situations.

Polycythaemia is highly likely to be absolute when haematocrit is greater than 0.56 in women and greater than 0.60 in men. Patients may present acutely with thromboembolic complications or hyperviscosity symptoms (e.g. blurred vision, headache, lethargy or weakness).

Patients with a raised haematocrit but normal RCM have an apparent polycythaemia that may relate to reduced plasma volume secondary to shock, dehydration (e.g. diuretics) or cigarette smoking. Absolute polycythaemia can be primary or secondary (Table 4.3).

Primary polycythaemia

Polycythaemia vera is an acquired clonal MPN arising from a bone marrow pluripotent stem cell. Patients may have erythromelalgia, pruritus (worse after a warm bath), gout, headaches or weakness. Splenomegaly is present in over two-thirds of patients. WBC and platelet count may be raised and erythropoietin level is usually low. The JAK2^{V617F} mutation can be found in blood or marrow

Table 4.3 Causes of polycythaemia.

Apparent polycythaemia
Dehydration, smoking, hypertension, shock
Absolute polycythaemia – primary
Polycythaemia vera (PV)
Absolute polycythaemia – secondary
Congenital
High oxygen affinity haemoglobin
Reduced 2,3-DPG mutase
Congenital methaemoglobinaemia
Erythropoietin receptor defect
Chuvash polycythaemia (VHL gene mutation)
Acquired
Hypoxia
  Cyanotic heart disease
  Chronic lung disease, sleep apnoea
  Smoking, carbon monoxide poisoning
  High altitude
Erythropoietin-producing lesions
  Renal cysts, renal artery stenosis
  Renal adenoma, haemangioma, carcinoma
  Uterine fibroids
  Cerebellar haemangioblastoma
  Hepatic lesions including carcinoma
  Phaeochromocytoma
Androgens
Erythropoietin administration (athletes)
Post-renal transplant erythrocytosis
Idiopathic polycythaemia

from approximately 95% of PV patients. A number of those testing negative for JAK2^{V617F} can be shown to have mutations in exon 12 of the JAK2 gene. Median survival for untreated PV is less than 2 years from diagnosis but greater than 15 years with treatment. Mortality is chiefly from thrombosis, but patients are also at increased risk of haemorrhage (mainly mucous membranes, skin and bowel, associated with high platelet count and acquired von Willebrand disease) and transformation to AML or myelofibrosis. Treatment typically involves:
• Venesection to a haematocrit less than 0.45
• Aspirin 75 mg/day (unless contraindicated)
• Aggressive management of conventional risk factors for atherosclerosis
• Consideration of cytoreductive therapies (e.g. intolerance of venesection, progressive splenomegaly or thrombocytosis)

Secondary polycythaemia

Erythrocytosis can be a physiological response to tissue hypoxia, to improve oxygen-carrying capacity. Although venesection may still be appropriate when thrombosis and symptoms of hyperviscosity occur, evidence of benefit is less certain, and target haematocrits are higher. Erythropoietin level may be normal or high.
• Cyanotic heart disease: patients may present perioperatively or as a consequence of their increased risk of paradoxical emboli causing stroke or brain abscess.
   ○ Multiple phlebotomies should be avoided since they may result in iron deficiency, reduced oxygen delivery and increase risk of stroke.
   ○ Venesection, which must be isovolaemic, is only recommended in such patients when haemoglobin greater than 20 g/dL, haematocrit greater than 0.65, dehydration has been excluded and hyperviscosity symptoms are present.
   ○ Pre-operative isovolaemic venesection to less than 0.65 may also be considered to reduce the risk of haemorrhage in noncardiac surgery [17].
   ○ Avoid bubbles in intravenous lines (risk of paradoxical air embolus), and consider fitting an air filter.
Post-renal transplant erythrocytosis develops in around 10% of patients, typically after 8–24 months. It is a risk factor for thromboembolic disease but usually responds to ACE inhibitors, although venesection is sometimes required.

Neonatal polycythaemia

This has been defined as a venous haematocrit greater than 65% (capillary samples will overestimate haematocrit). Haematocrit peaks approximately 4 h after birth, returning to the level seen at birth after approximately 18 h. Causes include:
- Dehydration (poor feeding, fluid loss)
- Transfusion (maternal–foetal, twin to twin, delayed cord clamping)
- Foetal hypoxia (intrauterine growth retardation, maternal diabetes or smoking, pregnancy-induced hypertension and acute perinatal asphyxia)
- Underlying disorder (e.g. Down syndrome, congenital adrenal hyperplasia)

Although not all newborns are symptomatic, increased viscosity may lead to irritability, tremor, lethargy, vomiting and poor feeding. They may have plethora, jaundice, thrombocytopenia, hypocalcaemia or hypoglycaemia. Other complications include seizures, intracerebral haemorrhage or infarction and respiratory and cardiac impairment. Longer-term neurodevelopmental impairment has been found in some studies.

Polycythaemic newborns should receive adequate hydration and be monitored for complications (including hypoglycaemia). Partial exchange transfusion (PET) is effective at reducing haematocrit and acute symptoms but does not appear effective in improving long-term neurodevelopmental outcome. PET may also be associated with an increased risk of necrotizing enterocolitis and is not currently recommended for asymptomatic newborns [18].

If PET is required:
- Aim for a target haematocrit of 0.55.
- Exchange

$$\text{volume } (\text{mL}) = \frac{\left(\text{observed} - \text{target haematocrit}\right)}{\text{observed haematocrit}} \times \text{blood volume}$$

- Blood volume is approximately 85–90 mL/kg body weight in the newborn.
- Venesect through an umbilical vein, peripheral vein or peripheral arterial catheter. Blood can be removed in smaller aliquots (e.g. 5–10 mL/kg).
- Infuse the same volume of normal saline by a peripheral vein.
- Keep nil by mouth during and for 4 h after the procedure.
- Carry out in neonatal intensive care with full monitoring.

Surgery

Patients presenting with acute thromboembolic complications may require emergency interventions such as coronary angioplasty or coronary artery bypass grafting. Surgery in patients with uncontrolled PV is known to result in greater morbidity and mortality due to thrombosis and haemorrhage. Elective surgery should therefore be deferred while polycythaemia is investigated and treated. PV should be treated with venesection to a haematocrit less than 0.45 and cytoreductive therapy may be required if thrombocytosis is present. Partial exchange transfusion should be considered for patients with a high oxygen affinity haemoglobin and haematocrit greater than 0.6, prior to major surgery [19]. If surgery cannot be deferred, consider pre-operative isovolaemic venesection (or isovolaemic erythropheresis if available). Haemorrhage may require platelet transfusion and investigation for acquired von Willebrand disease (see also approach to thrombocytosis in critical care).

Some potential pitfalls

- Pulse oximetry can be normal in carbon monoxide poisoning. If suspected, check carboxyhaemoglobin level.
- MPNs are a leading cause of venous thrombosis in the splanchnic circulation (Budd–Chiari syndrome, extrahepatic portal vein and mesenteric vein thrombosis). $JAK2^{V617F}$ mutation is positive in some patients despite a normal haematocrit and platelet count. A positive result may influence the length of anticoagulation and enable monitoring and early intervention with venesection or cytoreductive therapy.
- Haemoglobin S-containing red cells have poor flow characteristics and cause a higher blood viscosity than normal red cells at any given haematocrit. Increasing the haemoglobin can increase viscosity, even if transfusing with haemoglobin S-negative packed cells. Patients with sickle cell disease (SCD) should generally not be transfused above their baseline haemoglobin or above 100–110 g/L if carrying out exchange transfusion.

Approach to polycythaemia in critical care

If haematocrit is elevated, firstly, ensure the patient is adequately hydrated and repeat the FBC.
- History should include cardiac or respiratory symptoms, smoking and alcohol intake, medications (diuretics, oxygen therapy, testosterone replacement), occupation

(high performance athlete, time at high altitude, risk of carbon monoxide exposure), known fibroids, pruritus, erythromelalgia, haematuria, family history of polycythaemia or venesection.
• Examine for cardiorespiratory disease and organomegaly.
• Investigate with urine dipstick, liver and renal function, ferritin, JAK2 analysis and erythropoietin level. Arterial blood gases and chest X-ray may also be appropriate.

Subsequent investigation will be directed by the initial evaluation. Abdominal ultrasound is often helpful when an erythropoietin-producing lesion is suspected. Isovolaemic venesection (450–500 mL) can be carried out for symptoms of hyperviscosity or following acute thrombosis while diagnostic evaluation is underway.

References

1 Gurung AM, Carr B, Smith I. Thrombocytosis in intensive care. Br J Anaesth 2001;87(6):926–8.
2 Salim A, Hadjizacharia P, DuBose J et al. What is the significance of thrombocytosis in patients with trauma? J Trauma 2009;66(5):1349–54.
3 Valade N, Decailliot F, Rebufat Y, Heurtematte Y, Duvaldestin P, Stephan F. Thrombocytosis after trauma: incidence, aetiology, and clinical significance. Br J Anaesth 2005;94(1):18–23.
4 Aydogan T, Kanbay M, Alici O, Kosar A. Incidence and etiology of thrombocytosis in an adult Turkish population. Platelets 2006;17(5):328–31.
5 Griesshammer M, Bangerter M, Sauer T, Wennauer R, Bergmann L, Heimpel H. Aetiology and clinical significance of thrombocytosis: analysis of 732 patients with an elevated platelet count. J Intern Med 1999;245(3):295–300.
6 Buss DH, Cashell AW, O'Connor ML, Richards F, Case LD. Occurrence, etiology, and clinical significance of extreme thrombocytosis: a study of 280 cases. Am J Med 1994;96(3):247–53.
7 Bleeker JS, Hogan WJ. Thrombocytosis: diagnostic evaluation, thrombotic risk stratification, and risk-based management strategies. Thrombosis 2011;2011:536062.
8 Harrison CN, Bareford D, Butt N et al. Guideline for investigation and management of adults and children presenting with a thrombocytosis. Br J Haematol 2010;149(3):352–75.
9 Tiede A, Rand JH, Budde U, Ganser A, Federici AB. How I treat the acquired von Willebrand syndrome. Blood 2011;117(25):6777–85.
10 Bain B. Blood Cells: A Practical Guide. 3rd edition. London: Blackwell Science Ltd; 2002.
11 Ganzel C, Becker J, Mintz PD, Lazarus HM, Rowe JM. Hyperleukocytosis, leukostasis and leukapheresis: Practice management. Blood Rev 2012;26(3):117–22.
12 Porcu P, Cripe LD, Ng EW et al. Hyperleukocytic leukemias and leukostasis: a review of pathophysiology, clinical presentation and management. Leuk Lymphoma 2000;39(1–2):1–18.
13 Sanz MA, Grimwade D, Tallman MS et al. Management of acute promyelocytic leukemia: recommendations from an expert panel on behalf of the European LeukemiaNet. Blood 2009;113(9):1875–91.
14 Angelis M, Yu M, Takanishi D, Hasaniya NW, Brown MR. Eosinophilia as a marker of adrenal insufficiency in the surgical intensive care unit. J Am Coll Surg 1996;183(6):589–96.
15 Beishuizen A, Vermes I, Hylkema BS, Haanen C. Relative eosinophilia and functional adrenal insufficiency in critically ill patients. Lancet 1999;353(9165):1675–6.
16 Tefferi A, Patnaik MM, Pardanani A. Eosinophilia: secondary, clonal and idiopathic. Br J Haematol 2006;133(5):468–92.
17 Warnes CA, Williams RG, Bashore TM, et al. ACC/AHA 2008 Guidelines for the Management of Adults with Congenital Heart Disease: a report of the American College of Cardiology/American Heart Association Task Force on Practice Guidelines (writing committee to develop guidelines on the management of adults with congenital heart disease). Circulation 2008;118(23):e714–e833.
18 Mimouni FB, Merlob P, Dollberg S, Mandel D. Neonatal polycythaemia: critical review and a consensus statement of the Israeli Neonatology Association. Acta Paediatr 2011;100(10):1290–6.
19 McMullin MF, Bareford D, Campbell P et al. Guidelines for the diagnosis, investigation and management of polycythaemia/erythrocytosis. Br J Haematol 2005;130(2):174–95.

CHAPTER 5

The Abnormal Clotting Profile

Jecko Thachil

Department of Haematology, Central Manchester University Hospitals NHS Foundation Trust,
Manchester, UK

Introduction

The prothrombin time (PT) and activated partial thromboplastin time (APTT) are the commonly used screening tests for coagulation. These tests were developed to assess the coagulation system based on their classification into extrinsic (PT) or intrinsic (APTT) clotting pathways. For this reason, an abnormality in these tests would mean an abnormality in the clotting cascade, which does not always translate to clinical bleeding. At the same time, normal PT and APTT, although useful in ruling out most causes of bleeding disorders, cannot exclude some conditions including mild bleeding disorders and rare diseases like factor XIII deficiency (see Table 5.1 for an interpretation of basic coagulation tests).

The principle of coagulation screen

Prothrombin time and APTT tests are based on restarting the coagulation process, which has been inhibited by removal of calcium, complexed to the anticoagulant citrate in the coagulation tubes. To facilitate the coagulation process, which usually occurs on phospholipid membranes (of mainly platelets) *in vivo*, thromboplastin is added, which forms the source of phospholipids *in vitro*. Time taken for the clot to form is measured in seconds and compared with normal control.

Prothrombin time (PT)

This test measures the components of the extrinsic coagulation system (tissue factor; the initiator of this pathway was considered extrinsic to the body). Although it was originally devised to measure prothrombin (clotting factor II), it is now known to be affected by deficiencies of coagulation factors V, VII and X and fibrinogen, as well. The test involves adding an optimal concentration of thromboplastin (source of phospholipids) to the plasma, which has been recalcified. Thromboplastin or tissue extract used in PT was originally sourced from rabbit brain or lung, although more recently it is obtained by recombinant methods. The latter is highly sensitive to decrease in clotting factors since there is no contamination with any animal coagulation proteins.

A prolonged PT in ITU is most commonly due to the lack of vitamin K. Other causes in decreasing order of frequency include:
- Liver disease
- Warfarin
- Disseminated intravascular coagulation (DIC)
- Decrease in fibrinogen (abnormal APTT as well)
- High doses of heparin (abnormal APTT as well)
- Deficiency of clotting factor VII
- Deficiencies of clotting factors II, V and X (abnormal APTT as well)

In liver disease, the PT is often the first abnormality (before APTT), since factor VII has a short half-life and its deficiency is therefore the first to be detected. In DIC,

---

Haematology in Critical Care: A Practical Handbook, First Edition. Edited by Jecko Thachil and Quentin A. Hill.
© 2014 John Wiley & Sons, Ltd. Published 2014 by John Wiley & Sons, Ltd.

Table 5.1 Interpretation of clotting tests.

PT	APTT	Plt	Condition
N	N	N	Common – normal haemostasis, vascular abnormalities*
			Rare – platelet dysfunction, dysfibrinogenaemia, mild coagulation factor deficiency[†]
			Extremely rare – factor XIII deficiency, alpha 2-antiplasmin deficiency
Long	N	N	Common – coumarin anticoagulants, vitamin K deficiency, liver disease
			Rare – factor VII deficiency
N	Long	N	Common – antiphospholipid antibody, heparin, liver disease, factors VIII, IX, XI, XII deficiency, von Willebrand disease
			Rare – inhibitors to the aforementioned factors, high-molecular-weight kininogen (HMWK) or pre-kallikrein (PK) deficiency
Long	Long	N	Common – vitamin K deficiency[‡], oral anticoagulants[‡]
			Rare – factors V, VII, X and II deficiency
Long	Long	N	Heparin, liver disease, fibrinogen deficiency
			Hyperfibrinolysis
Long	Long	Low	DIC, acute liver disease

Plt, Platelet count; N, normal; DIC, disseminated intravascular coagulation.
*Vascular abnormalities include scurvy, Cushing's disease and Ehlers–Danlos syndrome.
[†]A mild coagulation disorder can be masked by the administration of blood products. This would include mainly mild factor VIII deficiency and some cases of von Willebrand disease.
[‡]PT is relatively more prolonged than APTT.

PT is more often abnormal than APTT since factor VIII levels, which can increase with conditions leading to DIC, can *correct* APTT. Very rarely, antibodies to factors VII, II, V and X can also prolong PT with special mention of factor V antibodies developing in those who had bovine thrombin as a haemostatic agent during surgery.

Prothrombin time is generally insensitive to unfractionated heparin since the PT reagent includes heparin neutralization agents. However, if there is contamination with concentrated heparin, the PT may be prolonged. Shortened PT is almost always seen with activated recombinant factor VII treatment.

INR

Since PT is based on tissue thromboplastin reagents, depending on the tissue of origin, variability in clotting times had been noted. The use of recombinant-derived thromboplastins did not completely eliminate this variability. For this reason, the international normalized ratio (INR) was developed mainly to standardize the widespread use of the oral anticoagulant warfarin. Warfarin exerts its anticoagulant action by inhibiting the function of Vitamin K-dependent coagulation factors, which

include factors II, VII, IX and X. INR uses a World Health Organization reference thromboplastin standard so that INRs measured anywhere in the world would yield similar results.

In this context, it is important to bear in mind that INRs are not reliable between laboratories for any other clinical conditions, which are normally associated with a prolonged PT (e.g. DIC or liver disease). In these situations, PT should be used instead of the INR. This is because the INR standardization is based on plasma from patients stably anticoagulated with warfarin or similar agents. However, for the other clinical conditions, INRs from the same laboratory can be used to follow the trend of coagulation abnormalities in individual patients.

Activated partial thromboplastin time (APTT)

This test measures the components of the intrinsic coagulation system (the factors measured by this test are intrinsic to the body). The PT was unable to reliably diagnose haemophilia, and further attempts by Langdell and colleagues identified that a reduction in thromboplastin reduces coagulation factor VII-mediated initiation of the coagulation process, making coagulation factor VIII more important. This formed the basis of *partial* thromboplastin (as opposed to complete thromboplastin in PT). Originally, there were wide variations in the PTT tests until the addition of kaolin was noted to stabilize the test but also *activated* it to comparatively shorter time.

The test involves incubation of plasma with the APTT reagent, which contains phospholipids, and an activator (suspension of negatively charged particle). This mixture is then recalcified, and the time taken for clot formation is measured and compared with the control. The APTT results are highly dependent on the reagents used with variable responses to factor deficiencies.

A prolonged APTT in ITU is most commonly due to the heparin. Heparin exerts its anticoagulant function by potentiating the effects of antithrombin, which is a natural anticoagulant. Other causes in decreasing order of frequency include:
- Lupus anticoagulant
- Liver disease
- DIC
- Decrease in fibrinogen (abnormal PT as well)
- Massive transfusion
- Deficiency of clotting factors VIII, IX, XI and XII; high-molecular-weight kininogen (HMWK); and pre-kallikrein (PK)
- Deficiencies of clotting factors II, V and X (abnormal PT as well)
- Antibodies to clotting factor VIII

Heparin contamination from central lines can affect the APTT result, and this is often overlooked. Peripherally accessed samples would avoid this error. Measuring thrombin time (TT) may also help in excluding heparin as a cause for prolonged APTT. TT will be prolonged by heparin, but not the deficiency of clotting factors. Low-molecular-weight heparins do not *usually* prolong APTT, while some of the newer anticoagulants (except fondaparinux) can have an effect on this test (see Chapter 8).

Lupus anticoagulant is notorious for causing an abnormal APTT and is usually of minor significance in patients with bleeding (except in those very rare cases of anti-prothrombin antibodies). Many clinical situations can lead to the development of lupus anticoagulant including, very commonly, infections. A positive lupus anticoagulant has to be differentiated from antiphospholipid syndrome where this test is persistently positive in the presence of thrombotic manifestations in the arterial or venous system. At the same time, the presence of lupus anticoagulant in isolation has been considered as a risk factor for venous thromboembolism. Further tests may be performed to identify or exclude this phenomenon as the cause of prolonged APTT including mixing studies and specific tests (dilute Russell viper venom and phospholipid neutralization). Mixing studies involve the addition of plasma from an individual who is known to have normal plasma coagulation factors to the patient plasma in a 50:50 mix. If the APTT performed after the mix has normalized, it suggests coagulation factor deficiency, but if it remains abnormal, it would suggest antibodies to coagulation factors or lupus anticoagulant. Further tests can differentiate these two categories although a discussion with haematologist is advised. Patients with multiple, mild factor deficiencies as in the case of liver disease may have disproportionately prolonged APTT compared to individual factor levels. In addition, individuals with deficiency of factor XII, HMWK or PK do not have bleeding tendency.

In recent years, APTT and its dynamic parameters have been suggested to represent a strong predictive marker for hypercoagulation. A shortening of APTT indicates a higher level of coagulation factors, especially factor VIII and fibrinogen, which occurs as an acute-phase reaction in inflammatory states. APTT value in the lower end of normal is useful although the parameter, maximum velocity of APTT-induced plasma clotting, is even better in identifying patients at risk of thrombosis. Despite its usefulness, short APTT is not a common parameter used in clinical practice.

Thrombin time

In this test, commercially available thrombin is added to plasma and the clotting time is measured. TT is a good measure of fibrinogen concentration and function although heparin can also affect TT.

A prolonged TT is noted in:
- Hypofibrinogenaemia (congenital or acquired in DIC)
- Elevated levels of fibrin/fibrinogen degradation products (DIC, liver disease or thrombosis)
- Presence of heparin (TT is prolonged in some cases to a large degree)
- Treatment with direct thrombin inhibitors
- Dysfibrinogenaemia

• Rarely low albumin or the presence of paraprotein
Indications for TT testing are:
• Detecting heparin – especially useful for the detection of heparin in patients who bleed after cardiac bypass surgery. If the TT is adjusted by altering the concentration of thrombin added, the test becomes highly sensitive to small quantities of heparin.
• Monitoring fibrinolytic therapy for ischaemic cardiovascular events.
• Hypofibrinogenaemia or dysfibrinogenaemia.

Fibrinogen assay

Most laboratories use a functional assay for measuring fibrinogen. The Clauss method involves using a high concentration of thrombin to clot diluted plasma (dilution will remove inhibitory substances like heparin or fibrin degradation products). The time taken for a clot to form is inversely proportional to the amount of fibrinogen in the plasma. The PT-derived fibrinogen is another method where fibrinogen concentration is determined based on the change in light scattering or absorbance during a PT measurement. This assay can be affected by the presence of fibrin degradation products. Clauss method, being functional and less affected by fibrinogen degradation products, may be preferred in the ITU patients.

Activated clotting time (ACT)

Activated clotting time (ACT) assay is used in the cardiac bypass surgery setting where very high concentrations of heparin are used. The conventional APTT method becomes insensitive at this high concentration of heparin. The ACT test is a modified form of whole blood clotting time where kaolin or celite is used to accelerate coagulation by activating the contact pathway. Tubes or cartridges are inserted into prewarmed ACT instruments and whole blood with or without heparin is added. After the blood is mixed, the tube is rotated automatically until a clot is formed. The ACT value obtained correlates linearly to the concentration of heparin in the blood specimen.

The normal (baseline) value is 120–140 s, while after heparinization, an ACT greater than 480 s is considered safe for cardiopulmonary bypass in the absence of aprotinin and greater than 700 s in the presence of aprotinin.

It is useful to bear in mind that ACT using kaolin and celite can give slightly different values. Despite its benefits in the cardiac peri-operative setting, ACT is probably not the most appropriate test for diagnosing heparin rebound in the post-operative state, since it is relatively insensitive to low heparin concentrations.

Heparin resistance

Heparin resistance is defined as the requirement for more than 35,000 U of heparin to prolong the APTT into the therapeutic range. In cardiac bypass procedures, the definition based on the ACT is the occurrence of at least one ACT less than 400 s after heparinization and/or the need for exogenous antithrombin administration. Anderson and Saenko have divided the causes of heparin resistance into biophysical and pharmacokinetic reasons. The former include the inability of the heparin-antithrombin complex to inactivate activated clotting factors bound to cells or cell membranes, while the latter is due to the binding of heparin to plasma proteins, which belong to acute-phase reactants group including platelet factor 4, fibrinogen and factor VIII. For this reason, it is not surprising that this phenomenon is most often encountered in acutely ill patients and peri-partum setting. Rarely, it has been associated with aprotinin. Although a commonly described reason is the deficiency of antithrombin, which is a natural anticoagulant required for the therapeutic effect of heparin, this has been debated. Despite this, patients with heparin resistance are usually treated with antithrombin replacement using concentrates or fresh frozen plasma. Alternative anticoagulants may also be tried in place of heparin. In some cases, alternative assays to measure heparin effectiveness may be employed (anti-factor Xa assay). In the intensive care, occasionally when patients receive unfractionated heparin, antithrombin deficiency associated with sepsis or inflammatory states may cause heparin resistance.

Anti-Xa assay

This assay is useful in monitoring heparins, both unfractionated and low-molecular-weight forms, although other anti-Xa agents including fondaparinux, rivaroxaban and apixaban can prolong anti-Xa levels. In this method, factor Xa in the specimen cleaves a chromogenic substrate and releases a coloured compound detected with a spectrophotometer. If any of the aforementioned therapeutic agents are present, it will variably affect this cleavage, resulting in decreased amounts of coloured compound generated. This can be extrapolated to *anti-Xa activity*. Local policies should be in place to determine the prophylactic and therapeutic targets for anti-Xa activity, bearing in mind that there is wide variability between different low-molecular-weight heparins for the same anti-Xa assay. Anti-Xa monitoring is useful in patients who receive low-molecular-weight heparin and are in extremes of weight and with moderate to severe renal impairment. It may be beneficial in the use of these agents in pregnancy.

Pre-analytical variables

While performing the tests for coagulation, it is crucial that the specimen is ideal for evaluation. Many pre-analytical factors can alter the results, which have impact on the interpretation of clinical conditions and guiding therapeutic strategies. This is especially so since the sample integrity can reflect on the *in vitro* stability of coagulation factors and platelets.

Narrow-gauge needles, prolonged tourniquet use (more than 1 min) and difficulties in venepuncture can activate clotting systems and give false results including shortening of PT and APTT and increase in fibrinogen and D-dimer. The order of blood collection has been considered important to avoid contamination with tissue factor in the first sample although this has been refuted. It is currently recommended that routine coagulation testing can be done on the first tube drawn. However, if a central venous access device is used, there is a potential for heparin contamination and sample dilution. The line should first be flushed with saline, and at least two dead space volumes of the blood should be discarded before obtaining sample for coagulation tests.

Sodium citrate is the anticoagulant often used for coagulation tests. The recommended ratio of blood to citrate ratio should be 9:1. Under-filled tubes will have more citrate and bind more calcium, leading to longer clotting times. Overfilling by adding more blood or combining samples from other tubes can also affect results. Another critical point is the haematocrit of the blood. Samples with haematocrit greater than 55% will spuriously prolong PT and APTT since this represents an under-filled tube due to the reduction of plasma volume in relation to the red cell volume (similar problems do not occur with severe anaemia). This can potentially be a problem in congenital cyanotic heart disease patients who may require anticoagulation. Specially prepared tubes are advised, or the removal of 0.1 mL of sodium citrate may be done since most high haematocrits fall between 55% and 65%. Since some of the coagulation tests are based on light transmittance in determining the clot formation, severe haemolysis and hyperlipidaemia can also affect the results.

Further reading

Anderson JA, Saenko EL. Heparin resistance. Br J Anaesth. 2002;88:467–9.

Favaloro EJ, Lippi G, Adcock DM. Preanalytical and postanalytical variables: the leading causes of diagnostic error in hemostasis? Semin Thromb Hemost 2008;34(7):612–34.

Kitchen S, Olson JD, Preston EF. In Kitchen S (ed), Quality in Laboratory Haemostasis and Thrombosis. 1st edition. Chichester: Wiley-Blackwell Publishers; 2009.

Laffan M, Manning R. In Bain BJ (ed), Practical Haematology. 11th edition. Churchill Livingstone Publishers; 2012.

Ng VL. Prothrombin time and partial thromboplastin time assay considerations. Clin Lab Med. 2009;29(2):253–63.

CHAPTER 6

Understanding the Blood Film

Stephen F. Hawkins[1] and Quentin A. Hill[2]

[1] Department of Haematology, Royal Liverpool University Hospital, Liverpool, UK
[2] Department of Haematology, Leeds Teaching Hospitals NHS Trust, Leeds, UK

A blood film is produced by smearing a small drop of blood on a glass slide, allowing it to dry and then applying a number of stains, which prepare it for examination by microscopy [1]. The most commonly used stain for routine blood films is May–Grünwald–Giemsa (MGG), but a number of additional stains are used in special circumstances (e.g. Giemsa at pH 7.2 for identification of malarial parasites).

A blood film may be prepared by laboratory staff in response to abnormal blood count parameters. Thresholds are usually determined locally (e.g. if the platelet count is <50 or leukocyte count >20). Additionally, a film can be requested by the clinician. Consider requesting a blood film during the investigation of suspected haemolysis, haematological malignancy, unexplained high blood counts or cytopenias and persistent or relapsing fever (especially with a relevant travel history or tick exposure). Blood films also have a role in monitoring the response to treatment of thrombotic microangiopathies.

The preparation of a blood film takes approximately 20 min, while the actual examination of it may take several minutes depending on the clinical scenario. It is important that the specific question being asked (e.g. 'mitral valve replacement with paravalvular leak, haemolysis?') is written on the request form, to ensure laboratory staff provide the most informative report.

The differential diagnosis and clinical approach to high and low blood counts are discussed in Chapters 1, 2, 3 and 4. How diagnosis of blood count abnormalities or suspected infection can be aided by the blood film will now be discussed. The meaning and possible causes of common blood film abnormalities are summarized in Table 6.1.

Red cells

Microcytic anaemia: in iron deficiency, there may be a thrombocytosis, especially if bleeding. Less frequently, severe iron deficiency may also result in a leukopenia and thrombocytopenia. The blood film may show hypochromic, microcytic red cells, polychromasia and pencil cell poikilocytes. Occasional target cells or basophilic stippling may also be seen. More frequent basophilic stippling and target cells favour an underlying thalassaemic condition but also consider lead poisoning where stippling is prominent. Dysplastic features (see macrocytic anaemia) suggest a primary bone marrow disorder while rouleaux points towards an anaemia of chronic disease [1].

Normochromic anaemia: although often multifactorial in a critical care setting, the blood film may indicate contributing factors such as renal impairment (acanthocytes) or blood loss (polychromasia). Inflammation may result in rouleaux, leukocytosis and thrombocytosis.

Macrocytic anaemia: megaloblastic anaemia (B12 and/or folate deficiency) causes oval macrocytes, anisocytosis, poikilocytosis and neutrophil hypersegmentation (right shift). There may be basophilic stippling and, if severe, microcytosis, red cell fragments, Howell–Jolly bodies, left shift, neutropenia, thrombocytopenia and reticulocytopenia [1]. Acute onset deficiency

Haematology in Critical Care: A Practical Handbook, First Edition. Edited by Jecko Thachil and Quentin A. Hill.
© 2014 John Wiley & Sons, Ltd. Published 2014 by John Wiley & Sons, Ltd.

Table 6.1 Common blood film terminology.

Blood film terminology	Meaning	Associated disorders
Red cells		
Acanthocytes	Cells with spicules of irregular size and spacing	High numbers associated with liver disease, some neuroacanthocytosis disorders and myelodysplasia. Smaller numbers if hyposplenic, hypothyroid, starvation or anorexia
Agglutination	Red cells form clumps	Cold agglutinins (autoantibodies most active below body temperature). May cause haemolysis
Anisocytosis	Variation in size	Present in haematinic deficiency and a variety of haematological disorders
Echinocytes (crenated or burr cells)	Short regular spicules	Storage artefact, renal failure, liver disease, vitamin E or pyruvate kinase deficiency, burn injury
Elliptocytes	Red cells with an elliptical, cigar or pencil shape	Hereditary elliptocytosis. Present in smaller numbers in thalassaemia, iron deficiency, megaloblastic anaemia, myelodysplasia or myelofibrosis
Fragments (schistocytes)	Red cell fragmentation due to intravascular destruction	Microangiopathic processes, malaria, paroxysmal nocturnal haemoglobinuria, ABO—mismatched blood transfusion
Irregularly contracted cells	Loss of central pallor, irregular shape	Disorders of haemoglobin (Hb) synthesis (e.g. Hb C, SC or H disease, β-thalassaemia trait), G6PD deficiency, drug-induced oxidative haemolysis
Macrocytic anaemia	Large red cells	Liver disease, hypothyroid, B12/folate deficiency, bleeding, haemolysis, myelodysplasia, medication, pregnancy, spurious (e.g. cold agglutinins)
Microcytic anaemia	Small red cells	Iron deficiency, thalassaemic disorders and traits, anaemia of chronic disease, sideroblastic anaemia, lead poisoning
Poikilocytosis	Variation in shape	Present in various disorders. If severe, consider myelofibrosis, hereditary pyropoikilocytosis, dyserythropoietic anaemia or storage artefact
Polychromasia	More reticulocytes: newly released red cells, larger and stain with a blue tint (higher RNA content)	Response to hypoxia, anaemia (e.g. bleeding or haemolysis) or haematinic replacement
Rouleaux	Red cells line up in stacks	Increased plasma proteins, e.g. inflammation, pregnancy
Spherocytes	Loss of membrane results in small cells without central pallor	Haemolytic conditions. Severe burns
Stomatocytes	Linear slit or mouthlike area of central pallor	Alcohol excess, chronic liver disease, chlorpromazine, inherited haemolytic conditions (e.g. hereditary stomatocytosis, cryohydrocytosis, Tangier disease). Small numbers can be normal
Target cells	An additional central area of dense staining	Liver disease, haemoglobinopathies, iron deficiency, hyposplenism
Teardrop poikilocytes (dacrocytes)	Teardrop shape	Myelofibrosis, myelodysplasia, marrow infiltration, thalassaemia, megaloblastic anaemia, some cases of acquired and Heinz body haemolytic anaemia
Red cell inclusions		
Basophilic stippling	Multiple small RNA deposits	Thalassaemia (major or trait), unstable Hb, iron deficiency (small numbers), megaloblastic anaemia, myelodysplasia, myelofibrosis, lead poisoning, pyrimidine 5′-nucleotidase deficiency
Howell–Jolly bodies	A round, usually solitary inclusion that is a nuclear remnant	Normally removed by the spleen; these are found in hyposplenic states including the neonatal period
Nucleated red cells	Early red cell forms in which the nucleus is still present	Abnormal outside the neonatal period. Response to anaemia, bone marrow disorder or infiltration, extramedullary haematopoiesis

Blood film terminology	Meaning	Associated disorders
Pappenheimer bodies	Iron-containing granules, usually 1–2 at the cells periphery	Sideroblastic anaemia, sickle cell disease, lead poisoning, post splenectomy
Ring forms, trophozoites, schizont	Intracellular stages of a parasitic life cycle. Varied morphology	Malaria or babesiosis
White cells		
Leukocytes	White cells	Normal subtypes of white cells are neutrophils, lymphocytes, monocytes, basophils and eosinophils
Cytosis (e.g. leukocytosis, thrombocytosis) or *philia* (e.g. neutrophilia)	An elevation above the normal range	See Chapter 4 for causes
Penia (e.g. neutropenia, thrombocytopenia)	A reduction below the normal range	See Chapters 1, 2 and 3 for causes
Atypical lymphocytes	Features may include increased size, irregular outline, basophilic or vacuolated cytoplasm, irregular or lobated nuclear outline, nucleoli	Viral infection (e.g. infectious mononucleosis, cytomegalovirus), tuberculosis, mycoplasma, toxoplasma, immunizations, drug hypersensitivity reaction, sarcoidosis
Auer rods	Azurophilic rodlike structures present in the cytoplasm of leukaemic blasts	Acute myeloid leukaemia and high-grade myelodysplasia
Hypogranular neutrophils	Reduced cytoplasmic granulation	Myelodysplasia
Large granular lymphocytes	Prominent cytoplasmic granules; nucleoli may be visible	Up to 10% of lymphocytes in healthy individuals
Large lymphocytes	Irregular outline, abundant cytoplasm, less condensed nuclear chromatin	Up to 10% of circulating lymphocytes in healthy individuals
Left shift	Presence of immature white cells, not normally seen in peripheral blood. Includes blasts, promyelocytes, myelocytes and metamyelocytes (in order of increasing maturity)	Infection, inflammation, pregnancy, bone marrow disorder, administration of growth factors (e.g. G-CSF)
Leukoerythroblastic film	Presence of immature red and white cells	Bone marrow disorders, marrow infiltration, severe anaemia, hypoxia or infection
Pelger–Huët anomaly	Neutrophils with a bilobed nuclei shaped like spectacles, a dumb-bell or peanut	Inherited or acquired (pseudo Pelger–Huët) due to myelodysplasia
Plasma cells	Antibody producing mature B lymphocytes	Myeloma, plasma cell leukaemia, reactive, e.g. infection
Right shift	An increase in percentage of neutrophils with five or more lobes	Megaloblastic anaemia. Occasionally seen with infection, iron deficiency, uraemia or myelodysplasia
Toxic granulation, vacuolated cytoplasm and Döhle bodies	Neutrophil cytoplasmic granulation is larger and more basophilic; cytoplasmic vacuolation and cytoplasmic blue-gray inclusions	Non-specific features usually associated with infection or inflammation
Platelets		
Platelet clumping	EDTA-dependent antibody-mediated formation of platelet clumps	Leads to a pseudothrombocytopenia

resulting in megaloblastic *arrest* may occur, usually in acutely unwell patients, resulting in pancytopenia but normal MCV and few or no macrocytes. Patients with haemolysis will usually have polychromasia due to the marrow releasing reticulocytes into the circulation [1]. In warm autoimmune haemolytic anaemia (AIHA), spherocytes (red cells which have lost their normal biconcave disc shape and become spherical) may be present. In cold-type AIHA, there is often agglutination of red cells. Microangiopathic haemolysis (e.g. disseminated intravascular coagulation [DIC] or thrombotic thrombocytopenic purpura) is accompanied by the mechanical fragmentation of red cells. These red cell fragments (or *schistocytes*) are usually associated with a thrombocytopenia. Occasional red cell fragments can be found in a normal blood film but are likely to be significant if greater than 1% of red cells. Liver disease can result in target cells and stomatocytes as well as acanthocytosis (red cells with a small number of spiky membrane protrusions) if advanced. Patients may have additional cytopenias, and those with acute alcoholic liver disease may develop haemolytic anaemia and hyperlipidaemia (Zieve's syndrome) as well as concomitant dietary haematinic deficiency. Finally, in patients with myelodysplasia, additional cytopenias may also be present as may anisocytosis, poikilocytosis, left shift, blast cells, basophilic stippling and dysplastic neutrophils (reduced granulation and/or abnormal-shaped nuclei).

Polycythaemia (raised haematocrit): thrombocytosis and leukocytosis may occur in primary or secondary polycythaemia although basophilia favours the former. Increased red cell turnover may exhaust iron stores in primary polycythaemia resulting in iron deficient indices (low MCV/MCH) and sometimes even anaemia.

White cells

Leukopenia: the blood film firstly confirms leukopenia by excluding artefact arising from an automated cell count. Leukopenia may be due to reduced production or increased consumption. Production is reduced in marrow failure, marrow suppression (e.g. drugs) or by deficiencies of B12 and/or folate. Blood film findings in B12 deficiency and myelodysplasia are outlined earlier under *macrocytic anaemia*. In most marrow failure syndromes, leukopenia is not an isolated finding. Leukoerythroblastic change (leukocyte precursors and nucleated red blood cells) may occur in myelofibrosis or malignant infiltration but can also be found in severe illness (hypoxia, sepsis or bleeding). Increased consumption of white cells can result from infection, hypersplenism or autoimmune destruction. Specific features will not be seen on the film (unless associated abnormalities, e.g. rouleaux from infection or acanthocytes in liver disease leading to hypersplenism).

Leukocytosis: this may be a primary bone marrow disorder or, more commonly, a secondary reactive leukocytosis.

Leukocyte morphology is usually sufficient for the provisional diagnosis of a primary disorder such as leukaemia, but specialist tests like bone marrow examination are required for confirmation and provide additional prognostic information. In acute leukaemia, blast cells

predominate while patients with chronic lymphocytic leukaemia usually have excess lymphocytes with relatively normal morphology but increased smear cells due to their greater mechanical fragility. Chronic myeloid leukaemia (CML) manifests as *left shift* of the myeloid series. Blast cells normally mature into promyelocytes then myelocytes and then metamyelocytes before being released into the blood as neutrophils. Left shift describes the appearance of myeloid precursors in the peripheral blood. In CML, myelocytes and neutrophils predominate and basophilia is typical. Various other haematological disorders can be suspected from the blood film, for example, the presence of large lymphocytes with abundant cytoplasm and irregular margins in hairy cell leukaemia.

Reactive leukocytosis in bacterial infection is predominantly a neutrophilia with increased granularity in the cytoplasm (toxic granulation) and blue-gray cytoplasmic inclusions (Döhle bodies). If infection is severe, neutrophil cytoplasm can be vacuolated and there may be left shift. Viral infection (e.g. infectious mononucleosis) usually results in a lymphocytosis often with more frequent reactive or *atypical* lymphocytes (large pleomorphic lymphocytes with abundant cytoplasm and visible nucleoli). A marked reactive leukocytosis with left shift can follow infection but also growth factor administration, haemorrhage and as a paraneoplastic reaction. Unlike leukaemia, reactive leukocytosis is self-limiting and rarely greater than 100×10^9/L, but peripheral blood immunophenotyping can be helpful where there is diagnostic uncertainty.

Platelets

Thrombocytopenia: in the most common scenario of increased platelet consumption or destruction, platelet turnover is increased, resulting in platelet anisocytosis and giant platelets on the blood film. If there is an underlying bone marrow disorder, additional features may be seen (e.g. blast cells, dysplastic changes and teardrop poikilocytes). Concomitant red cell fragments suggest an underlying microangiopathy. Pseudothrombocytopenia may be identified from the film when it is due to platelet clumping (an artefact caused by antibodies against the EDTA anticoagulant used for sample collection) or platelet satellitism (an immune-mediated platelet adherence to neutrophils). Rarely, thrombocytopenia may be the presenting feature of a congenital platelet disorder, some of which also result in platelet dysfunction and a bleeding tendency. Very small platelets are seen in X-linked thrombocytopenia and Wiskott–Aldrich syndrome. Consistently, large platelets may be found in Bernard–Soulier syndrome, von Willebrand disease 2B, platelet type von Willebrand disease, gray platelet syndrome (gray appearance due to lack of α-granules) and the MYH9 disorders (Döhle body-like inclusions are seen in neutrophils, e.g. May–Hegglin anomaly).

Thrombocytosis: a concomitant leukocytosis does not discriminate between a reactive cause and a primary disorder such as a myeloproliferative neoplasia (MPN). In patients with an MPN, there may also be a raised haematocrit, anaemia, leukoerythroblastic change, teardrop poikilocytes, basophilic stippling or dysplasia. Patients for whom the thrombocytosis is reactive to severe illness may have inflammatory changes (rouleaux) or left shift. Other reactive causes with typical blood film findings are iron deficiency and hyposplenism.

Infection

Infection can have diverse effects on the blood and may increase or reduce leukocyte or platelet counts. It can result in anaemia through inflammation (anaemia of chronic disease), triggering of autoimmune haemolysis, microangiopathic haemolysis, secondary splenomegaly or direct bone marrow suppression. Sepsis may cause reactive changes in neutrophils, rouleaux, left shift, red cell fragmentation (DIC), leukoerythroblastic change or pancytopenia (bone marrow suppression or haemophagocytosis).

Blood film examination remains central to the diagnosis of blood-borne parasites including *Plasmodium*, *Babesia*, *Trypanosoma* species and filarial nematodes (*Brugia*, *Loa loa* (Figure 6.1), *Mansonella* and *Wuchereria*) [2]. Adequate clinical details and travel history on the request are needed to inform film stain selection, preparation and interpretation. Thin and thick films are usually made if a parasite is suspected. A buffy coat film may also be prepared to concentrate the nucleated cells and improve test sensitivity.

Severe cases of malaria may present to critical care with renal failure, seizures, coma, hypotension, pulmonary oedema, DIC or a metabolic acidosis. Films

should be prepared with Giemsa although Field or Wright–Giemsa stains may also be used. In thick films, red cells are lysed prior to examination to enable rapid detection of a parasite. The thin film aids identification of a particular species (*Plasmodium falciparum* (Figure 6.2), *Plasmodium vivax*, *Plasmodium malariae*, *Plasmodium ovale* or *Plasmodium knowlesi*) and determines the level

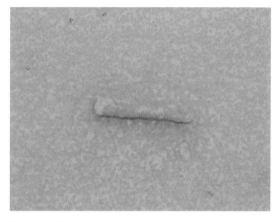

Figure 6.1 Microfilaria of *Loa loa*. Peripheral blood (×20 magnification) from a woman returning from Cameroon with aching joints. Source: Image taken from UK NQAS general haematology blood films for parasite identification survey material. Copyright UK NQAS. Reproduced with permission.

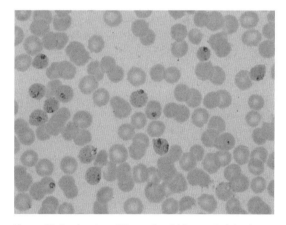

Figure 6.2 Trophozoites of *Plasmodium falciparum*. Peripheral blood (×100 magnification) from a safari tourist returning ill from South Africa. The parasites are small and often adherent to the red cell membrane (accolé forms) with coarse irregular red cell stippling (Maurer's clefts), all characteristic features of *falciparum*. Source: Image taken from UK NQAS general haematology blood films for parasite identification survey material. Copyright UK NQAS. Reproduced with permission.

of parasitaemia. Blood films may be negative due to low parasitic loads, tissue sequestration of parasitized cells or the periodicity of the disease. Serial blood films may therefore be required where clinical suspicion remains. Rapid diagnostic tests are also available and may be used in parallel with microscopy by some laboratories. These usually combine detection of a non-specific plasmodium antigen like lactate dehydrogenase with a *falciparum*-specific antigen such as histidine-rich protein 2.

African (sleeping sickness) or American (Chagas disease) trypanosomiasis may involve critical care due to cardiac or neurological involvement. These slender motile extracellular parasites can be visualized in the acute phase of Chagas disease by microscopy, but tissue culture or serology is required in latent and chronic phases. Diagnosis in the acute phase of sleeping sickness is by microscopy of thin and thick films, CSF or tissue aspirates.

Babesiosis is a rare tick-borne protozoal parasite occurring in the USA and Europe. Severe infection is more likely in hyposplenic or immunosuppressed patients and may result in fever, myalgia, haemolysis, thrombocytopenia, hepatomegaly, DIC, acute respiratory distress and cardiac or renal failure. Diagnosis is by microscopy of Giemsa-stained thick and thin films although serological and PCR assays have been developed. Trophozoites most often appear as small rings within red cells and can be confused with *P. falciparum*. They can also be pear shaped or occur in pairs or tetrads (*Maltese cross* forms).

Bacteria or fungi can be observed between cells or within leukocytes. This rare but significant finding occurs most frequently in patients who are hyposplenic, immunosuppressed or have an indwelling venous line [1].

Bartonellosis, a bacillus spread by sandflies in some Andean regions of South America, invades red cells and the reticuloendothelial system, resulting in fever (Oroya fever), malaise, anaemia, lymphadenopathy and hepatosplenomegaly. It can be visualized within red cells on a Giemsa-stained blood film and is associated with haemolytic changes. Finally, various species of the *Borrelia* genus are tick- or louse-borne spirochetes that result in relapsing fever. Consider in patients with a recurrent fever, travelling from an endemic area. Thin and thick films are a first-line investigation, and organisms can be seen between cells during the febrile episode.

In summary, the blood film can add considerable information to the full blood count. Although often automatically performed in response to abnormal results, it can also be requested. Consider this when haemolysis or haematological malignancy is suspected. Also consider a film for unexplained high blood counts, cytopenias or persistent fever (in a hyposplenic patient or if tick exposure or relevant travel history). Being familiar with blood film terminology aids its interpretation. Discuss with a haematologist if the report isn't understood, the findings can't be reconciled with the clinical picture or haematological input is needed for the patient's ongoing diagnosis and management.

References

1 Bain BJ. Blood Cells: A Practical Guide. 3rd edition. Oxford: Blackwell Science Ltd; 2002.
2 Rosenblatt JE. Laboratory diagnosis of infections due to blood and tissue parasites. Clin Infect Dis 2009;49(7):1103–8.

SECTION 2

Approach to Coagulation Problems

CHAPTER 7

Venous Thromboembolism in Intensive Care

Sarah A. Bennett and Roopen Arya

King's Thrombosis Centre, Department of Haematological Medicine, King's College Hospital NHS Foundation Trust, London, UK

Introduction

Risk factors for venous thromboembolism (VTE) in intensive care unit (ICU) patients are more heterogeneous than in other care groups but frequent due to the nature of critical illness. Different clinical presentations of VTE like haemodynamic instability, episodes of desaturation and limb swelling are common signs in these patients, which may also be attributed to thrombosis. Concurrently, bleeding risk can be high for a number of reasons, including trauma, recent surgery, organ dysfunction and the associated coagulopathy. The importance of preventing VTE in this patient group however should not be underestimated. Omission of early thromboprophylaxis (within 24 h of admission to ICU) is associated with more severe episodes of VTE and increased mortality [1].

Epidemiology

Venous thromboembolism in the ICU patient group is often asymptomatic, and rates are therefore difficult to estimate. Cross-sectional studies have demonstrated that up to 10% of patients have pre-existing deep vein thrombosis (DVT) on admission to ICU. Clinicians should therefore be vigilant and consider the diagnosis in all patients admitted to their unit and prescribe thromboprophylaxis in the absence of any absolute contraindications. In this respect, studies have shown that up to one-third of patients who do not receive thromboprophylaxis in ICU will develop a DVT [2]. The estimation of PE incidence has been more difficult to ascertain since even when PE leads to death, diagnosis is not often confirmed due to reduced post-mortem rates – patients who were ventilated or treated for other pulmonary conditions as well as trauma victims are less likely to have post-mortems. Six studies in critically ill patients over the past three decades revealed PE on post-mortem examination in up to 27% of patients, the majority of which were unsuspected. PE either caused or contributed to death in 10% of these patients.

Risk factors for development of VTE in intensive care

The increased susceptibility to the development of VTE results from numerous factors and can be helpfully thought of as those that are present before ICU admission and those that are acquired during the ICU admission (see Table 7.1). While the relative contribution of each is unknown, patients with multiple risk factors should be deemed at the highest risk and receive thromboprophylaxis

---

Haematology in Critical Care: A Practical Handbook, First Edition. Edited by Jecko Thachil and Quentin A. Hill.
© 2014 John Wiley & Sons, Ltd. Published 2014 by John Wiley & Sons, Ltd.

Table 7.1 Risk factors for VTE in intensive care patients.

Present prior to intensive care unit (ICU) admission:
Age (>60 years)
Personal (or first-degree relative with) history of venous
    thromboembolism (VTE)
Known thrombophilias
Intimal injury (e.g. trauma, surgery)
Hypercoagulability (active cancer or cancer treatment, sepsis,
    dehydration)
Obesity (BMI > 30 kg/m^2)
Reduced mobility (e.g. spinal cord injury, bed rest for ≥ 3 days,
    stroke)
Hormonal factors (pregnancy or up to 6 weeks postpartum)
Significant co-morbidities (e.g. heart disease, endocrine and
    respiratory pathology, acute infectious diseases and inflammatory
    conditions)
Acquired during ICU admission:
Use of sedation and muscle relaxant infusion
Invasive/non-invasive positive pressure ventilation
Intravascular catheter device
Sepsis
Renal replacement therapy
Vasopressor requirement
Haemostasis support (e.g. platelet transfusion and recombinant
    factor VIIa)

Source: Adapted from Geerts et al. [3]. Copyright Elsevier.
Reproduced with permission.

as appropriate. Efforts should be made to minimize cumulative risk where possible, such as the use of minimal sedation and shorter periods of central venous catheters.

Thromboprophylaxis

All patients in critical care are at high risk of VTE, and thromboprophylaxis should be given routinely. There is evidence to suggest that by doing so the incidence of proximal DVT can be reduced by around 50% [4–6].

Pharmacological

Prophylactic dose heparin (unfractionated heparin (UFH) and low-molecular-weight heparin (LMWH)) has been compared to placebo in a handful of studies examining the efficacy of DVT prevention in general ICU patients. Pharmacological thromboprophylaxis reduced the rate of VTE by at least 55%. Whether one type of heparin is superior in preventing VTE than the other remains unknown in this group of patients.

The PROTECT study provides the only direct comparison between UFH and LMWH in preventing VTE in critical care patients [7]. This multicentre study involving 3764 randomized ICU patients (with the exception of trauma, orthopaedic and neurosurgical patients) showed no significant difference in the rate of proximal DVT (5.8% UFH and 5.1% dalteparin) between the two groups. Fewer patients receiving dalteparin developed PE (1.3% vs. 2.3%) although the hospital mortality rate did not differ between the groups. Major bleeding rates were comparable, and there were fewer cases of heparin-induced thrombocytopenia (HIT) in the dalteparin cohort.

Low-molecular-weight heparin is increasingly favoured over UFH due to the reduced incidence of HIT and osteoporosis and the high bioavailability and largely predictable anticoagulant effects. LMWHs do not require routine monitoring or dose adjustments, but serum anti-factor Xa levels may offer guidance and have been successfully used in certain patient groups where the pharmacokinetics are more unpredictable. Although trials often focus on laboratory parameters such as anti-Xa levels as surrogate markers for anticoagulant effectiveness, the interpretation of these tests in ICU patients has not been extensively studied. It is also useful to bear in mind that increased body weight, multi-organ dysfunction and high vasopressor requirements with the resulting impairment to cutaneous blood flow may all lead to underdosing of heparins. Besides, medications administered subcutaneously in patients with shock may not be reliably absorbed. In those patients with antithrombin deficiency (e.g. severe sepsis), heparin administration without monitoring can lead to underdosing as well. Conversely, bioaccumulation (particularly with repeated administration) may occur in patients with renal insufficiency, leading to overdosing and haemorrhagic complications.

Mechanical

There is very little evidence to guide clinicians on the use of mechanical measures to prevent VTE in medical as well as in ICU patients. Anti-embolism stockings (AES), intermittent pneumatic compression (IPC) and foot impulse devices are the main modalities (see Table 7.2). Mechanical devices should be considered in conjunction with pharmacological prophylaxis in high-risk patients when the clinical condition allows. Immobility is a

Table 7.2 Guidance for use of thromboprophylaxis measures and therapeutic anticoagulation.

	Guidance for use	Contraindications
Unfractionated heparin (UFH)	Prophylactic dose: 5000 U two to three times daily Therapeutic anticoagulation requires an intravenous infusion (refer to BNF or local guidelines for regime)	If heparin-induced thrombocytopenia (HIT) is strongly suspected or confirmed, heparin should be stopped and an alternative anticoagulant (such as fondaparinux) should be given (see Chapter 10)
Low-molecular-weight heparin (LMWH)	Monitoring not routinely required, but anti-Xa measurement may be useful in certain patient groups to rule out bioaccumulation: aim for trough levels in those with renal impairment of 0.2–0.4 U/mL To ensure appropriate therapeutic dosing in obese, pregnant patients or those with high renal clearance, aim for peak levels taken 3–4 h post subcutaneous injection of 0.4–1.0 U/mL Prophylactic doses should be prescribed according to weight; for enoxaparin, we suggest: <50 kg → 20 mg OD 50–99 kg → 40 mg OD 100–149 kg → 40 mg BD >150 kg → 60 mg BD (see BNF for alternative LMWH agent dosing)	Switch to UFH if creatinine clearance (CrCl) is <30 mL/min If HIT is strongly suspected or confirmed, heparin should be stopped and an alternative anticoagulant (such as fondaparinux) should be given (see Chapter 10)
Anti-embolism stockings (AES): compression of the deep venous system promotes increased blood flow velocity with reduction in venous dilatation	These should be thigh or knee length and measured to fit Maximum benefit is gained if worn at all times, day and night, providing adequate monitoring of underlying skin is undertaken twice in every 24-h period	Acute stroke patients Suspected or confirmed peripheral arterial disease or neuropathy Local leg conditions (e.g. severe dermatitis, recent skin graft, allergy) Congestive cardiac failure Massive leg oedema Deformity of leg preventing correct fit Patient refusal
Intermittent pneumatic compression (IPC) *devices*: blood is emptied from behind valves to reduce venous stasis	Optimal benefit is likely only when these devices are *in situ* If removed, check manufacturer instructions for guidance on reapplication. If unworn for a period of time, exclusion of DVT may be required prior to continued use	Suspected or confirmed acute deep vein thrombosis (DVT) (due to risk of clot embolization) As for AES
Foot impulse devices: promotes emptying of blood from the plexus of veins in the sole of the foot (venae comitantes), which occurs as part of normal weight bearing	May be used in patients with external fixators or where access to the leg is restricted Evidence in non-lower extremity trauma patients suggests that they may be less effective than IPC	Pre-existing venous thromboembolism (VTE) or thrombophlebitis As for AES

universal risk factor for critically ill patients, and the main aim with these methods is to reduce the resultant venous stasis. At times, the bleeding risk for the patient may be increased such that the risk/benefit ratio dictates that pharmacological thromboprophylaxis is relatively or absolutely contraindicated.

Diagnosis of VTE

Diagnosis is difficult because the usual signs and symptoms cannot be easily relied upon. Most patients in ICU are unable to report the characteristic symptoms of PE such as dyspnoea and chest pain due to sedation and mechanical ventilation. Furthermore, physical examination may be limited to the obvious swelling, erythema and warmth of affected limbs. There is no validated VTE prediction tool available for this patient group. D-dimers being invariably raised have very limited utility in these patients. The investigations of choice would be duplex ultrasonography for DVT and CT pulmonary angiography for patients with suspected PE. For those who are unable to transfer for imaging, duplex ultrasonography with or without bedside echocardiography is a readily available alternative. Right ventricular enlargement and hypokinesis, paradoxical interventricular septal motion, tricuspid regurgitation and pulmonary hypertension may all be suggestive of PE. More recently, NT pro-BNP has been suggested as a useful biomarker, which if negative may exclude a significant PE [8].

Treatment of VTE

There are two main objectives: the first is to provide definitive treatment in case of haemodynamic compromise, and the second is to prevent progression or recurrence of VTE. In most cases, the primary treatment would constitute anticoagulation, with LMWH or UFH in the first instance, and commencement on oral anticoagulation when appropriate. LMWH is the anticoagulant of choice for use in intensive care; however, there are times when UFH may be more appropriate (see Table 7.2). Patients with severe renal impairment and those at high risk of bleeding requiring short-acting therapeutic anticoagulation may be better managed with an intravenous infusion of UFH until oral anticoagulation is established or a switch to LMWH can be made.

If the bleeding risk is high, for example, following trauma or in the immediate post-operative situations, an IVC filter might be inserted as a temporary measure. Haemodynamically unstable patients with PE should be thrombolysed; in case of failure of thrombolysis or high bleeding risk, embolectomy might be required.

Special considerations

Kidney disease

Acute and/or chronic kidney disease in ICU patients is important to consider; approximately one-third have severe disease (creatinine clearance (CrCl) < 30 mL/min), and a further third have mild or moderate disease (CrCl 51–80 mL/min and CrCl 30–50 mL/min, respectively). In addition to nephrotoxic drugs, mean arterial pressure and circulating blood volume both affect renal function and may fluctuate significantly in this patient group. Bioaccumulation is often a concern with repeated dosing of LMWH and is an issue that has not been adequately investigated in the ICU setting. Kidney disease is common in the elderly, affecting more than 60% of those aged greater than or equal to 70 years. As such, caution should be taken when prescribing LMWHs. A normal creatinine (80–120 µmol/L) in such patients may be misinterpreted as indicative of normal renal function; however, it should be considered that creatinine levels fall with age as muscle mass decreases.

Line-related clots and superficial vein thrombosis

Routine thromboprophylaxis has limited efficacy in preventing line-related thrombosis. ICU patients have multiple risk factors for VTE, and common usage of indwelling central venous catheters further predisposes them to upper limb thrombosis and lower limb DVT. Line-related thrombosis should be treated with anticoagulation. The indwelling catheter can be safely left *in situ* most cases if still functional and required [9]. Superficial vein thrombosis secondary to central lines may also warrant anticoagulation if symptomatic, and extensive in size, to prevent post-thrombotic syndrome (PTS). As a guide, 6 weeks of therapeutic dose, LMWH can be given, following which a review should be carried out to determine whether further treatment is necessary.

IVC filters

IVC filters should not be used for primary thromboprophylaxis [10]. The only indications for their use are to prevent PE in patients with proximal DVT or PE who cannot be anticoagulated or in whom PE has recurred despite adequate anticoagulant therapy. When the contraindication to pharmacological therapy is no longer present, all patients with an IVC filter (which should always be a retrievable filter) should be considered for anticoagulation, and the filter should be removed as soon as possible. Complications of filters left *in situ* include extracaval extension and caval thrombosis. In addition, they may lead to recurrent DVT and PTS, hence the need for anticoagulation. Free-floating thrombus is not an indication for IVC filter insertion. Studies have shown that more than half of free-floating clots either reattach to the vascular wall or decrease in size/resolve within the first few weeks of anticoagulation. The incidence of PE is also no greater in patients with free-floating thrombus compared to those with adherent clots.

Trauma, burns and neurosurgical patients

Trauma patients often have complex injuries or ongoing haemorrhage and consequently are at high risk of both VTE and bleeding. In addition, injuries to the lower limbs (including fractures, immobilization with plaster casts or external fixators), which preclude the use of mechanical measures, make this a difficult patient group to manage. Daily review of clinical condition will assist the team regarding appropriate thromboprophylaxis. Once the bleeding risk is reduced, pharmacological anticoagulation should be commenced without delay.

Patients with thermal injuries represent a group at high risk of VTE; increasing total body surface area (TBSA) has been identified as an independent risk factor for thrombosis. Moreover, the physiological response to thermal injury is the development of a hyperdynamic circulation, which may facilitate clearance of heparin from the body. The potential for underdosing should be considered and may be particularly relevant for patients requiring therapeutic anticoagulation. Measurement of peak anti-Xa activity 3–4 h post dose may assist the clinician with appropriate dosing.

Neurosurgical patients represent another challenging group at high risk of VTE due to factors such as limb paralysis, stroke and immobility. Analogous to trauma patients who are often at high risk of bleeding, daily review of clinical condition will aid decision-making regarding appropriate thromboprophylaxis.

Procedures and temporary interruption of anticoagulation

Any interruption to anticoagulation should be minimized as far as possible, but care should be taken not to expose patients to the complications of bleeding. Patients in ICU often require lumbar punctures and spinal or epidural anaesthesia; if procedures are performed too close to an anticoagulant administration, there is a risk of peri-spinal haematoma with subsequent spinal cord ischaemia and paraplegia. All patients should be assessed by a senior clinician, but as a general rule, any intervention, including central venous access, chest drain insertion and placement or removal of a spinal catheter, should be delayed for 12 h after administration of prophylactic LMWH. Similarly, heparin should not be administered sooner than 4 h following these procedures. Patients on treatment dose LMWH may benefit from morning administration; under normal circumstances, elective procedures can be safely undertaken by omitting the heparin on the morning of the procedure. A prophylactic or split full dose can be given 4 h following the procedure with resumption of the full daily dose the next morning as appropriate. Patients receiving treatment dose heparin who are deemed to be at the highest risk of VTE might be best managed with a continuous intravenous UFH infusion to allow for minimal interruption of anticoagulation.

Asymptomatic and incidental VTE

The clinical relevance of incidental VTE is uncertain even outside the ICU setting. However, subclinical DVTs still have the potential to propagate and embolize, making it unethical to withhold treatment. Furthermore, it is well recognized that a large proportion of patients with DVT also have asymptomatic PE. In critically ill patients with limited cardiopulmonary reserve, even a small PE could have severe or even fatal consequences. The majority of deaths from PE occur within hours of the embolic event and are often secondary to asymptomatic DVT. Sudden episodes of haemodynamic instability or hypoxaemia may be the only clues to diagnosis in mechanically ventilated patients. Difficulty in weaning from mechanical ventilation should also raise suspicion of underlying PE. Patients who have incidental subsegmental PE should undergo screening for DVT in order to facilitate treatment decisions. If DVT is present, then therapeutic anticoagulation is required unless contraindications exist. No definitive recommendation can be made for those with isolated subsegmental PE, and treatment decisions should be made on an individual basis.

Summary

Venous thromboembolism is a very significant patient safety issue in hospitals, and intensive care patients are at particularly high risk. All patients should be risk assessed for VTE on admission to ICU, and reassessment should occur on a daily basis or more frequently if the clinical condition of the patient is changing rapidly. This is especially pertinent as contraindications to pharmacological thromboprophylaxis may be transient. Multimodality prophylaxis should be used for those at highest risk. Unless there is a contraindication, all patients should receive pharmacological thromboprophylaxis. When this is unsuitable, mechanical measures should be put in place, with pharmacological anticoagulation commenced as soon as the bleeding risk is reduced.

References

1 Ho KM, Chavan S, Pilcher D. Omission of early thromboprophylaxis and mortality in critically ill patients: a multicentre registry study. Chest 2011;140(6):1436–46.

2 Kapoor M, Kupfer YY, Tessler S. Subcutaneous heparin prophylaxis significantly reduces the incidence of venous thromboembolic events in the critically ill [abstract]. Crit Care Med 1999;27(Suppl.):A69.

3 Geerts W, Cook D, Selby R, Etchells E. Venous thromboembolism and its prevention in critical care. J Crit Care 2002;17(2):95–104.

4 Hirsch DR, Ingenito EP, Goldhaber SZ. Prevalence of deep venous thrombosis among patients in medical intensive care. JAMA 1995;274:335–7.

5 Marik PE, Andrews L, Maini B. The incidence of deep venous thrombosis in ICU patients. Chest 1997;111:661–4.

6 Schonhofer B, Kohler D. Prevalence of deep-venous thrombosis of the leg in patients with acute exacerbations of chronic obstructive pulmonary disease. Respiration 1998; 65:173–7.

7 The PROTECT Investigators. Dalteparin versus unfractionated heparin in critically ill patients. N Engl J Med 2011;364:1.

8 Vuilleumier N, Le Gal G, Verschuren F et al. Cardiac biomarkers for risk stratification in non-massive pulmonary embolism: A multicenter prospective study. J Thromb Haemost 2009;7(3):391–8.

9 Guyatt GH, Akl EA, Crowther M et al. Executive Summary: Antithrombotic Therapy and Prevention of Thrombosis. 9th edition. American College of Chest Physicians Evidence-Based Clinical Practice Guidelines. Chest 2012;141 (2 Suppl):7–47S.

10 British Committee for Standards in Haematology. Guidelines on use of vena cava filters. Br J Haematol 2006;134:590–5.

CHAPTER 8

Reversal and Monitoring of Anticoagulants

Joost J. van Veen

Department of Haematology, Sheffield Haemophilia and Thrombosis Centre, Sheffield Teaching Hospitals NHS Foundation Trust, Sheffield, UK

Introduction

Anticoagulants are increasingly used in a variety of clinical settings, and their most important adverse event is bleeding. Major haemorrhage was an independent predictor of mortality in various studies and occurs in 1–4% of patients depending on the type of anticoagulant used, its dose and indication. In such instances, urgent reversal of anticoagulant effects should be considered. Whereas vitamin K antagonists (VKA) and heparin have specific antidotes, newer anticoagulants do not have specific agents available as yet.

Reversal of anticoagulation is usually considered in cases of major bleeding or the need for emergency surgery. Options include withholding the anticoagulant, applying general/supportive measures and using specific antidotes or general pro-haemostatic drugs. The preferred option is dependent on the patient characteristics (indication for anticoagulation/thrombotic risk of immediate reversal, co-morbidities including renal/hepatic dysfunction and cardiovascular reserve), the pharmacological properties of the anticoagulant (half-life/clearance mechanism) and the strength of evidence for the reversal agent used.

In this chapter, general measures to stop bleeding, individual anticoagulants and their reversal methods, route of elimination and laboratory monitoring are discussed and summarized in Table 8.1.

General measures

General measures should be applied to all instances of haemorrhage. These include:

- Stopping all anticoagulation (and concomitant antiplatelet agents if patients are on them)
- Identification of the bleeding source and applying local measures (pressure, endoscopic or radiological procedures and surgery)
- Supportive measures (intravenous (IV) fluids, red cell transfusions, maintaining body temperature and correction of pH/electrolyte imbalances)

Whereas local measures including packing and pressure bandages are often applied in minor bleeding, more aggressive measures (activated or non-activated prothrombin complex concentrate) should not be withheld in clinical situations of major bleeding as their benefits, even in fully anticoagulated patients, are likely to outweigh the risks associated with uncontrolled bleeding. A full blood count and coagulation screen including activated partial thromboplastin time (APTT), prothrombin time (PT) and fibrinogen should be performed in these cases, bearing in mind the fact that they cannot always be used in assessing the degree of anticoagulation, where specialist assays may be required (discussed in the following text).

Haematology in Critical Care: A Practical Handbook, First Edition. Edited by Jecko Thachil and Quentin A. Hill.
© 2014 John Wiley & Sons, Ltd. Published 2014 by John Wiley & Sons, Ltd.

Table 8.1 Characteristics of anticoagulants and possible reversal agents.

Anticoagulant (route of administration)	Elimination route (half-life)	Laboratory monitoring	Reversal agent	Evidence base	Notes
1. Warfarin	1. Hepatic (35–45 h)	INR	1. Vitamin K	Randomized controlled trials and prospective studies for warfarin reversal	1. 5 mg IV vitamin K significantly reduces INR in 6–8 h. 1–3 mg oral will partially correct high INR at 24 h (avoid in acenocoumarol)
2. Acenocoumarol	2. Hepatic (8–12 h)	INR	2. PCC		2. 25–50 U/kg PCC will fully correct INR within 10 min. 5 mg IV vitamin K must be given simultaneously
3. Phenprocoumon (oral)	3. Hepatic (4–5 days)	INR	3. Fresh frozen plasma (FFP)		3. FFP should only be used in the absence of PCC
Dabigatran (oral)	1. Creatinine clearance (CrCl) >80 mL/min 13 h; 2. CrCl 50–80 mL/min 15 h; 3. CrCl 30–50 mL/min 18 h; 4. CrCl <30 mL/min 27 h	Normal thrombin time excludes significant anticoagulation. Normal activated partial thromboplastin time (APTT) excludes high levels of dabigatran	Consider (A)PCC or rFVIIa*; Haemodialysis; Activated charcoal may be used in overdose within 2 h of ingestion	No clinical data. Conflicting animal and *in vitro* studies	PCC partially effective in animal model of intracranial haemorrhage but not in controlled trial in healthy non-bleeding volunteers
1. Rivaroxaban; 2. Apixaban (oral)	1. 7–9 h; 2. 9–14 h (75% hepatic, 25% renal)	Anti-Xa levels with specific standard. Prolong the prothrombin time (PT) (INR)/ APTT but cannot be used to monitor anticoagulation	Consider (A)PCC or rFVIIa*	No clinical data. Conflicting animal and *in vitro* studies	Controlled trial in healthy non-bleeding volunteers suggested an effect of PCC in rivaroxaban reversal
Unfractionated heparin (UFH) (IV (S/C))	Rapid cellular mechanism. Renal at high doses (60–90 min. Longer at high doses)	APTT†	Protamine sulphate; Infusion may be required for reversal of S/C UFH	Extensive clinical experience	1 mg protamine reverses 100 U given in the last 15 min. For a typical infusion of 1250 U/h: 30 mg. Maximum protamine dose: 50 mg
LMWH (S/C)	Renal (4 h)	Anti-Xa levels with LMWH standard. The APTT may be prolonged but cannot be used for monitoring	Protamine sulphate (IV); rFVIIa (20–120 µg/kg)*	One small clinical case series, animal and *in vitro* studies	Partial reversal only. 1 mg for 100 U LMWH given in the previous 8 h (maximum single dose 50 mg). Further 0.5 mg/100 U if unsuccessful. Lower doses if LMWH given over 8 h ago
				Anecdotal registry data and case report	rFVIIa to be tried only in life-threatening bleeding unresponsive to general measures and protamine

Drug	Elimination (half-life)	Monitoring	Reversal	Evidence	Comments
Fondaparinux (S/C)	Renal (17–21 h, longer in renal impairment)	Anti-Xa levels with fondaparinux standard	rFVIIa 90 µg/kg*	Clinical case series and controlled study in non-bleeding healthy volunteers	1 small clinical case series with 50% success rate
Danaparoid (IV/SC)	Renal (25 h)	Anti-Xa levels with danaparoid standard	Consider (A)PCC or rFVIIa* Plasmapheresis	No clinical or animal data	
Bivalirudin (IV)	80% proteolysis, 20% renal (25 min (3.5 h in dialysis-dependent renal failure))	APTT†, ACT	Consider (A)PCC or rFVIIa* Haemodialysis Haemofiltration	Case report for rFVIIa, no clinical data for (A)PCC	Given its short half-life, general measures are likely to be sufficient
Argatroban (IV)	Hepatobiliary (45 min)	APTT†	Consider (A)PCC or rFVIIa* Haemodialysis	2 case reports without effect of rFVIIa, conflicting ex vivo study	Given its short half-life, general measures are likely to be sufficient

(A)PCC, activated prothrombin complex concentrate; PCC, prothrombin complex concentrate; rFVIIa, recombinant factor VIIa (NovoSeven®); LMWH, low-molecular-weight heparin; IV, intravenous; S/C, subcutaneous.

*rFVIIa and (A)PCC are experimental reversal agents. rFVIIa has been associated with an increased risk of arterial thrombosis, and the summary of product characteristics states that it should not be used in unlicensed indications. There are no good data on a possible thrombotic tendency of (A)PCC in these situations. All should be avoided unless in case of life-threatening bleeding unresponsive to other measures with the exception of PCC in vitamin K antagonist (VKA) reversal.

†Baseline prolongation of the APTT (DIC or presence of lupus anticoagulant) can result in overestimation of the anticoagulant effect.

General pro-haemostatic agents

Fresh frozen plasma

The APTT/PT is often prolonged in patients on antico-agulants, but this usually reflects inhibition of coagulation factors by the anticoagulant and not a coagulation factor deficiency. The common practice of fresh frozen plasma (FFP) administration is therefore unlikely to correct the bleeding unless if used as part of a massive transfusion protocol when coagulation factor replacement may be beneficial. An exception is the use of FFP in the reversal of VKA-induced bleeding if prothrombin complex concentrate (PCC) is unavailable (see following text).

Recombinant factor VIIa and (activated) prothrombin complex concentrate

Recombinant factor VIIa (rFVIIa) is licensed for the treatment of inherited/acquired haemophilia and anti-bodies to coagulation factors VIII and IX and inherited factor VII deficiency and in Europe for the treatment of Glanzmann's thrombasthenia.

(Activated) Prothrombin complex concentrate ((A) PCC) is licensed for the treatment of bleeding/cover of surgery in congenital/acquired haemophilia A and anti-bodies to FVIII or as prophylaxis in congenital haemo-philia A with high responding inhibitors and frequent joint bleeding. (A)PCC contains several coagulation factors as well as small amounts of activated coagulation factors, whereas rFVIIa contains activated coagulation factor VII only. PCC is licensed in the UK as a four-factor concentrate containing factors II, VII, IX and X for the emergency reversal of VKA and does not contain acti-vated coagulation factors. Some preparations do not con-tain factor VII (three-factor concentrate).

All three agents have been suggested for reversal of anticoagulant-related bleeding when no specific reversal agents are available. The data in this setting is sparse and mostly limited to animal studies, studies in healthy (non-bleeding) volunteers, single case reports and in vitro studies, which raises the risk of publication bias.

An additional concern relates to thrombogenicity. rFVIIa is well tolerated in licensed indications, but it's off-licence use for life-threatening bleeding in surgical and other situations has been associated with an overall risk of arterial thrombosis of 5.5% versus 3.2% in placebo and 10.8% versus 4.1% in placebo at age over 75 years [1]. The cur-rent summary of product characteristics of rFVIIa states that it should not be used in unlicensed indications [2]. A meta-analysis of PCC for emergency reversal of VKA showed a thrombotic risk of 1.4% [3], but no data for its use in other (unlicensed) indications are available.

Because of these limitations, rFVIIa and (A)PCC should only be used in life-threatening bleeding when other measures have failed and after full discussion and documentation of the risks and benefits involved. The evidence for their use in the reversal of individual antico-agulants is discussed in the following text.

Reversal of individual anticoagulants

Vitamin K antagonists

Vitamin K antagonists reduce the functional levels of fac-tors II, VII, IX and X. The most widely used drug in the UK and North America is warfarin. Others including phenprocoumon, acenocoumarol and phenindione differ in their half-life (phenprocoumon 4–5 days and aceno-coumarol 8–12 h). Major bleeding with VKA occurs in 1–3% of patients. All these agents can be reversed with the use of vitamin K, PCC or FFP. A detailed review on the reversal of warfarin using these different agents was recently published [4].

Whether vitamin K alone may be used or additional PCC is required depends on the urgency of the situation. Both products are required in major/life-threatening bleeding or emergency surgery (see following text). The IV administration of 5 mg vitamin K reverses the INR with a significant effect at 6–8 h. Oral vitamin K takes longer with reversal at 24 h. In life-threatening bleeding or emergency surgery, reversal can be achieved within 10 min by administration of 25–50 U/kg PCC, preferably be with a four-factor concentrate and combined with 5 mg vitamin K as the half-life of the administered coagu-lation factors is finite [4]. FFP should only be used if PCC is not available as large volumes (15–30 mL/kg) are needed to supply sufficient coagulation factors with the risk of fluid overload. Other disadvantages compared to PCC include the time needed for thawing and adminis-tration, a small risk of transfusion-related lung injury and it may carry infective agents [4]. The effect of reversal is judged by INR measurements. rFVIIa is not recom-mended for warfarin reversal. In non-major bleeding or elective surgery, vitamin K by itself can be used. There is a small risk of anaphylactoid reactions with IV vitamin K, and it should be given slowly, diluted in IV fluids. For partial correction of high INRs (>8.0) into the therapeutic range, without bleeding, 1–3 mg oral vitamin K may be used, but it should be avoided for acenocoumarol because of its short half-life and risk of subtherapeutic INRs [4]. In the latter case, omitting a dose and dose adjustment are sufficient.

Heparins and indirect factor Xa inhibitors

These include unfractionated heparin (UFH), low-molecular-weight heparins (LMWH), danaparoid and fondaparinux. UFH has a complex mode of action but mainly dependent on inhibition of factors IIa (thrombin) and Xa. LMWH have higher anti-Xa than anti-IIa activity, whereas danaparoid has predominantly an anti-Xa effect. Major bleeding occurs in 1–4% of patients on LMWH depending on the dose and indication. The characteristics and differences between these agents were recently reviewed [5]. All require the presence of a specific pentasaccharide that binds to antithrombin, potentiating its effect. Fondaparinux is a synthetic pentasaccharide with anti-Xa activity only.

Reversal of UFH is well established using protamine, given slowly to avoid adverse reactions. One milligram will reverse 100 U UFH given in the previous 15 min, and doses vary between 25 and 50 mg (Table 8.1). Higher doses are routinely used in UFH reversal following cardiac surgery. Protamine has a short half-life, and infusions may be necessary after subcutaneous (S/C) UFH administration. As the half-life of IV UFH is short (60–90 min but longer if large doses are given), general measures may be sufficient. The APTT is used to monitor the effect of protamine [5].

Protamine only partially reverses the anti-Xa effect of LMWH based on *in vitro* data and animal studies. The clinical effectiveness is unclear with the largest case series describing a partial effect in 18 patients only [6]. The half-life is relatively short (4 h), but significant accumulation and longer half-lives occur in renal failure. The reversal recommendations for LMWH using protamine [5] are given in Table 8.1. LMWH can be monitored with anti-Xa measurements using a LMWH standard, but this is unsuitable to assess the effect of protamine administration [6]. The APTT cannot be used to monitor LMWH. rFVIIa for LMWH reversal has been described in a registry study and case report, but its use is not recommended [5, 6].

Danaparoid is used in the treatment of heparin-induced thrombocytopenia (HIT), is renally excreted and has a long half-life (25 h). There is no reversal agent for danaparoid, and protamine is ineffective. Plasmapheresis has been used to remove danaparoid from the circulation. There are no clinical data on the use of rFVIIa or (A)PCC in bleeding associated with danaparoid [5]. Danaparoid can be monitored by anti-Xa levels using a danaparoid standard. The APTT is unsuitable for this purpose.

Fondaparinux is used at prophylactic doses (2.5 mg) in prevention of venous thrombosis and treatment of acute coronary syndrome. It is used at therapeutic doses (5–10 mg) in the treatment of venous thrombosis. The half-life is 17 h, but significant accumulation and prolongation of the half-life occur in renal failure (72 h if creatinine clearance (CrCl) < 30 mL/min). There is no specific antidote and protamine is ineffective. The only reversal agent with limited clinical experience is rFVIIa. This was found to be effective in four of eight patients with major bleeding at a dose of 90 μg/kg [7]. A placebo-controlled study in healthy volunteers treated with therapeutic doses of fondaparinux and 90 μg/kg rFVIIa demonstrated reversal of laboratory markers of coagulation [8]. Fondaparinux can be monitored by anti-Xa measurements using a fondaparinux standard but are not expected to correlate with the bleeding risk after reversal attempts with rFVIIa. The APTT cannot be used to monitor fondaparinux. The indications and pharmacology of fondaparinux were recently reviewed [5].

Intravenous direct thrombin inhibitors

These agents directly block the enzymatic activity of thrombin and include argatroban and bivalirudin.

Argatroban is a reversible direct thrombin inhibitor with hepatobiliary excretion and a half-life of 45 min. Dose reductions are needed in moderate hepatic impairment, multiple organ failure and hepatic congestion. It is licensed for the treatment of HIT [5]. The bleeding risk is estimated at approximately 1%/day. Given its short half-life, general measures may be sufficient in bleeding associated with argatroban. There are no data on the use of (A)PCC in argatroban-related bleeding. There are two case reports in uncontrolled bleeding where rFVIIa was given together with blood products without immediate effect, but one *ex vivo* study suggested that rFVIIa improved coagulation parameters assessed by thromboelastography [9]. Therefore, no recommendations can be made on the reversal agent to be used, but it can be removed using haemodialysis [5]. The effect of argatroban is monitored by APTT, but the dose response is not linear with a plateau at higher APTT values. It also prolongs the PT (INR), making the introduction of warfarin in HIT patients difficult [5].

Bivalirudin forms a reversible bond with thrombin and is cleared through proteolysis by thrombin itself (80%), and only 20% is excreted renally. The half-life is 25 min but 3.5 h in dialysis-dependent patients. It is licensed for percutaneous coronary interventions (PCI) and patients with HIT or who are at high risk of HIT undergoing PCI. The characteristics and use of bivalirudin were recently reviewed [5]. Given its short half-life, stopping the drug and applying general measures are likely to be sufficient, but the drug can be removed using haemodialysis/haemofiltration. There is minimal evidence for the use of rFVIIa and no clinical data on the use of (A)PCC. The effect of bivalirudin can be monitored by APTT and activated clotting time (ACT).

New oral anticoagulants

These include the direct thrombin inhibitor dabigatran and the direct factor Xa inhibitors rivaroxaban and apixaban.

Dabigatran is licensed for the prevention of venous thrombosis following total hip/knee replacement and stroke prevention in atrial fibrillation (SPAF). Maximum levels are reached within 2–3 h. Dabigatran is renally cleared and the half-life is strongly dependent on the creatinine clearance (CrCl) (see Table 8.1). Based on the half-lives, the manufacturer recommends omission of dabigatran for 2–4 days (CrCl > 80 mL/min and 30–50 mL/min, respectively) before surgery with high bleeding risk is undertaken. Bleeding was found in 2.71–3.11% depending on the dose used (see [11] for a review on dabigatran) but may be higher outside trial situations in elderly patients with multiple co-morbidities. There is no antidote for dabigatran and no reports yet on the use of rFVIIa or (A)PCC in a clinical setting. PCC was reported useful in an animal study of intracranial haemorrhage [10], whereas rFVIIa was not effective. PCC however was ineffective in a controlled study on healthy, non-bleeding volunteers [11]. Animal studies have also been conflicting. Haemodialysis reduces plasma levels of dabigatran, and preliminary evidence indicates that

activated charcoal binds dabigatran and may be tried within 2 h of ingestion. Routine coagulation tests cannot be used to monitor dabigatran, but a normal thrombin time excludes significant anticoagulation, and a normal APTT makes high levels of dabigatran unlikely but does not exclude these [12]. More specialized assays such as the Haemoclot® assay can be used to monitor plasma drug concentrations but are not widely available.

Both rivaroxaban and apixaban have a licence for thromboprophylaxis following total hip/knee replacement and SPAF. Rivaroxaban also has a licence for the treatment of venous thrombosis. Both reach peak levels at 3 h and have half-lives of 7–9 and 9–14 h, respectively. Clearance is hepatic (75%) and renal (25%). The risk of bleeding with rivaroxaban was 3.4% (SPAF), and the annual rate of bleeding on apixaban was 2.13%. Similar to dabigatran, these numbers may be higher in *real-life experience*. There is no specific antidote, but a controlled trial in healthy non-bleeding volunteers suggested an effect of PCC in reversal of rivaroxaban [11]. In animal studies, the data of (A)PCC and rFVIIa have been conflicting, and there are no reports on their clinical effectiveness. Both drugs have high plasma protein binding, making it unlikely that haemodialysis will be effective. Although both prolong the PT and APTT, routine coagulation tests cannot be used to estimate the amount of circulating drug. A normal PT makes therapeutic anticoagulation with rivaroxaban unlikely but does not exclude this, and anti-Xa assays using specific calibrators are recommended but not widely available [12].

Conclusion

Life-threatening bleeding on anticoagulants is infrequent, but management is difficult when no specific reversal agents are available. General measures should be applied in all cases, but specific antidotes only exist for VKA and UFH. For others, general pro-haemostatic agents may be used after careful assessment of the risks and benefits. Coagulation screens should be performed in these patients but may not always be useful in assessing the degree of anticoagulation, and specialist assays may be required.

References

1 Levi M, Levy JH, Andersen HF, Truloff D. Safety of recombinant activated factor VII in randomized clinical trials. N Engl J Med 2010;363(19):1791–800.

2 Sorour Y, Van Veen JJ, Makris M. Recombinant factor VIIa for unlicensed indications – a definite no or a cautious maybe in selected patients? Int J Clin Pract 2010;64(11):1468–71.

3 Dentali F, Marchesi C, Pierfranceschi MG, Safety of prothrombin complex concentrates for rapid anticoagulation reversal of vitamin K antagonists. A meta-analysis. Thromb Haemost 2011;106(3):429–38.

4 Makris M, Van Veen JJ, Maclean R. Warfarin anticoagulation reversal: management of the asymptomatic and bleeding patient. J Thromb Thrombolysis 2010;29(2):171–81.

5 Garcia DA, Baglin TP, Weitz JI, Samama MM. Parenteral anticoagulants: antithrombotic therapy and prevention of thrombosis, 9th edition: American College of Chest Physicians Evidence-Based Clinical Practice Guidelines. Chest 2012;141(2 Suppl.):e24S–e43S.

6 van Veen JJ, Maclean RM, Hampton KK et al. Protamine reversal of low molecular weight heparin: clinically effective? Blood Coagul Fibrinol 2011;22(7):565–70.

7 Luporsi P, Chopard R, Janin S et al. Use of recombinant factor VIIa (NovoSeven®) in 8 patients with ongoing life-threatening bleeding treated with fondaparinux. Acute Card Care 2011;13(2):93–8.

8 Bijsterveld NR, Moons AH, Boekholdt SM et al. Ability of recombinant factor VIIa to reverse the anticoagulant effect of the pentasaccharide Fondaparinux in healthy volunteers. Circulation 2002;106(20):2550–4.

9 Young G, Yonekawa KE, Nakagawa PA, Blain RC, Lovejoy AE, Nugent DJ. Recombinant activated factor VII effectively reverses the anticoagulant effects of heparin, enoxaparin, fondaparinux, argatroban, and bivalirudin ex vivo as measured using thromboelastography. Blood Coagul Fibrinol 2007;18(6):547–53.

10 Zhou W, Schwarting S, Illanes S et al. Hemostatic therapy in experimental intracerebral hemorrhage associated with the direct thrombin inhibitor dabigatran. Stroke 2011;42(12):3594–9.

11 Eerenberg ES, Kamphuisen PW, Sijpkens MK, Meijers JC, Buller HR, Levi M. Reversal of rivaroxaban and dabigatran by prothrombin complex concentrate: a randomized, placebo-controlled, crossover study in healthy subjects. Circulation 2011;124(14):1573–9.

12 van Veen, Smith J, Kitchen S, Makris M. Normal prothrombin time in the presence of therapeutic levels of rivaroxaban. Br J Haematol 2013;160(6):859–61.

Further reading

Makris M, van Veen JJ, Tait CR, Mumford AD, Laffan M, On Behalf of the British Committee for Standards in Haematology. Guideline on the management of bleeding in patients on antithrombotic agents. Br J Haematol 2013;160(1):35–46.

CHAPTER 9

Disseminated Intravascular Coagulation

Jecko Thachil

Department of Haematology, Central Manchester University Hospitals NHS Foundation Trust, Manchester, UK

Introduction

Disseminated intravascular coagulation (DIC) has probably afflicted mankind from the very beginning, since it often arises as a consequence of severe sepsis or trauma. It can be described as an overexaggerated pathological response to triggering factors which in the physiological phase would have been beneficial to the host. The natural process of DIC is illustrated by its definition provided by the International Society on Thrombosis and Haemostasis, that is, 'An acquired syndrome characterized by the intravascular activation of coagulation with loss of localization arising from different causes. It can originate from and cause damage to the microvasculature, which if sufficiently severe, can produce organ dysfunction' [1].

Pathophysiology

The characteristic pathophysiological feature of DIC is the unregulated and excessive generation of thrombin (see Figure 9.1). Normal haemostatic plug formation involves regulated, localized and limited generation of thrombin. Thrombin is a master regulator, balancing both procoagulant and anticoagulant activities and the profibrinolytic and antifibrinolytic pathways. When the inciting insult (e.g. sepsis) is persistent or severe, the

amount of thrombin generated becomes excessive. The normal mechanisms which control this excess thrombin production (anticoagulant mechanisms) become overwhelmed, leading to dissemination of the clot into the systemic circulation. The thrombin-orchestrated fibrinolytic pathway tries frantically to deal with the excess fibrin formed. This generates a large amount of fibrin degradation products through plasmin, the key enzyme in this regard. The parallel and concomitant activation of the inflammatory cascade and the perturbation of the endothelial microvasculature add to the heterogeneity of this process. Thus, DIC is a complex coagulation disorder where accelerated thrombosis occurs in tandem with increased fibrinolysis and thus can present with bleeding and thrombotic manifestations occurring simultaneously or at various times during the course of a clinical episode.

Clinical features

Disseminated intravascular coagulation is a syndrome and not a diagnosis in itself. It is always seen in the presence of an underlying disorder like sepsis or trauma, which initiates the process of intravascular coagulation. Also, the features associated with the primary illness frequently obscure the clinical manifestations of DIC.

The symptoms specific to DIC can range from occasional bleeding episodes to severe haemorrhagic diathesis,

Haematology in Critical Care: A Practical Handbook, First Edition. Edited by Jecko Thachil and Quentin A. Hill.
© 2014 John Wiley & Sons, Ltd. Published 2014 by John Wiley & Sons, Ltd.

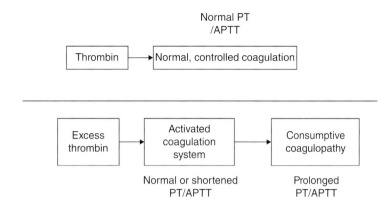

Figure 9.1 Top of the figure shows physiological state and the bottom of the figure shows coagulation changes in disseminated intravascular coagulation (DIC).

which can coexist with thrombosis and complications arising from organ dysfunction. Although the pathogenesis of DIC is extensive thrombin generation and widespread fibrin deposition, the clinical manifestation often recognized and associated with DIC is bleeding, reported in up to 70% of patients. This excess bleeding in DIC has been attributed to the depletion of coagulation factors and platelets, which are consumed during the large amount of thrombus formation. However, there are several other factors, which can also lead to this bleeding state including abnormal platelet function and fibrinolysis due to renal dysfunction, decreased clotting synthesis due to liver impairment and depletion of nitric oxide from endothelial dysfunction leading to uninhibited platelet activation and consumption.

Bleeding when it occurs is observed initially in the skin, where spontaneous ecchymoses and petechiae can develop and become widespread due to dermal ischaemia and necrosis, as in the case of meningococcal septicaemia. Venepuncture and indwelling catheter or needle sites and wounds from recent surgeries or other procedures can also demonstrate excessive blood oozing. Mucosal bleeding arises due to the excess fibrinolysis, in the gastrointestinal and genitourinary tracts, leading to sometimes life-threatening haemorrhage.

The thrombotic manifestations of DIC may affect practically all parts of the body, although the severity and localization of the thrombi can vary considerably depending on several factors, including the nature of the underlying trigger mechanism. The following organ dysfunctions have been related solely to DIC in a decreasing order of frequency: renal (24%), liver (18%), lungs (16%) and

central nervous system (1.7%). An experimental animal study mapping fibrin distribution in organs affected by DIC was done by Regoeczi and Brain, who demonstrated that the maximum fibrin recoverable was from the kidneys. This observation would explain the preponderance of renal dysfunction among all the organs affected by DIC despite the different aetiologies. Cerebral involvement in DIC can manifest in non-specific ways depending on the extent and location of thrombi, haemorrhage or both in its vasculature. The most common neurological complications of DIC described are large vessel occlusion, obtundation and coma, subarachnoid haemorrhage and multiple cortical and brainstem haemorrhages and infarction. A higher incidence of nervous system haemorrhagic complications is noted in DIC associated with acute promyelocytic leukaemia, without early treatment with antileukaemic agents. Pulmonary manifestations in DIC can vary from transient hypoxia in mild cases to alveolar haemorrhage or emboli and ARDS in severe cases. It is difficult to distinguish whether the ARDS developed due to the DIC itself or the underlying illness such as septicaemia, amniotic fluid embolism or severe trauma.

Underlying aetiology may influence the pattern of organ involvement seen in DIC. Those with underlying infection have more frequent liver and renal dysfunction, while respiratory dysfunction is more frequent in trauma cases. This variability indicates that the clinical manifestations are determined not only by the process of intravascular coagulation but also by the underlying clinical disorders. For example, while DIC due to obstetric disorders mainly present as bleeding with less common organ dysfunction, those who develop DIC due to sepsis mainly have organ impairment compared to haemorrhagic problems.

This clinical heterogeneity of DIC may be explained by the variable expression of molecules participating in DIC processes, which in turn depends on the organs and tissues affected. Also, the underlying disorders that initiate DIC may trigger different pathways of thrombin and plasmin generation, resulting in predominantly thrombosis or haemorrhage. All the same, if the uncontrolled intravascular coagulation continues unabated, multi-organ failure is often a common outcome in any of these conditions.

Diagnosis

Disseminated intravascular coagulation should be considered in any patient with progressive thrombocytopenia (usually gradual) and worsening prothrombin time (PT), APTT, fibrinogen and D-dimer levels. Several experts have established composite scoring systems to assist in the correct diagnosis of DIC, and these are summarized in Table 9.1. Guidelines and consensus reports summarizing the diagnostic process for DIC stress the fact that there is no single laboratory test currently

available for an accurate and a precise diagnosis of DIC due to their non-specific nature:

• For example, despite fibrinogen reduction being the consequence of excess thrombin generation in the clinical states leading to DIC, a low fibrinogen level is only seen in approximately one-third of cases. In most of the underlying cases, this is secondary to the initial increase in the fibrinogen level from the inflammatory state, which accompanies the underlying disorder. Hence, a drop in fibrinogen may only bring it to within normal range, making the physicians unsuspicious of the non-overt DIC state.

• Similarly, abnormal PT and APTT may only be noted in approximately half of the patients. In this context, it needs to be borne in mind that prolonged PT is very common in intensive care units in patients who may have vitamin K deficiency.

• Thrombocytopenia is however very common, observed in over 90% of the cases. Once again, a normal platelet count should not deter from the diagnosis of DIC, while a drop in the count should be taken into consideration.

• A rise in fibrin-related markers including D-dimer would mean that thrombin has acted on fibrinogen to make fibrin and can be helpful in combination with the other markers to diagnose DIC.

Table 9.1 Currently available diagnostic criteria to diagnose disseminated intravascular coagulation (DIC).

	ISTH criteria	JMWH criteria	JAAM criteria
Underlying clinical condition predisposing to DIC	Essential	1 point	Essential
Clinical symptoms	Not used	Bleeding – 1 point Organ failure – 1 point	SIRS score >/= 3 – 1 point
Platelet count (in × 10⁹/L)	50 to 100 – 1 point <50 – 2 points	80 to 120 – 1 point 50 to 80 – 2 points <50 – 3 points	80 to 120 or >30% reduction – 1 point <80 or >50% reduction – 2 points
Fibrin-related marker	Moderate increase – 2 points Marked increase – 3 points	Fibrin degradation products (FDP) (µg/mL) 10 to 20 – 1 point 20 to 40 – 2 points >40 – 3 points	FDP (µg/mL) 10 to 25 – 1 point >25 – 3 points
Fibrinogen	<1 – 1 point	1 to 1.5 – 1 point <1 – 2 points	Not used
Prothrombin time (PT)	Prolongation 3 to 6 s – 1 point >6 – 2 points	PT ratio 1.25 to 1.67 – 1 point >1.67 – 2 points	PT ratio ≥1.2 – 1 point
DIC diagnosis	≥5 points	≥7 points	≥4 points

ISTH, International Society on Thrombosis and Haemostasis; JMWH, Japanese Ministry of Health and Welfare; JAAM, Japanese Association for Acute Medicine.

• For the aforementioned reasons, serial testing, if possible, should be undertaken to aid in the diagnosis of DIC in the setting of a clinical condition known to trigger this complication. This would also be beneficial in trying to judge whether excess thrombin generation is persisting or has ceased. Besides repeated analysis, a combination of results of the routinely performed blood tests should be considered to make a diagnosis of DIC.

Differential diagnosis

Disseminated intravascular coagulation can be confused with several other conditions:
• Catastrophic antiphospholipid syndrome – usually, the presentation is acute with multisystem thrombosis which includes micro- and macro-vasculature. Bleeding is unusual in this condition. PT and APTT are usually normal although if prolonged ischaemia occurs, this can result in secondary DIC.
• Thrombotic thrombocytopenic purpura – in this condition, the thrombocytopenia is usually abrupt. There is haemolytic anaemia as well. Schistocytes or fragmented red cells in the blood film are usually numerous (in DIC, these may be seen but not in large amounts). Again, PT and APTT are usually normal unless DIC develops from tissue ischaemia.
• Liver disease – an underlying chronic liver disease is probably one of the most difficult situations to be differentiated from DIC. Serial worsening of the laboratory parameters may be helpful to point towards DIC.
• Septicaemia without DIC – progressive thrombocytopenia can occur in the absence of DIC due to sepsis. Elevated D-dimer levels can be a non-specific finding in these cases. Fibrinogen levels usually are high, however. Once again, serial testing of a combination of tests can provide the clues for DIC.
• Heparin-induced thrombocytopenia (HIT) – increasing use of thromboprophylaxis and awareness has led to increased suspicion of this diagnosis on the critical care units. Thrombocytopenia here is often acute with normal PT and APTT. Fibrinogen levels are not usually low. Secondary DIC can develop with HIT.
• Systemic vasculitis – multi-organ failure can develop in the context of progressive thrombocytopenia in systemic vasculitis. D-dimer can be high although a low fibrinogen is not characteristic.

Treatment

Since DIC develops secondary to other diseases, the cornerstone of therapy is the treatment of the underlying disorder. If the inciting process cannot be halted, the treatment of DIC with any available measure is likely to be futile. The classical example is obstetrical DIC, where the best treatment would be the delivery of the placenta (or the foetus), which is the triggering factor for DIC. In addition, ancillary measures have to be taken into consideration to ensure a good outcome. For example, in trauma-related DIC, the appropriate early management of severe hypotension and related acidosis and hypothermia is crucial for a successful outcome despite aggressive blood product administration, which may be considered as the treatment for DIC. Additional strategies are required to *support* these patients until adequate control of the triggering disease process is achieved. These may be divided into blood product support and specific drug therapies.

Transfusion support

Blood product support for patients with DIC includes platelets, fresh frozen plasma and fibrinogen replacement in the form of cryoprecipitate or fibrinogen concentrates [2]. Since DIC is a procoagulant process, it is important that any of these blood components are *only* administered in patients who have bleeding manifestations. Platelets should be considered in the bleeding patient if the platelet count is less than 50×10^9/L although this is only a guide and the threshold platelet count should be based on the patients' clinical situation. Bleeding in DIC can also be due to platelet dysfunction necessitating platelet transfusions in those who may have higher platelet count. Fresh frozen plasma is given if there is bleeding and prolonged PT and APTT (more than 1.5 times the upper limit of normal range). The recommended dose is 15–20 mL/kg although a higher dose may be necessary if volume overload is permissible in patients with severe bleeding. Prolongation of the clotting screen in this context may also be related to the interference by fibrinogen or fibrin degradation products (FDP), reaffirming the notion that plasma transfusion should be reserved for patients with bleeding. Prothrombin complex concentrates are not advisable in such patients in lieu of fresh frozen plasma since it can aggravate thrombosis due to the associated decrease in antithrombin. Cryoprecipitate (two pools) or fibrinogen concentrate (3 g) can be considered in patients with bleeding and fibrinogen levels less than 1.5 g/L. Although a lower threshold (1.0 g/L) has been suggested, in a patient with active bleeding, early replacement of fibrinogen is beneficial. It should however be borne in mind that platelets, coagulation factors and fibrinogen levels may all decrease rapidly in tandem with the continuing thrombin generation and a single set of blood results may only provide a snapshot of the situation. It is also necessary that a prolonged PT in all cases is not automatically attributed to DIC, but vitamin K deficiency is excluded in such critically ill patients who may not have received adequate nutrition but several antibiotics affecting vitamin K metabolism.

Specific drug therapies

Heparin, in the unfractionated form, has been historically used a treatment of DIC related to purpura fulminans, intrauterine foetal death, giant haemangiomas and some cases of aortic aneurysms. In recent years, there is a trend towards using low-molecular-weight heparin (LMWH) in place of the unfractionated heparin due to its predictive pharmacokinetics and lesser bleeding risks. The Japanese Ministry of Health and Welfare approved the LMWH dalteparin for use in DIC after a multicentre trial showed significantly reduced organ failure. In addition, LMWH prophylaxis should be considered highly necessary in patients with DIC in the critical care unit where the incidence of venous thromboembolism is extremely high. In those with a high risk of bleeding, unfractionated heparin may still be considered due to its short action and ease of reversibility.

Low levels of antithrombin, one of the natural anticoagulants depleted early in DIC, have been shown to be a predictor of adverse clinical outcome and 28-day mortality in DIC. On the contrary, antithrombin replacement significantly shortened duration of symptoms and allowed rapid normalization of coagulation parameters in DIC patients. However, in the KyberSept trial, antithrombin therapy did not show any survival advantages over placebo although a *post hoc* analysis could attribute this failure to co-administered heparin. Currently, antithrombin use is restricted to clinical trials.

Thrombomodulin is an endothelial surface cofactor, which in the presence of thrombin, potentiates activated protein C, a natural anticoagulant. Recombinant, soluble thrombomodulin demonstrated significantly better DIC resolution rates (66% vs. 50%) and mortality (28% vs. 35%) in a randomized, double-blind clinical trial in comparison with heparin. Lower 28-day mortality and a rapid decrease in the Sequential Organ Failure Assessment (SOFA) score on day 1 in sepsis-related DIC have also been observed with this agent.

Activated protein C had been until recently hailed as a major advancement in the treatment of patients with severe sepsis and DIC based on the Protein C Worldwide Evaluation in Severe Sepsis (PROWESS) trial. However, the inherent bleeding risks with this agent were considered significant, and the recent PROWESS–SHOCK trial failed to identify any survival advantage, and activated protein C has been withdrawn from the market.

Synthetic protease inhibitors (gabexate mesilate), agents noted to have antithrombin activity, have been recommended by the Japanese experts for use in patients with haemorrhage immediately after an operation or where there is a marked decrease in platelet count.

Since hyperfibrinolysis is common with DIC, antifibrinolytics would be a natural choice for its treatment. However, hyperfibrinolysis in DIC is secondary to excess thrombin generation and is a natural reactionary process to deal with the uncontrolled thrombin generation. For this reason, inhibiting excessive fibrinolysis with antifibrinolytic agents can prove deleterious in the setting of DIC. In acute coagulopathy of trauma, however, where hyperfibrinolysis predominates (this situation has been termed DIC with fibrinolytic phenotype as opposed to DIC with coagulopathic phenotype), antifibrinolytic agents may be beneficial for those with persistent bleeding in the very early stages. Another clinical situation is massive postpartum haemorrhage where fibrinolysis is excessive, and tranexamic acid has been demonstrated to be hugely beneficial (see chapter 15 on massive transfusion/trauma). Whether this clinical situation should be considered as DIC is controversial.

In summary, the treatment of DIC is varied based on the diverse causes and clinical manifestations associated with DIC; a given therapeutic approach may only be suitable for one aetiology and not the other. Even in the same clinical situation, the management strategy should be personalized depending on the clinical picture of thrombosis or haemorrhage.

References

1 Taylor Jr FB, Toh CH, Hoots WK, Wada H, Levi M. Towards definition, clinical and laboratory criteria, and a scoring system for disseminated intravascular coagulation—on behalf of the Scientific Subcommittee on DIC of the ISTH. Thromb Haemost 2001;86:1327–30.

2 Gando S, Saitoh D, Ogura H et al. Natural history of disseminated intravascular coagulation diagnosed based on the newly established diagnostic criteria for critically ill patients: results of a multicenter, prospective survey. Crit Care Med 2008;36: 145–50.

Further reading

Levi M, Toh CH, Thachil J, Watson HG. Guidelines for the diagnosis and management of disseminated intravascular coagulation. British Committee for Standards in Haematology. Br J Haematol 2009;145:24–33.

Regoeczi E, Brain MC. Organ distribution of fibrin in disseminated intravascular coagulation. Br J Haematol 1969;17:73–81.

Thachil J, Toh CH. Disseminated intravascular coagulation in obstetric disorders and its acute haematological management. Blood Rev 2009;23:167–76.

Wada H, Asakura H, Okamoto K et al. Expert consensus for the treatment of disseminated intravascular coagulation in Japan. Thromb Res. 2010;125:6–11.

CHAPTER 10

Heparin-Induced Thrombocytopenia

Jerrold H. Levy[1] and Anne M. Winkler[2,3,4]

[1] Department of Anesthesiology and Critical Care, Duke University School of Medicine, Durham, NC, USA
[2] Department of Pathology and Laboratory Medicine, Emory University School of Medicine, Atlanta, GA, USA
[3] Grady Health System Transfusion Service, Atlanta, GA, USA
[4] Emory Special Coagulation Laboratory, Atlanta, GA, USA

Introduction

Heparin-induced thrombocytopenia (HIT) is an immune-mediated coagulopathy that can occur in critically ill patients following heparin exposure that is associated with thrombotic complications. HIT is a clinicopathologic diagnosis that requires stopping heparin and initiating alternative anticoagulation therapy if a thrombotic event occurs or for thromboembolic prophylaxis [1]. This chapter will discuss the pathophysiology, diagnosis, treatment and alternative anticoagulation strategies for HIT in the intensive care unit (ICU).

Pathogenesis/frequency

The prothrombotic events occurring with HIT are caused by antibodies that develop to a complex of heparin and platelet factor 4 (PF4), a basic protein stored in the alpha granules of platelets. Following platelet activation, especially after surgery, immunoglobulin G (IgG) antibodies form against the complexes of heparin and PF4 in certain susceptible individuals. There is a stoichiometric ratio at which this complex formation occurs since excess amounts of either heparin or PF4 may not allow the complex to develop. Once the antibodies are formed, they activate platelets through their Fc domain and FcγIIa receptors. The activated platelets generate microparticles and activate monocytes and endothelial cells, which express tissue factor, all resulting in a procoagulant state.

Although 7–50% of heparin-treated patients form low titres of heparin–PF4 antibodies, clinical HIT is estimated to occur in approximately 1–5% of patients receiving unfractionated heparin and less than 1% of patients receiving low-molecular-weight heparin [2, 3]. In the ICU setting with complex critically ill patients, the incidences may be higher. The incidence in cardiac transplant and neurosurgical patients is reported to be 11% and 15%, respectively [1]. In this context, it is important to bear in mind that positivity for HIT antibodies, by itself, does not translate into clinical HIT. The iceberg model proposed by Warkentin illustrates this point, wherein only few patients with antibody positivity will have clinical HIT, and of these, only few will develop thrombosis.

Post-operative cardiac surgery patients are at an increased risk of antibody development, in part due to platelet activation that occurs following surgery and cardiopulmonary bypass (CPB) and the higher doses of heparin administered. HIT antibodies are usually cleared in approximately 3 months [4]. The presence and the level of the antibodies, irrespective of thrombocytopenia, are associated with increased adverse events. HIT increases the odds of thrombosis (odds ratio, 37) with an overall thrombotic risk of 38–76%. Thrombosis appears coincident with, or slightly before, the decline in platelet count [5].

Haematology in Critical Care: A Practical Handbook, First Edition. Edited by Jecko Thachil and Quentin A. Hill.
© 2014 John Wiley & Sons, Ltd. Published 2014 by John Wiley & Sons, Ltd.

Thrombocytopenia in the ICU

The diagnosis of HIT in the ICU is often difficult due to competing causes of thrombocytopenia including post-operative dilutional changes, sepsis, disseminated intravascular coagulation, intra-aortic balloon pump (IABP) with mechanical destruction, extracorporeal life support (ECLS) or other drug-induced causes of thrombocytopenia (see Chapter 3) [6]. In cardiac patients, glycoprotein IIb–IIIa inhibitors are important causes of drug-induced thrombocytopenia, and thienopyridines have been associated with rare cases of thrombotic thrombocytopenic purpura (TTP).

An important cause of thrombocytopenia in the ICU is volume resuscitation after haemorrhagic shock and CPB where a 40–60% decrease in platelet count occurs. HIT after CPB often has a biphasic pattern that decreases after CPB-related thrombocytopenia corrects or a persistently low/decreasing platelet count greater than 4 days postoperatively. HIT can manifest acutely within minutes–hours of heparin exposure (rapid-onset HIT) associated with hypotension or shock caused by pre-existing antibodies due to prior exposure, manifesting as anaphylaxis, and include hypotension, pulmonary hypertension and/or tachycardia 2–30 min after intravenous administration [1]. HIT can also occur days to weeks after exposure (delayed-onset HIT) in patients presenting with thrombosis.

Laboratory testing

Current laboratory testing for HIT includes (i) antigen–antibody assays and (ii) functional platelet activation assays. The enzyme-linked immunosorbent assay (ELISA) and rapid particle gel immunoassay detect polyclonal antibodies to complexes of PF4 and heparin or complexes of PF4 and other polyanions. The most commonly used commercial ELISAs detect IgG, IgM and IgA antibodies and while sensitive are not specific for HIT; however, newer assays detect IgG antibodies and improve clinical specificity. It is crucial that ELISA results are not reported as positive or negative, but rather as the level of optical density (OD) and/or antibody titre, which is important for clinical decision-making. The likelihood of a positive serotonin release assay (SRA) increases with higher OD. An important study reported that most HIT cases were associated with an ELISA OD greater than 1.40 U.

A positive ELISA is considered to be an OD greater than 0.4 or greater than 0.5, dependent upon the assay manufacturer, but weak positive results (0.4–1.00 OD) excluded a diagnosis of HIT in most cases with only an approximately 5% chance of positive SRA [7]. However, *high-titre negative* ELISA results may become positive on retesting if heparin is continued or due to antibody formation. An additional step in the laboratory evaluation may involve neutralization of the antibody tests with higher heparin concentrations. This also can be helpful in suggesting the specificity of the antibody tests. We believe functional tests are important to determine if the antibody positivity is clinically relevant. The functional tests include the SRA and heparin-induced platelet activation test. These tests detect heparin-dependent, platelet-activating antibodies and are considered the gold standard for the laboratory diagnoses of HIT because of high sensitivity/specificity, but the disadvantage is that they require specialized laboratories.

Diagnosing HIT in the ICU

Diagnosing HIT in ICU patients can be difficult as previously described, especially in cardiothoracic surgical patients. Because the sensitivity of readily available antibody immunoassays is high but specificity is quite low, we have used both a clinical probability score and laboratory immunoassay to increase specificity, which is of particular importance in the ICU setting [8]. We reported testing of ICU patients with both the heparin–PF4 immunoassay and SRA assigning a high, intermediate or low clinical *4Ts* probability score that quantifies thrombocytopenia, timing of platelet decrease and thrombotic complications in each patient. The 4Ts score is a useful clinical estimate to determine if HIT is present and includes (i) thrombocytopenia with a platelet count fall greater than 50% and platelet nadir greater than or equal to 20 (2 points) or platelet count fall 30–50% and platelet nadir 10–19 (1 point); (ii) timing of platelet fall with clear onset between days 5 and 10 or platelet fall less than or equal to 1 day (2 points) or onset after day 10 (1 point); (iii) new confirmed thrombosis (2 points) or progressive, recurrent or suspected thrombosis (1 point); and (iv) no other likely cause for thrombocytopenia (2 points) or possible other cause (1 point). The resulting clinical probability scores are divided into high (6–8 points), intermediate (4–5 points) and low (≤3 points) groups [9].

In our ICU study, we compared the clinical score and the heparin–PF4 immunoassay against the *gold standard* diagnostic test, the SRA. The sensitivity and specificity for heparin–PF4 OD greater than 0.4 were 100% and 26%, respectively. Sensitivity and specificity for the diagnosis of HIT with a combination of heparin–PF4 OD greater than 0.4 and high/intermediate 4Ts score were 100% and 70%, respectively. The negative predictive value was 100% for low 4Ts score. We demonstrated that the use of the 4Ts clinical score combined with the heparin–PF4 immunoassay for HIT diagnosis increases the sensitivity and specificity of HIT testing compared with the heparin–PF4 immunoassay alone. Furthermore, with an intermediate 4Ts score and positive heparin–PF4 antibody test, a confirmatory platelet activation assay such as the SRA is necessary. Physicians treating patients in the ICU and after cardiothoracic surgery should recognize the need for an antibody test and confirmation with a platelet activation assay with even moderate clinical probability of HIT. As an attempt to expedite SRA results and improve diagnostic accuracy, our institution automatically reflexes positive HIT ELISAs to SRA, which has resulted in faster turnaround times, decreased alternative anticoagulation exposure and decreased diagnosis due to unconfirmed false-positive ELISA results.

Treatment

The recommended treatment for patients with strongly suspected or confirmed HIT is discontinuation of heparin and initiation of a non-heparin, alternative anticoagulant such as a direct thrombin inhibitor (e.g. argatroban, bivalirudin, desirudin and lepirudin). Documentation of the patient's HIT status including a sign on the patient's bed and/or chart stating "No heparin: HIT" may help prevent unintended heparin exposure. Different direct thrombin inhibitors are approved in different countries for use in HIT patients without thrombosis (argatroban), HIT patients with thrombosis (lepirudin, argatroban) and patients with or at risk of HIT undergoing percutaneous coronary intervention (PCI) (argatroban, bivalirudin). The direct thrombin inhibitors do not resemble heparin, do not cross-react with heparin–PF4 antibodies and cannot promote HIT. Danaparoid, a heparinoid with minimal cross-reactivity with heparin–PF4 antibodies, was one of

the first agents approved but is not widely available. Fondaparinux is a selective factor Xa inhibitor with a low risk for antibody formation; however, fondaparinux has a long half-life that is prolonged with renal failure.

Managing HIT should include stopping heparin and continued alternative anticoagulant coverage to prevent thrombotic complications. In patients with thrombotic complications, an alternative anticoagulant needs to be started. However, for the patient with thrombocytopenia with suspected HIT but without thrombotic complications, stopping the heparin is critical, and awaiting ELISA results should be considered. The risk of excessive bleeding especially recently after surgery should be carefully considered since bleeding is also associated with adverse outcomes. Low-molecular-weight heparins should be avoided because they cross-react with heparin–PF4 antibodies. Heparin should be avoided, at least as long as heparin–PF4 antibody testing is positive; however, it can be used if SRA is negative.

Alternative anticoagulation therapies: Argatroban

Argatroban is perhaps the only agent readily used in patients with renal dysfunction because it is the only intravenous agent hepatically metabolized. It is also a small molecule (molecular weight 526 Da) developed from l-arginine, which minimizes risk for sensitization and antibody formation. The recommended initial dose is an infusion of 2 mcg/kg/min that is too high in the ICU, and lower doses such as that for hepatic impairment (0.5 mcg/kg/min) should be started to achieve an activated partial thromboplastin time (APTT) prolongation 1.5–3 times the baseline. Argatroban will also prolong the prothrombin time (PT)/international normalized ratio (INR), and methods for monitoring the argatroban-to-coumarin transition using the INR or chromogenic factor Xa assay should be followed.

We reported the safety and efficacy of argatroban in the post-operative cardiothoracic surgical patient in the ICU using argatroban as a therapeutic agent for the treatment of suspected HIT by comparing thrombotic and bleeding events, platelet dynamics, antiplatelet factor 4/heparin antibody titre and clinical probability score between patients who did and did not receive argatroban. In 87 patients with suspected HIT, 47 patients (54%) were treated with argatroban, and 40 patients (46%) were not treated with argatroban [10]. There was no association between argatroban therapy and bleeding, mortality, length of stay or pretreatment thrombotic events. We believe that clinical suspicion of HIT as detected by clinical probability score and thrombotic complications should prompt immediate cessation of heparin and initiation of an alternative anticoagulant such as argatroban. The results from this study demonstrate that argatroban should be considered without increased risk for adverse events, including bleeding, in the cardiothoracic ICU after surgery [10].

Alternative anticoagulation therapies: Fondaparinux

Fondaparinux is a synthetic pentasaccharide with minimal *in vitro* cross-reactivity with HIT sera. It is approved for prophylaxis and treatment of venous thromboembolism. Prospective, controlled studies in HIT with small numbers have recently been reported; however, it has a long half-life with once a day dosing and should be avoided with renal dysfunction.

Alternative anticoagulation therapies: New oral anticoagulants

In the ICU, DVT prophylaxis is important but often a management issue in patients with HIT. Current studies suggest the new agents including dabigatran, a direct thrombin inhibitor, and rivaroxaban or apixaban, antifactor Xa inhibitors, can potentially be used for DVT prophylaxis as they are approved for different indications depending on the country. Because these agents require enteric absorption, the dabigatran capsule cannot be modified for enteric tube placement although other agents can. Although anecdotal reports have suggested the use of these agents for HIT, they cannot be recommended until prospective studies confirm their efficacy and safety.

Conclusion

Heparin-induced thrombocytopenia is a prothrombotic disorder that can occur in the ICU and should be considered an important differential diagnosis in the thrombocytopenic patient, although other causes of thrombocytopenia should be ruled out. Heparin should be discontinued if HIT is suspected, confirmatory laboratory testing should be performed, and parenteral alternative anticoagulation should be commenced. Heparin should be avoided as long as the antibody test is positive; however, the titre of the antibody is important and patients with positive antibodies should undergo functional platelet testing.

References

1 Levy JH, Tanaka KA, Hursting MJ. Reducing thrombotic complications in the perioperative setting: an update on heparin-induced thrombocytopenia. Anesth Analg 2007;105(3):570–82.

2 Martel N, Lee J, Wells PS. Risk for heparin-induced thrombocytopenia with unfractionated and low-molecular-weight heparin thromboprophylaxis: a meta-analysis. Blood 2005;106(8):2710–5.

3 Greinacher A. Heparin-induced thrombocytopenia. J Thromb Haemost 2009;7(Suppl. 1):9–12.

4 Warkentin TE, Kelton JG. Temporal aspects of heparin-induced thrombocytopenia. N Engl J Med 2001;344(17): 1286–92.

5 Greinacher A, Farner B, Kroll H, Kohlmann T, Warkentin TE, Eichler P. Clinical features of heparin-induced thrombocytopenia including risk factors for thrombosis. A retrospective analysis of 408 patients. Thromb Haemost 2005;94(1):132–5.

6 Rice TW, Wheeler AP. Coagulopathy in critically ill patients: part 1: platelet disorders. Chest 2009;136(6):1622–30.

7 Warkentin TE, Sheppard JI, Moore JC, Sigouin CS, Kelton JG. Quantitative interpretation of optical density measurements using PF4-dependent enzyme-immunoassays. J Thromb Haemost 2008;6(8):1304–12.

8 Demma LJ, Winkler AM, Levy JH. A diagnosis of heparin-induced thrombocytopenia with combined clinical and laboratory methods in cardiothoracic surgical intensive care unit patients. Anesth Analg 2011;113(4):697–702.

9 Lo GK, Juhl D, Warkentin TE, Sigouin CS, Eichler P, Greinacher A. Evaluation of pretest clinical score (4 T's) for the diagnosis of heparin-induced thrombocytopenia in two clinical settings. J Thromb Haemost 2006;4(4):759–65.

10 Demma LJ, Paciullo CA, Levy JH. Recognition of heparin-induced thrombocytopenia and initiation of argatroban therapy after cardiothoracic surgery in the intensive care unit. J Thorac Cardiovasc Surg 2012;143(5):1213–8.

CHAPTER 11
Thrombotic Microangiopathies

Mari Thomas[1] and Marie Scully[2]

[1]Haemostasis Research Unit, University College London, London, UK
[2]Department of Haematology, University College Hospital London, London, UK

Introduction

Thrombotic microangiopathies (TMAs) represent a spectrum of disorders characterized by thrombosis in small vessels. Thrombocytopenia is usually present, and review of the blood film confirms the microangiopathic process, with red cell fragmentation and often polychromasia. Considerable developments have been made in the field of TMA in recent years, and new genetic and autoimmune causes have been identified for the two major forms: haemolytic uraemic syndrome (HUS) and thrombotic thrombocytopenic purpura (TTP). However, the differential diagnosis of TMA may be difficult and remains a clinical one in the first instance. Differential diagnoses include disseminated intravascular coagulation (DIC); autoimmune disease e.g. lupus; severe hypertension; infections such as endocarditis; catastrophic antiphospholipid syndrome (CAPS); and malignancy (Figure 11.1).

Thrombotic thrombocytopenic purpura

Thrombotic thrombocytopenic purpura is a rare, acute, life-threatening disorder with an incidence of approximately six cases per million per year. There is no age limit, but TTP typically affects females between 30 and 40 years. TTP is characterized by thrombocytopenia, microangiopathic haemolytic anaemia (MAHA) and clinical features related to microvascular thrombosis. It occurs as a result of deficiency of the VWF-cleaving protease ADAMTS13, leading to the accumulation of ultralarge VWF multimers (ULVWF), increased platelet adhesion and aggregation and microthrombus formation. Most cases are acquired idiopathic, antibody-mediated TTP, but TTP may be precipitated by HIV infection, pregnancy, connective tissue disorders, pancreatitis or certain drugs [1]. In congenital TTP, ADAMTS13 deficiency results from recessive bi-allelic mutations in the ADAMTS13 gene.

Clinical features of TTP

Thrombotic thrombocytopenic purpura is a clinical diagnosis and must be considered in any patient with MAHA and low platelet counts in the absence of another cause. Clinical features are variable, and the classical pentad of MAHA, thrombocytopenia, fever, neurological involvement and renal failure is rarely seen.

In a recent study, 15 out of 40 patients required ITU admission, and 15% of cases were intubated and ventilated [2]. Neurological impairment is present in up to 80% of cases and may be fluctuating. Neurological features include headache, behavioural changes, transient ischaemic attacks, seizures or coma. Renal involvement is variable, resulting in reversible impairment. Cardiac

Haematology in Critical Care: A Practical Handbook, First Edition. Edited by Jecko Thachil and Quentin A. Hill.
© 2014 John Wiley & Sons, Ltd. Published 2014 by John Wiley & Sons, Ltd.

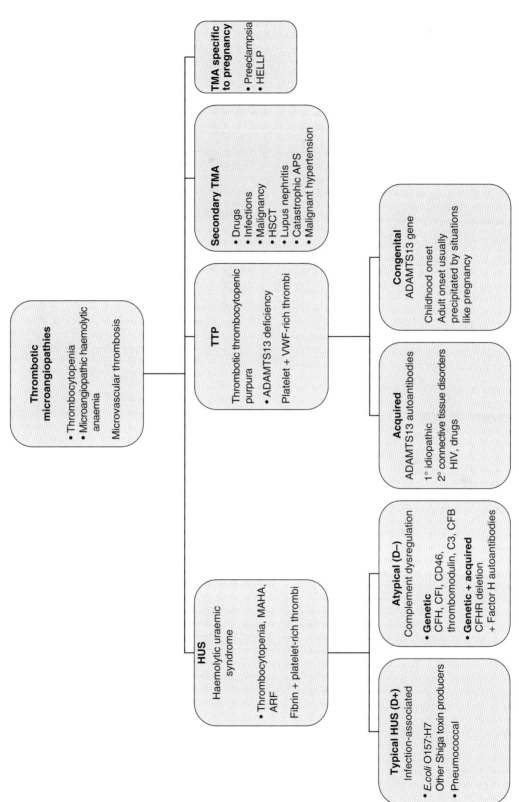

Figure 11.1 Subtypes of thrombotic microangiopathies (TMA). MAHA, microangiopathic haemolytic anaemia; ARF, acute renal failure; VWF, von Willebrand factor; APS, antiphospholipid syndrome; HELLP, haemolysis, elevated liver enzymes and low platelets; CFH, complement factor H; CFI, complement factor I; CFB, complement factor B; CFHR, complement factor H-related protein.

features may include infarction, arrhythmias and sudden cardiac arrest. Elevated troponin-T levels at presentation are an accurate predictor of disease severity [3]. Gastrointestinal features occur in a third of cases [1]. Patients may present with symptoms of thrombocytopenia such as bruising and petechiae. Autopsy studies confirm multi-organ involvement in TTP, with platelet and VWF-rich microthrombi (in contrast to the fibrin deposits seen in HUS or an inflammatory component in DIC or autoimmune disease).

Laboratory features in TTP

The blood film shows red cell fragmentation, polychromasia, anaemia and low platelets (below 150×10^9 but usually $<50 \times 10^9$). The reticulocyte count is increased and bilirubin is raised due to haemolysis. The clotting screen is typically normal. Lactate dehydrogenase (LDH) is disproportionately increased relative to the degree of haemolysis, due to associated tissue ischaemia. Virology screen pretreatment is necessary to exclude HIV-associated TTP and prior to therapy with large volumes of plasma.

Management of TTP
Plasma exchange (PEX)

Prompt diagnosis and treatment is the key to survival in TTP. Without therapy, mortality is 90% – reduced with plasma exchange (PEX) to 15–20%. Plasma is a source of the missing/dysfunctional enzyme ADAMTS13, and PEX allows delivery of large volumes of plasma and assists in the removal of ULVWF and anti-ADAMTS13 antibodies in the case of acquired TTP.

Plasma exchange must be started as soon as the diagnosis of TTP is suspected. If not, high-dose plasma infusions should be started as a holding measure, e.g. while awaiting transfer to a tertiary referral centre. Intensive PEX regimes are required in severe cases such as those with new/progressive neurological or cardiac symptoms. PEX should continue for at least 2 days after normalization of the platelet count. The UK guidelines recommend the use of solvent–detergent-treated FFP (Octaplas, Octapharma) to minimize pathogen exposure [4]. Complications of PEX include those related to the central venous catheter such as sepsis and reactions to plasma.

Immunosuppression

As the majority of TTP cases are acquired antibody-mediated, immunosuppression is used to attain complete

remission and/or prevent relapse. Steroids such as pulsed intravenous methylprednisolone or high-dose oral therapy are widely used in the treatment of TTP.

Rituximab, a monoclonal anti-CD20 antibody, acting on B lymphocytes, results in depletion of antibody-producing B cells. Initially used in patients' refractory to first-line therapy or with relapse, its use during acute presentation has also been demonstrated [2]. The first dose may be given over a longer period, e.g. 6–8h, to minimize allergic-type symptoms although subsequent doses can be infused more quickly. Typical rituximab dosing is $375 \, mg/m^2$ weekly, although in patients undergoing concomitant PEX, it may be given every 3–4 days.

Other immunosuppressive therapies

Vincristine and cyclophosphamide (both pulsed and daily dosing) have been used with some success, although the reported numbers are extremely low. The use of ciclosporin has led to high rates of clinical and haematological response, but relapses are documented after cessation of therapy.

Supportive therapy

Red cell transfusion may be required for rapid haemolysis, and all patients should receive folic acid supplementation. Platelet transfusions are contraindicated unless there is life-threatening haemorrhage as they are associated with disease exacerbation. Occult infection may prevent response to PEX or precipitate early relapse. An underlying infection should be actively sought. Low-dose aspirin (75 mg daily) and thromboprophylaxis are started with platelet count greater than 50×10^9/L and graduated elastic compression stockings used from admission.

Role of ADAMTS13 assays

Samples for ADAMTS13 activity and antibody status should be taken before PEX, but therapy must commence immediately before results are known. Severe ADAMTS13 deficiency and anti-ADAMTS13 IgG antibodies identify a specific group of patients with idiopathic TTP, but severe ADAMTS13 activity does not identify all patients who may respond to PEX. Some patients with moderate ADAMTS13 deficiency may have other disorders, and different assay methods vary in their detection of patients with severe deficiency [5].

The presence of inhibitory autoantibodies against ADAMTS13 at diagnosis confirms acquired deficiency and excludes congenital TTP and provides a rationale for increasing therapy, e.g. PEX frequency, and/or intensifying immunosuppression, e.g. using rituximab. Suboptimal response to PEX, ADAMTS13 activity greater than 10% and no measurable anti-ADAMTS13 IgG should prompt consideration of alternative diagnoses, e.g. atypical HUS (aHUS) or secondary TMA.

ADAMTS13 assays also have a role in patients in remission: severely reduced levels of ADAMTS13 during clinical remission are associated with a higher risk of relapse [6].

Pregnancy-associated TMA
Thrombocytopenia and MAHA may be found in a number of conditions in pregnancy or the postpartum period. Pre-eclamptic toxaemia (PET) is defined by hypertension, proteinuria and oedema. It may be complicated by renal impairment, eclampsia (convulsions) or abnormal coagulation. Prompt delivery, control of hypertension and use of magnesium sulphate are standard therapies. Complications require further supportive care. Haemolysis, elevated liver enzymes and low platelets (HELLP) can be complicated by DIC, placental abruption, acute renal failure (ARF), pulmonary oedema and liver failure that may require transplantation. Steroids may have a role, but management centres on prompt delivery and symptomatic therapy for complications, e.g. blood product/organ support. It is important to bear in mind that 20–30% of PET and HELLP cases occur after delivery. Failure of PET/HELLP to resolve with standard therapy, worsening thrombocytopenia or deteriorating clinical symptoms, should lead to consideration of PEX. Indeed, PET may be a presenting feature of TTP.

More than half of TTP patients are women of childbearing age and pregnancy is a precipitating cause of TTP in about 10% all female cases. TTP can present in any trimester but typically in the third or postpartum and is managed with standard therapy, i.e. PEX and steroids. A severe reduction in ADAMTS13 activity appears specific for TTP. Pregnancy-associated HUS is a rare disorder accounting for only 20% of all aHUS cases. Ninety percent of cases occur postpartum, and it can be differentiated by significant renal impairment and proteinuria. aHUS is associated with complement-mediated abnormalities (see following text), and therefore, prompt PEX +/− eculizumab is the treatment of choice.

Haemolytic uraemic syndrome (HUS)

Haemolytic uraemic syndrome is characterized by ARF, thrombocytopenia and MAHA. TMA affects predominantly the renal microvasculature, but the brain, heart, lungs and gastrointestinal tract may also be involved. HUS is divided into infection-induced (typical) HUS and aHUS.

Infection-induced HUS (typical HUS)
Typical HUS is frequent in children and is often associated with diarrhoea and termed D+HUS. D+HUS results from infections with Shiga and Shiga-like toxin-producing bacteria. The most common pathogen is *Escherichia coli* O175:H7, but other non-O157:H7 strains are endemic in other countries, and *Shigella*, *Salmonella* and *Campylobacter* species have also been implicated. Typical sources of infections are contaminated food such as uncooked meat: additional infections are mediated by person-to-person contact.

Mechanism of Shiga toxin (Stx)
All Shiga toxins (Stx) consist of an enzymatically active A subunit and a pentameric binding subunit (B). Stx A-mediated enzymatic cleavage of ribosomal RNA leads to a ribotoxic cellular stress response, resulting in apoptosis, loss of endothelial antithrombotic properties and cytokine release. Tissue injury may be caused directly by apoptosis or indirectly by thrombosis and ischaemia.

Clinical features
D+HUS presents as a sudden clinical deterioration 2 days to 2 weeks after seeming improvement of a diarrhoeal illness. Diagnosis is usually straightforward and based on the full blood count, blood film, serum creatinine and urinalysis. Determining the aetiology is important as therapy and prognosis of typical HUS and aHUS differ.

D+HUS is usually an acute self-limiting disease. Although ARF is part of the triad of HUS, only about half of all children with typical HUS require dialysis. Classical childhood HUS has a relatively good prognosis, and greater than 90% of childhood cases recover independent renal function spontaneously. However, about one-third of patients have severe defects such as hypertension and proteinuria [7], with longer-term renal damage in some cases.

Management

Management of typical HUS requires careful supportive therapy. Early parenteral volume expansion during *E. coli* O157:H7 infection appears to be associated with decreases in the rates of oliguria/anuria, the need for dialysis and the length of hospitalization. There is no evidence for the use of loop diuretics which do not prevent ARF, shorten recovery period or improve survival. Antibiotics do not improve outcomes and should not routinely be used. Glucocorticoids are not recommended, and there is no role for plasma therapy, anticoagulation, antiplatelet therapy or thrombolysis. Intestinal STX binders have been used in an attempt to reduce toxin absorption but have not shown improvement in mortality or dialysis rates [8].

Pneumococcal HUS (about 5% of cases of infection-related HUS) is a disease of young children occurring about a week after the onset of infection. Invasive *Streptococcus pneumoniae* produces neuraminidase that cleaves sialic acid residues from various glycoproteins and exposes the T antigen on red cell surfaces. Desialation is thought to predispose to a TMA [9]. The development of multi-organ failure is recognized and managed with supportive care, with approximately 70% of patients requiring renal dialysis. Mortality rates have improved but remain up to 12% primarily from sepsis. Renal outcome remains less favourable than in STEC-HUS [10]. The incidence of streptococcal-associated infections has decreased since the introduction of childhood immunization.

Atypical HUS (aHUS)

About 10% of HUS patients develop the atypical form. aHUS is a rare disease (~2 cases/million/year), affecting all ages but primarily children and young adults. About 20% cases of aHUS have a familial background, and some patients have recurrent disease. aHUS has a poor prognosis with mortality rates close to 25%, and 50% of patients do not recover renal function [9].

Pathophysiology

It is now recognized that aHUS is a disorder of complement regulation. The alternative complement pathway is constitutively activated to ensure defence against pathogens. Host cells are normally protected by regulators including factor H, CD46 (previously termed membrane cofactor protein (MCP)) and factor I. In aHUS, uncontrolled complement activation leads to generation of the inflammatory anaphylotoxin C5a and formation of the terminal complement membrane attack complex (MAC) with resulting tissue damage.

Mutations and copy number variation have been found in genes encoding the inhibitors of the complement system: factor H (*CFH* in 30% of patients), CD46 (*CFI* in 10%), factor I (10%) and thrombomodulin (5%). Factor H antibodies occur in 10% of aHUS cases (mainly children), associated with deficient factor H-related protein. Activating mutations have also been reported in the alternative complement cascade factor B (*CFB*) and C3 in a small number of patients [9].

Investigations

Serum levels of C3 and C4 may be reduced but are not diagnostic. Identification of the underlying molecular abnormality can guide future management. CD46 expression on peripheral blood mononuclear cells should be assessed, and mutation screening of *CFH*, CD46, *CFI*, *CFB* and C3 undertaken, as well as screening for autoantibodies against factor H [9]. ADAMTS13 levels should be measured to exclude an unusual presentation of congenital TTP with end-stage renal failure after recurrent episodes – severe ADAMTS13 deficiency is not a feature of HUS. Patients with MCP abnormalities can have a relapsing course, often triggered by infections, with mild renal impairment initially, and may be misdiagnosed as TTP. However, ADAMTS13 activity is not reduced, i.e. less than 5%, and there are no associated antibodies to ADAMTS13.

Management

Atypical HUS should be treated with PEX, the duration and frequency being determined by clinical response. This removes both hyperfunctional complement components (e.g. gain-of-function C3 mutants) and factor H autoantibodies and helps replace non-functioning complement regulators.

Eculizumab (*Soliris*) is a high-affinity humanized monoclonal antibody that binds to and blocks cleavage of C5, thereby preventing formation of the MAC. It has been shown to be safe and effective in aHUS and can reverse renal damage following an acute episode or following renal transplantation and is the likely treatment of choice in acute cases. Length of therapy and financial implications need to be further defined. Patients treated with complement inhibitors are at risk of increased microbial infection, particularly meningococcal infections, and it is therefore recommended to vaccinate patients prior to treatment.

Renal transplantation is associated with an overall 50% recurrence rate of HUS in the allograft, with the outcome depending on the underlying genetic abnormality [9]. 80% of patients with a mutation in the soluble regulators *CFH* or *CFI* lose their graft to recurrent disease within 2 years. In contrast, patients whose only defect is in the MCP *CD46* (while less likely to be dialysis dependent requiring transplantation) usually have a good outcome as the defective protein is replaced with the transplant. Patients with *CFB* or *C3* mutations are thought to have a significant risk of recurrence post transplant, and patients with anti-factor H autoantibodies should be treated to reduce the antibody titre before renal transplantation [9].

Secondary TMAs

Secondary TMAs are associated with a precipitant. Supportive care and treatment of the underlying cause are the mainstays of therapy. Platelet transfusions are not contraindicated.

Lupus nephritis: SLE is a multi-organ disorder and presentation with a TMA is typically associated with lupus nephritis. A confirmed diagnosis (following immunological investigations and renal biopsy) requires immunosuppressive therapy, such as steroids, cyclophosphamide or rituximab.

Catastrophic antiphospholipid syndrome (CAPS)

This is characterized by thrombosis in three or more organs, systems or tissues, developing simultaneously or within a week, in the presence of antiphospholipid antibodies. The hallmark is small vessel occlusion. Historically, mortality was greater than 50% but is reduced with the use of anticoagulation and immunosuppressives, e.g. steroids. Patients also receive PEX and more recently rituximab.

Malignant hypertension

Thrombocytopenia, MAHA and elevated serum LDH characterize TMA associated with malignant hypertension. There is normalization of the platelet count, and LDH after adequate blood pressure control is achieved.

Transplant-associated microangiopathy (TAM)

Transplant-associated microangiopathy (TAM) results from endothelial toxicity associated with chemotherapy, infections (usually viral or fungal), immunosuppressives such as ciclosporin and GVHD. Systemic microthrombi are not formed; ADAMTS13 activity is normal or only mildly reduced and the condition does not respond to PEX. Treating underlying infections, reducing the dose or altering the type of immunosuppression and using defibrotide may be of benefit.

Malignancy-associated TMA

Transplant-associated microangiopathy may be the presenting or terminal feature of adenocarcinomas. Treatment of the underlying cancer is the mainstay of therapy. PEX has not shown to be beneficial.

Conclusion

Increased understanding of the disease mechanisms underlying the TMAs is allowing more accurate diagnosis, which should translate into improved therapy and better patient outcomes. Despite this, the initial diagnosis of TTP remains a clinical one and a haematological emergency. PEX must be instituted promptly in any patient with thrombocytopenia and MAHA in the absence of another defined cause.

References

1 Scully M, Yarranton H, Liesner R et al. Regional UK TTP registry: correlation with laboratory ADAMTS 13 analysis and clinical features. Br J Haematol 2008;142(5):819–26.

2 Scully M, McDonald V, Cavenagh J et al. A phase 2 study of the safety and efficacy of rituximab with plasma exchange in acute acquired thrombotic thrombocytopenic purpura. Blood 2011;118(7):1746–53.

3 Hughes C, McEwan JR, Longair I et al. Cardiac involvement in acute thrombotic thrombocytopenic purpura: association with troponin T and IgG antibodies to ADAMTS 13. J Thromb Haemost 2009;7(4):529–36.

4 Allford SL, Hunt BJ, Rose P, Machin SJ. Guidelines on the diagnosis and management of the thrombotic microangiopathic haemolytic anaemias. Br J Haematol 2003;120(4):556–73.

5 Hovinga JA, Vesely SK, Terrell DR, Lammle B, George JN. Survival and relapse in patients with thrombotic thrombocytopenic purpura. Blood 2010;115(8):1500–11; quiz 662.

6 Ferrari S, Scheiflinger F, Rieger M et al. Prognostic value of anti-ADAMTS 13 antibody features (Ig isotype, titer, and

inhibitory effect) in a cohort of 35 adult French patients undergoing a first episode of thrombotic microangiopathy with undetectable ADAMTS 13 activity. Blood 2007;109(7):2815–22.

7 Zipfel PF, Wolf G, John U, Kentouche K, Skerka C. Novel developments in thrombotic microangiopathies: is there a common link between hemolytic uremic syndrome and thrombotic thrombocytic purpura? Pediatr Nephrol 2011;26(11):1947–56.

8 Bitzan M, Schaefer F, Reymond D. Treatment of typical (enteropathic) hemolytic uremic syndrome. Semin Thromb Hemost 2010;36(6):594–610.

9 Taylor CM, Machin S, Wigmore SJ, Goodship TH. Clinical practice guidelines for the management of atypical haemolytic uraemic syndrome in the United Kingdom. Br J Haematol 2010;148(1):37–47.

10 Loirat C, Saland J, Bitzan M. Management of hemolytic uremic syndrome. Presse Med 2012;41(3 Pt 2):e115–35.

CHAPTER 12
Critical Care of Patients with a Congenital Bleeding Disorder

Vanessa Martlew

Department of Haematology, Royal Liverpool Hospital, Liverpool, UK

Introduction

Individuals diagnosed with inherited bleeding disorders in the UK are registered centrally by the United Kingdom Haemophilia Centre Doctors' Organisation (UKHCDO) and are provided with a card indicating their diagnosis and the contact details of their local haemophilia centre where further information is available about their precise diagnosis and appropriate haemostatic support. Their advice should be sought as soon as possible about the usual haemostatic strategy and products for the patient concerned.

The most frequently occurring inherited bleeding disorders include von Willebrand disease, haemophilia A, haemophilia B and disorders of platelet function as well as the much less frequently occurring rare disorders of other coagulation factors and hereditary thrombocytopenias.

von Willebrand disease

This is the most frequently occurring bleeding disorder in Western Europe being detected in 1% of the population when routine screening is undertaken although only a fraction of these are symptomatic. Its inheritance is autosomal and usually dominant, occurring equally in males and females.

It is characterized by a quantitative and/or qualitative defect of von Willebrand factor and is classified into three types:
- Type 1 (85% cases) is associated with a mild to moderate deficiency of normally functioning von Willebrand factor.
- Type 2 is characterized by a functional defect of von Willebrand factor and is further subdivided into four types:
  - Type 2A (10%) individuals have significant reduction of von Willebrand activity caused by an absence of high-molecular-weight von Willebrand multimers.
  - Type 2 B (5%) is characterized by increased avidity for platelets so individuals may present with thrombocytopenia.
  - Type 2 M (rare) individuals exhibit decreased platelet binding to the vascular sub-endothelium with normal amounts of high-molecular-weight von Willebrand multimers.
  - Type 2 N (rare) is associated with selectively impaired binding of factor VIII.
- Type 3 (rare) is associated with a severe deficiency (<1%) of von Willebrand factor.

von Willebrand factor is produced in platelets and by the vascular endothelium. This is required for both normal platelet–platelet interaction and platelet binding to the vascular sub-endothelium as well as binding to factor VIII to prevent the proteolysis of this important coagulation factor in the circulation. It is an acute-phase reactant, which is increased in inflammation.

Haematology in Critical Care: A Practical Handbook, First Edition. Edited by Jecko Thachil and Quentin A. Hill.
© 2014 John Wiley & Sons, Ltd. Published 2014 by John Wiley & Sons, Ltd.

The majority of people with the disorder (type 1) have a quantitative defect of functionally normal von Willebrand factor (normal range of 50–150%). Haemostatic support is, therefore, directed at increasing the amount of available von Willebrand factor either by boosting native values using DDAVP (a synthetic vasopressin) or supplementation with intermediate purity plasma-derived factor VIII concentrate rich in von Willebrand factor (e.g. Haemate P, Wilate). There is as yet no recombinant products available to replenish von Willebrand factor. Those with type 2 and type 3 von Willebrand disease will usually require the latter to restore normal von Willebrand function.

The dose of DDAVP is 0.3 μg/kg to a total not in excess of 30 μg administered intravenously in 100 mL normal saline over 30 min. It may also be given intranasally 150 μg in each nostril. Common side effects which may make it less suited to use in critical care include flushing, hypertension and hyponatraemia. The low sodium is as a consequence of retention of free water necessitating fluid restriction to 1500 mL in the 24 h following administration of DDAVP in order to avoid severe headache. On second and subsequent dosing in a short period of time (<7 days), DDAVP is associated with a degree of tachyphylaxis. Supplementary treatment with concentrate may, therefore, be required when normal levels of von Willebrand activity must be maintained for a period of days, especially in the post-operative setting after major surgeries. In the event of bleeding, the antifibrinolytic agent tranexamic acid may be a useful addition although this must be carefully considered in the presence of a consumptive coagulopathy.

Monitoring of von Willebrand factor replacement is different based on different indications. In most cases, a factor VIII and ristocetin cofactor levels of 100 U/dL if not at least 50 U/dL (in minor cases) will be required to prevent bleeding. Specialized laboratories should be performing these tests since quality checks are crucial in obtaining accurate and reliable results.

The haemophilias

The haemophilias are the best known of the hereditary bleeding disorders. They are inherited in an X-linked recessive manner. They are classified according to the level of coagulant factor deficiency as follows: mild is less than 50% but greater than 5%, moderate is less than 5% but more than 1% and severe is less than 1%. The normal range is 50–150%.

Haemophilia A is associated with a deficiency of factor VIII and occurs in 1 in 5000 of all live male births, while factor IX deficiency or haemophilia B (Christmas disease) is much less frequently occurring in 1 in 30,000 of all live male births. Even in the absence of overt bleeding, patients with inherited bleeding disorders who need critical care management require prophylactic treatment to ensure adequate background levels of coagulant factor throughout their stay. It is considered beneficial to continue to prescribe their usual brand of factor concentrate wherever possible as inhibitors to transfused product are more likely to occur on first exposure.

Haemophilia B

Individuals with haemophilia B are deficient in factor IX and benefit from normal levels of factor IX coagulant protein while receiving intensive care. This should be prescribed as a recombinant factor IX concentrate, e.g. BeneFIX (Wyeth), to maintain factor IX in the normal range, i.e. greater than 50%. The dose of factor IX required may be calculated as desired rise in factor IX × weight in kg and is measured in international units (IU). Factor IX levels should be checked 30 min after administration to ensure adequate levels have been achieved. When invasive therapeutic procedures are planned, the factor IX target may need to be raised to greater than 100%. Also after major surgery, this level should be maintained for a minimum of 5 days. Although the half-life of factor IX is longer than factor VIII, top-up doses of recombinant factor IX concentrate are likely to be required every 12–24 h.

In contrast to haemophilia A, DDAVP is ineffective in boosting factor IX levels for persons with Christmas disease, although tranexamic acid may be prescribed to good effect to minimize mucosal bleeding.

Haemophilia A

Individuals with haemophilia A are deficient in factor VIII and will also benefit from normal levels of factor VIII coagulant protein while receiving intensive care. Although individuals with mild haemophilia may achieve normal levels of factor VIII after a single dose of DDAVP, its half-life is of the order of 8–12 h, and treatment may be required twice daily. As DDAVP is known to be associated with tachyphylaxis on repeated administration over a short period of time, its use will be limited in the critical care setting. The majority of patients with haemophilia A will, therefore, require recombinant factor VIII concentrate, e.g. Kogenate (Bayer) and ReFacto AF (Wyeth), to maintain their factor VIII levels within the normal range throughout their intensive care admission. The dose of factor VIII concentrate may be calculated as (desired rise in factor VIII × weight in kg) × 0.5. Factor VIII levels should be checked 30 min after administration to ensure adequate levels have been achieved. As the half-life of factor VIII is 8–12 h, top-up doses of recombinant factor VIII concentrate are likely to be required every 12 h. Tranexamic acid may be prescribed to good effect to minimize mucosal bleeding at any site outside the urinary tract – the latter being contraindicated because of the potential for its antifibrinolytic action producing clots in the ureters. When invasive therapeutic procedures are planned, the factor VIII target should be raised to greater than 100% and after surgery maintained at this level for a minimum of 5 days.

The use of continuous infusion has become more common particularly in the post-operative setting and where staffing ratios permit close control. This maintains a stable and continuous level of factor activity and levels out *peaks and troughs* usually leading to lower usage of factor concentrate and allows laboratory monitoring with random blood samples for factor VIII assay.

Rare bleeding disorders

Factor XI deficiency (haemophilia C)

Factor XI deficiency is inherited in an autosomal recessive manner, but the bleeding tendency does not correlate well with the factor XI – personal and family history of bleeding being a better guide to the haemostatic defect in the kindred concerned. It usually presents as a mild bleeding tendency, but this may be troublesome after surgery or in intensive care, and more bleeding may be expected with levels of factor XI less than 20%.

Where haemostatic support is indicated for surgery on invasive procedures, those mildly affected may be supplemented using a virally inactivated fresh frozen plasma, e.g. Octaplas (Octapharma), at a dose of 15–20 mL/kg, whereas those with a severe deficiency less than 2% may benefit from factor XI concentrate. As the latter is potentially prothrombotic unlike other concentrates, its dosage

should be gauged to increase factor XI to the lower end of the normal range around 70%. With a long half-life of 22 h, supplementation may only be needed every 24–48 h.

Tranexamic acid may be prescribed to good effect to minimize mucosal bleeding at any site outside the urinary tract – the latter being contraindicated because of the potential for its antifibrinolytic action producing clots in the ureters.

Disorders of fibrinogen

In common with von Willebrand disease, these may either be quantitative (afibrinogenaemia/hypofibrinogenaemia) or qualitative (dysfibrinogenaemia) or sometimes include a mixture of both. In the critical care setting, this must be distinguished from the more frequently occurring acquired hypofibrinogenaemias, the latter usually being associated with a thrombocytopenia and features of microangiopathy in the peripheral blood.

Afibrinogenaemia is a very autosomal rare disorder with no fibrinogen detectable in either plasma or platelets. In recessive cases, patients have a severe bleeding phenotype, while the heterozygotes have low levels of normal fibrinogen. Replacement therapy is provided as a plasma-derived fibrinogen concentrate (CSL Behring), the standard initial haemostatic dose being 2 g. Fibrinogen assays post dose should aim to maintain the circulating fibrinogen above 1 g/L, and with a long half-life, further supplements may only be required every other day in the absence of increased consumption.

A number of functional defects of fibrinogen are described in dysfibrinogenaemia, and some individuals also have a quantitative defect. The inheritance is autosomal and variable. The clinical phenotype may be either haemorrhagic or thrombotic or a mixture of both. Hence, its management in the critical care setting presents a considerable therapeutic challenge. Fibrinogen supplements are required as for afibrinogenaemia for those with concomitant deficiency and a bleeding phenotype, while the risk of thrombosis may require either thromboprophylaxis or treatment in addition to haemostatic supplementation as assessed on an individual basis.

Factor VII deficiency

This is usually a mild bleeding disorder of autosomal recessive inheritance. There is a poor correlation between plasma levels of factor VII above 10%, but below this value, bleeding is more common. For invasive procedures in critical care, normal levels may be restored by the administration of recombinant activated factor VII (rFVIIa) (Novonordisk) *at a much lower* dose of 20 µg/kg than that used to procure haemostasis in those either with acquired inhibitors of coagulation or massive haemorrhage. rFVIIa (NovoSeven) has a short half-life, and prolonged period of treatment may be required 4–6 hourly.

Factor XIII deficiency

This disorder is characterized by a significant bleeding diathesis and delayed healing in an individual with normal coagulation profile, platelet count and bleeding time. The diagnosis is confirmed on a clot solubility test. A plasma-derived factor XIII concentrate (Fibrogammin P from Aventis Behring) is available for supplementation and with a long half-life may only be required every 5–6 weeks in the steady state. On admission to a critical care unit this supplementation should be continued.

Coagulation factor deficiencies supplemented by virally inactivated fresh frozen plasma

There remain a number of isolated coagulation deficiencies for which no specific supplement is available as well as the combined deficiencies for which virally inactivated fresh frozen plasma, e.g. Octaplas (Octapharma), is the appropriate haemostatic agent.

This is usually started at a dose of 20 mL/kg and maintained at 3–6 mL /kg daily thereafter. These factors include:

Factor deficiency	Target maintenance factor value*
II (prothrombin)	20–30%*
V	25%
X	10–15%*
V + VIII	V = VIII > 50%

*In the event of major surgery or bleeding, a prothrombin complex concentrate, e.g. Octaplex (Octapharma), may be administered.

Disorders of platelet function

These are usually associated with a variable degree of mucocutaneous bleeding. There are two well-recognized rare autosomal recessive disorders associated with

structural anomalies of membrane glycoprotein and a group of disorders, which is categorized under platelet storage pool defects.

In Glanzmann's thrombasthenia, failure of platelet aggregation occurs in the absence of platelet membrane GpIIb–IIIa. Unfortunately, the latter is one of the most immunogenic of the platelet glycoproteins, and the majority of affected individuals exhibit refractoriness to random platelet concentrate on second and subsequent transfusion as a consequence of anti-HPA-1A alloantibodies. Adequate platelet increments after this may be procured by careful selection of HLA- and HPA-matched platelets with the assistance of the National Blood and Transplant Service. In the event of severe and uncontrollable bleeding, rFVIIa (NovoSeven) at a dose of 90–120 µg/kg has been used to good effect. In Bernard–Soulier syndrome, failure of platelet adhesion occurs in the absence of platelet membrane GpIb–IX–V. Transfusion of unselected platelets will be required to maintain haemostasis regularly and at weekly intervals throughout the intensive care admission in the absence of consumption. GpIb–IX–V deficiency is not usually associated with platelet refractoriness. In individuals with a platelet storage pool defect,, the bleeding tendency is usually attributable to granular deficiency or dysfunction. They respond to platelet transfusion, but as a proportion represent a variant of von Willebrand dysfunction, they may, therefore, respond to DDAVP in shortening the bleeding time. Those already registered may already have their response to DDAVP determined, and thus, a therapeutic challenge information may be obtained from the registered hospital.

Transfusion-transmitted agents

The screening of donor blood for hepatitis B was introduced in the 1970s, HIV in October 1984 and hepatitis C in September 1991. All those registered with inherited bleeding disorders have been treated with virally inactivated plasma products since January 1985 in the UK. All patients in receipt of pooled plasma products prepared from British plasma between 1980 and 2001 are considered to be at risk of transmission of variant CJD, and special procedures must be undertaken to prevent transmission when they require invasive procedures involving lymphoid and neurological tissues.

Thromboprophylaxis

Provided haemostasis is restored to normal as previously recommended for all those with inherited disorders of coagulation who require intensive care, their risks of thrombosis will be similar to normal. They may therefore be considered for pharmacological thromboprophylaxis in the usual way.

Further reading

Bolton-Maggs PH, Perry DJ, Chalmers EA et al. The rare coagulation disorders – review with guidelines for management from the United Kingdom Haemophilia Centre Doctors' Organisation. Haemophilia 2004;10:593–628.

Bolton-Maggs P, Chalmers EA, Collins PW et al. A review of inherited platelet disorders with guidelines for their management on behalf of the UKHCDO. Br J Haematol 2006;134:603–33.

Keeling D, Tait C, Makris M. Guideline on the selection and use of therapeutic products to treat haemophilia and other hereditary bleeding disorders. Haemophilia 2008;14:671–84,

Lee CA, Chi C, Pavord SR et al. The obstetric and gynaecological management of women with inherited bleeding disorders-review with guidelines produced by a taskforce of UK Haemophilia Centre Doctors' Organization. Haemophilia 2006;12:301–36.

Murphy M, Brown M, Carrington P et al. Guidelines for platelet transfusion. Br J Haematol 2002;122:10–23.

Pasi KJ, Collins PW, Keeling D et al. Management of von Willebrand's disease: a guideline from the UK Haemophilia Centre Doctors' Organisation. Haemophilia 2004;11:218–31.

SECTION 3
Approach to Transfusion Problems

CHAPTER 13

Blood Components and Their Contents

Shubha Allard

Clinical Haematology, Barts and the London NHS Trust, NHS Blood and Transplant, London, UK

Introduction

Careful donor selection followed by stringent testing by the blood service is essential to ensure a safe blood supply. In developed countries, blood is processed into its component parts such as red cells, platelets, fresh frozen plasma (FFP) and cryoprecipitate and granulocytes for clinical use and not transfused as *whole blood*. Donated blood is a limited resource, and hospital blood transfusion practice must focus on ensuring safe and appropriate use including the use of clinical guidelines supported by education and training with regular audit of practice. Robust systems are essential for accurate patient identification throughout the transfusion process and include the final bedside check to minimize errors.

Blood transfusion and the regulatory framework

Transfusion medicine must be practised within a strict regulatory framework – the European Union (EU) blood directives have been transposed into the UK law with the Blood Safety and Quality Regulations (BSQR) 2005 setting standards for quality and safety in the collection, testing, processing, storage and distribution of human blood components [1]. The regulations affect both the national blood services (called *blood establishments* in the BSQR) and hospital transfusion laboratories.

Donor selection and testing

All donors in the UK are voluntary and unpaid. They are carefully selected using a donor health questionnaire to ensure that they are safe to donate and to exclude anyone at risk of transmitting infection. Donors can give around 450 mL of whole blood three to four times a year, which is separated into red cells, platelets and plasma. These individual components can also be collected by separate component donation using apheresis [2].

The UK plasma is no longer used for fractionation for manufacture of blood products such as albumin, intravenous immunoglobulin, anti-D or factor concentrates (see succeeding text).

Microbiological testing of donor blood

Transfusion transmitted infection. In the UK, all donations are tested for syphilis, hepatitis B, hepatitis C, HTLV1 and HIV. The tests used and the estimated risk [3] are summarized in Table 13.1.

Some donations are also tested for cytomegalovirus (CMV) antibody to help provide CMV-negative blood for particular patient groups. The Specialist Advisory Committee on the Safety of Blood, Tissues and Organs (SaBTO) in the UK has reviewed evidence [4] available and recommended that leucodepletion of all blood

Haematology in Critical Care: A Practical Handbook, First Edition. Edited by Jecko Thachil and Quentin A. Hill.
© 2014 John Wiley & Sons, Ltd. Published 2014 by John Wiley & Sons, Ltd.

Table 13.1 Transfusion transmitted infection in UK: Estimated risk in 2010–2013 [3].

Test	Testing introduced	Examples of testing methods used	Approximate risk of infection
Syphilis	1940s	Antibody	
Hepatitis B	1970/2009 onwards	Surface antigen/(HBsAg)/Nucleic acid testing	1 in 1 million
HIV	1985/2001 onwards	Antibody/nucleic acid testing	1 in 7 million
HCV	1991/1999 onwards	Antibody/nucleic acid testing	1 in 29 million
HTLV	2002	Antibody	

components (other than granulocytes) provides adequate CMV risk reduction for various patients requiring transfusion (haemopoietic stem cell transplant patients, organ transplant patients and immune-deficient patients, including those with HIV) without the requirement for CMV-seronegative components in addition. However, CMV-seronegative red cell and platelet components should be provided for intrauterine transfusions and for neonates and for pregnant women requiring repeat elective transfusions during the course of pregnancy.

Donors are tested for malaria and *T. cruzi* antibodies when indicated by their travel history. Other discretionary tests include anti-HBc (e.g. after body piercing).

Variant Creutzfeldt–Jakob disease (vCJD). To date, there have been four cases in the UK where blood transfusion may have been implicated in transmission of new variant Creutzfeldt–Jakob disease (vCJD). A further transmission of variant CJD prions was described in February 2009 in a patient with haemophilia who had received batches of factor VIII (FVIII) to which a donor who subsequently developed variant CJD had contributed plasma. The patient died of other causes but was found to have evidence of prion accumulation in his spleen. There is no blood test at present readily available for detecting prions, although there is active international research ongoing in this field. The full risk of vCJD in the UK population remains uncertain, and accordingly, the UK blood services have taken a number of precautionary measures to reduce the potential risk of transmission of prions by blood, plasma and blood products, the latter requiring fractionation of very large volumes of plasma [5].

These include:
- Universal leucocyte depletion (removal of white cells) of all blood donations since 1998
- Importation of plasma for countries other than the UK for fractionation to manufacture plasma products
- Importation of FFP for use in children born after January 1996
- Exclusion of blood donors who have received a transfusion in the UK since 1980

Processing of blood

Donor blood is collected into plastic packs containing citric phosphate dextrose and then transported without delay to the blood centre for processing. All units undergo initial leucodepletion to remove white cells. Further processing (see Figure 13.1) is then undertaken to produce red cells, platelets and plasma or cryoprecipitate under stringent standards of quality control as mandated by the BSQR 2005.

Red cells in additive solution

During processing, the majority of plasma is removed and replaced with an optimal additive solution comprising saline, adenine, glucose and mannitol (SAG-M). Citrate binds calcium and acts as an anticoagulant, and the glucose and adenine support red cell metabolism during storage.

A standard red cell component in additive solution contains red cells (Hct 0.50–0.70 and Hb content > 40 g/U), 5–30 mL of plasma and 100 mL of SAG-M solution in a total volume of 220–340 mL [3]. Standard red cells contain no functional platelets, granulocytes or coagulation factors and are stored at 4 °C with a shelf life of 35 days.

Platelets

An adult therapeutic dose (ATD) or 1 U of platelets can either be produced by single-donor apheresis or by centrifugation of whole blood followed by separation and pooling of the platelet-rich layer from four donations suspended in plasma. Platelets can be stored for 5 days at 20–24 °C with constant agitation. Bacterial testing of platelets prior to release now introduced by some of the blood services such as NHS Blood and Transplant can reduce the risk of bacteriological contamination and with an extension of the shelf life of platelet units to 7 days. Platelet components must not be placed in a refrigerator.

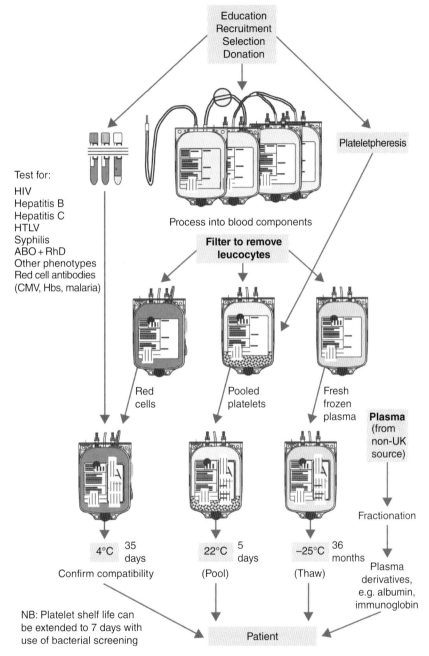

Test for:

HIV
Hepatitis B
Hepatitis C
HTLV
Syphilis
ABO + RhD
Other phenotypes
Red cell antibodies
(CMV, Hbs, malaria)

NB: Platelet shelf life can
be extended to 7 days with
use of bacterial screening

Figure 13.1 Processing of blood components. Source: Reproduced with permission from Handbook of Transfusion Medicine [6]. Crown Copyright .

Fresh frozen plasma

Fresh frozen plasma is a source of coagulation factors and is produced by separation and freezing of plasma at −30 °C. Single donation units, sourced from non-UK plasma and treated with methylene blue to reduce microbial activity, are indicated for all children born after 1996. Solvent–detergent plasma is prepared commercially from pools of 300–5000 plasma donations that have been

Table 13.2 Comparisons of standard fresh frozen plasma (FFP) with solvent–detergent FFP.

	Standard adult FFP	SD-FFP
Source	Single donor for each unit of FFP	60–1500 donors contributing to plasma pool
Supplier	Supplied by blood service	Supplied by commercial manufacturer
Volume	250–300 mL	200 mL
Product licence	Not required	Licensed, batch product
Thawing needed	Yes	Yes
Coagulation factor content	Variable between units: 75% of units have FVIII >0.7 IU/mL	Constant within batch: all factors >0.5 IU/mL
Viral inactivation	No	Yes

sourced from non-UK donors and treated with solvent and detergent to reduce the risk of viral transmission (Table 13.2).

Cryoprecipitate

Cryoprecipitate is prepared by undertaking controlled thawing of frozen plasma to precipitate high-molecular-weight proteins including FVIII, von Willebrand factor and fibrinogen. Cryoprecipitate consists of the cryoglobulin fraction of plasma containing the major portion of FVIII and fibrinogen. It is obtained by thawing a single donation of FFP at $4°C \pm 2°C$. The cryoprecipitate is then rapidly frozen to $-30°C$. In the UK, it is available as pools of 5 U.

Clinical and laboratory transfusion practice

Blood Safety and Quality Regulations: Impact on hospital transfusion practice

The chief executive of each hospital with a transfusion laboratory needs to submit a formal annual statement of compliance to the Medicines and Healthcare products Regulatory Agency (MHRA). Hospital transfusion laboratories can be inspected by the MHRA [5] and in the event of significant deficiencies can be given the order to *cease and desist from activities*. The key requirements for hospital transfusion laboratories include:
• A comprehensive quality management system based on the principles of *good practice*, including stringent

requirements for storage and distribution of blood and components, with emphasis on *cold chain* management
• Traceability, requiring all hospitals to trace the fate of each unit of blood/blood component (including name and patient ID) with records being kept for 30 years
• Education and training of staff involved in blood transfusion, with maintenance of all training records
• Haemovigilance, with reporting of all adverse events

Hospital transfusion laboratories undertaking any processing activities such as irradiation must have a licence from the MHRA indicating blood establishment status.

Better Blood Transfusion

A series of three *Better Blood Transfusion* health service circulars published in 1998, 2002 and 2007 promote safe transfusion practices within hospitals with emphasis on the appropriate use of blood and components in all clinical areas [7].

All hospitals must have Hospital Transfusion Committees (HTCs), with multidisciplinary representation. These committees are responsible for overseeing implementation of guidelines and the audit and training of all staff involved in transfusion. The HTC has an essential role within the hospital clinical governance framework and must be accountable to the chief executive.

The smaller Hospital Transfusion Team (HTT), including the transfusion nurse specialist, transfusion laboratory manager and consultant haematologist in transfusion, undertakes various activities on a day-to-day basis to achieve the objectives of the HTC.

Patient Blood Management

Many of the aforementioned principles of *Better Blood Transfusion* are now encompassed in Patient Blood Management (PBM), an evidence-based, patient-focused initiative involving an integrated multidisciplinary multimodal team approach with the aim of optimizing the patient's own blood volume (especially red cell mass), minimizing the patient's blood loss and optimizing the patient's physiological tolerance of anaemia and therefore reducing unnecessary transfusion [8].

Guidelines and training

All hospitals must have a transfusion policy with clear guidance on correct patient identification and the safe administration of blood and components, including the detection and management of adverse reactions.

The National Patient Safety Agency has issued a safe practice notice entitled *Right Patient, Right Blood*, which states that all hospital staff involved in the transfusion process, including phlebotomists, porters and medical and nursing staff, must undergo training and competency testing [9].

There must be clear guidelines for safe and appropriate use of red cells and components in all clinical specialties, including medicine, surgery, paediatrics and obstetrics and intensive care. Hospitals must have local major haemorrhage protocols that need to be adapted for specific clinical areas. All medical, nursing, laboratory and support staff should know where to find the major blood loss protocol in relevant areas and be familiar with the contents, supported by training and regular drills. All hospitals must have also a policy for management of patients who refuse blood, e.g. Jehovah's Witnesses (see Chapter 21).

The various guidelines and protocols should be developed in collaboration with relevant clinical teams involved and must be ratified by the HTC.

Blood group and compatibility testing

The patient's blood group must be tested to determine ABO and RhD type, and an antibody screen must be undertaken. The majority of laboratories in the UK now use automated testing with advanced information technology systems for documentation and reporting of the results.

The updated BCSH compatibility guidelines emphasize the need for having a second group and screen (G&S) sample for confirmation of the ABO group where there is no previous record in the laboratory of a previous blood group result and where this does not impede the delivery of urgent red cells or other components [10]. The timing of the G&S sample prior to issue of blood is dependent on whether or not a patient has been recently transfused or pregnant. Where there has been no transfusion or pregnancy within the preceding 3 months, the G&S blood sample is valid for up to 7 days [10].

The hospital transfusion laboratory can readily provide red cells that are ABO and RhD compatible using electronic issue (or *computer crossmatch*), with no further testing needed provided the patient does not have any antibodies and that there are robust automated systems in

place for antibody testing and identification of the patient. In this setting, since blood can be readily issued, there is no need to reserve units for individual cases. In patients with red cell antibodies, crossmatch is essential between the patient's blood and the red cell units to be transfused to ensure compatibility.

Where electronic issue is not available, a locally agreed Maximum Surgical Blood Ordering Schedule (MSBOS) should be used for surgery to decide how many red cell units should be reserved and available for particular cases based on the procedure.

The hospital transfusion laboratory also needs to ensure that appropriate blood and components are provided for patients with special requirements such as CMV-negative blood or irradiated blood. The latter is needed for immunocompromised patients to minimize the risk of transfusion-associated graft-versus-host disease.

Clinical use of blood and components

The decision to transfuse must be based on a thorough clinical assessment of the patient and their individual needs, and the indication for transfusion should be documented in the patients' clinical records. The initial assessment should include an evaluation of the patient's age, body weight and any co-morbidity that can predispose to transfusion-associated circulatory overload (TACO) such as cardiac failure, renal impairment, hypoalbuminaemia and fluid overload [11, 12]. These factors should be considered when prescribing the volume and rate of the transfusion and in deciding whether diuretics should be prescribed. Patients identified at risk of TACO should be monitored for signs of circulatory overload, including fluid balance with careful attention to the rate of transfusion as TACO can occur after only one unit of red cells in at-risk patients. As a general guide, transfusing 1 U of red cells typically gives a Hb increment of 1 g/dL but only if applied as an approximation for a 70–80 kg patient. For patients of lower body weight, the total volume transfused should be reduced, and for paediatric patients, the transfusion should be prescribed in millilitres (see Chapter 34). Single unit red cell transfusions are recommended where possible, especially in non-bleeding adult patients, and further units should not be prescribed without further clinical assessment and monitoring the patient's haemoglobin [13].

Errors in the requesting, collection and administration of blood components (red cells, platelets and plasma components) can lead to significant risks for patients. The Serious Hazards of Transfusion (SHOT) scheme launched in 1995 has repeatedly shown that *wrong blood into patient* episodes are an important reported transfusion hazard and these are mainly due to human error that can lead to life-threatening haemolytic transfusion reactions and other significant morbidity.

A patient identification band (or risk assessed equivalent) must be worn by all patients receiving a blood transfusion with the minimum patient identifiers including last name, first name, date of birth and unique patient identification. Positive patient identification is essential at all stages of the blood transfusion process including blood sampling, collection of blood from storage and delivery to the clinical area and administration to the patient.

Observation and monitoring of the patient during a transfusion is essential if adverse reactions to the transfusion are to be quickly identified and managed. Many serious reactions are apparent within 30 min of starting the transfusion of a blood component unit [11], and close observation during this period is essential [12].

The detection and clinical management of acute transfusion reactions [14] is covered in Chapter 14. Any adverse events or reactions related to the transfusion should be appropriately investigated and reported to local risk management, SHOT and the MHRA via the Serious Adverse Blood Reactions and Events (SABRE) system.

Hospitals must have a clear policy detailing how transfusion traceability or *fate of unit* is achieved by robust electronic or manual systems as mandated by the BSQR.

Use of red cells

Red cells are indicated to increase the haemoglobin and hence the oxygen-carrying capacity of blood following acute haemorrhage or in chronic anaemia.

There has been a trend for lowering the haemoglobin threshold used as a *trigger* for red cell transfusion, but individual patient factors must be taken into account [15]. Management of anaemia in critical care together with transfusion triggers and strategies for transfusion avoidance is covered in Chapter 17.

Routine autologous donation and storage of blood prior to surgery is no longer recommended in the UK.

Use of platelets

A unit of platelets should be infused over a period of 30 min in an adult using a standard blood administration set [6, 16].

ABO and RhD identical platelets should be used as far as possible, but ABO non-identical units may be given, especially at times of shortage or in emergency situations, where no ABO identical platelets are immediately available or when HLA-matched platelets are required (see succeeding text).

If an RhD-negative woman of childbearing potential has been given RhD-positive platelets, then anti-D administration as per BCSH guidelines [16] is recommended to reduce the risk of developing alloimmune anti-D antibodies.

Platelets are indicated for the treatment or prophylaxis of bleeding in patients with thrombocytopenia or with platelet dysfunction in a number of situations (see Table 13.3). The lack of evidence base supporting platelet transfusion practice has come under scrutiny with increasing research in this area [17].

Platelet refractoriness resulting in a failure to obtain a satisfactory increment to platelet transfusions may be due

Table 13.3 Indications for use of platelets.

Bone marrow failure	To prevent spontaneous bleeding when platelet count $<10 \times 10^9$/L or $<20 \times 10^9$/L if there is an additional risk, e.g. sepsis
Prior to invasive procedures	Minor surgery or procedures – raise platelet count to $>50 \times 10^9$/L Major surgery $>80 \times 10^9$/L Eye surgery or neurosurgery $>100 \times 10^9$/L
Massive blood transfusion	Platelet count $<50 \times 10^9$/L anticipated after 1.5–2 × blood volume replacement Aim to maintain platelet count $>75 \times 10^9$/L
Disseminated intravascular coagulation (DIC)	Platelet transfusion indicated in acute DIC if low platelets and bleeding but not in chronic DIC without bleeding
Platelet dysfunction	Inherited – Glanzmann's thrombasthenia Acquired – antiplatelet drugs, e.g. aspirin and clopidogrel
Autoimmune thrombocytopenia	Platelet transfusions should only be used if major haemorrhage is present

Platelet transfusions are contraindicated in thrombotic thrombocytopenic purpura (TTP).

to immune or non-immune causes. The main immune cause is HLA alloimmunization, which occurs following previous pregnancy or transfusion, but its incidence in relation to the latter has declined as a result of leucocyte depletion of blood components. Non-immune clinical factors include infection (and its treatment with antibiotics and antifungal drugs), disseminated intravascular coagulation (DIC) and splenomegaly. HLA-matched platelet transfusions are indicated if no obvious non-immune causes are present and if HLA antibodies are detected.

Use of fresh frozen plasma and cryoprecipitate

In adults, the therapeutic dose of FFP is 12–15 mL/kg body weight FFP. Thawed FFP is best used immediately but may be stored at 4 °C and infused within 24 h [18].

In the UK, all children born after 1996 should receive methylene blue-treated FFP with the volume being transfused based on weight. Solvent–detergent-treated plasma is indicated for large volume replacement in patients being plasma exchanged for thrombotic thrombocytopenic purpura (TTP).

There is a relative lack of good evidence to support the clinical use of FFP, and practice is therefore often empirical in relation to many situations [19]. FFP is indicated in patients with acute DIC in the presence of bleeding and abnormal coagulation results. The aetiology of coagulopathy associated with massive haemorrhage is multifactorial and will depend on the clinical scenario with many contributory factors including activation of fibrinolysis, dilutional and consumptive coagulopathy, DIC exacerbated by hypothermia and hypocalcaemia. FFP used early may pre-empt the development of significant coagulopathy. However, studies investigating the use of early FFP in traumatic massive haemorrhage in a ratio of 1:1 with red cells have all been retrospective, often in the military situation, and are hampered by the effect of survivor bias [20]. Also, while traditional practice entails the use of FFP with the aim of maintaining the prothrombin time (PT) and activated partial thromboplastin time (APTT) to be at a ratio of less than 1.5 X normal, in practice, there are often significant delays in the availability of laboratory-based coagulation testing. An empirical approach pending further clinical studies includes the administration of FFP early in the resuscitation process at

a dose of 15–20 mL/kg (pragmatically 4 U) and before coagulation investigation results are known (although baseline tests should have been taken). Further treatment should then if possible be guided by the results of laboratory-based (e.g. PT/APTT) or if available near-patient tests of coagulation (e.g. TEG/ROTEM).

Fresh frozen plasma should not be used for reversal of oral anticoagulation where the use of prothrombin complex concentrate is indicated [21]. The coagulopathy of liver disease is also complex with many studies showing the lack of evidence of clinical benefit of prophylactic FFP transfusion in this setting.

A study of the use of FFP in critical care units in the UK showed a wide variation in practice [22]. In particular, it was noted that where FFP has a higher probability of patient benefit, namely, in a bleeding patient with deranged coagulation, inadequate doses were given to correct the clotting defect. On the contrary, a large number of FFP transfusions were given to patients without bleeding with little or no derangement of coagulation raising key questions around appropriate use and unnecessary exposure to blood components.

Use of cryoprecipitate

Low fibrinogen levels commonly occur in massive haemorrhage. FFP may help improve fibrinogen levels, but if bleeding continues and the fibrinogen levels are greater than 1.5 g/L or as guided by TEG, fibrinogen replacement is indicated. The adult dose of cryoprecipitate is 10 donor units produced as two pools of 5 U in each pool. Fibrinogen concentrate while available in the UK for replacement in congenital hypofibrinogenaemia is not licensed for massive haemorrhage but is used extensively in Europe as an alternative to cryoprecipitate at a dose of 3–4 g.

Cryoprecipitate must not be used for replacement of coagulation factors in inherited conditions such as haemophilia or von Willebrand disease, since specific factor concentrates are available for treatment.

Clinical audit

There should be regular multidisciplinary audits of transfusion practice, with feedback of the results to all relevant staff and with re-audit to ensure that changes in practice have been undertaken where needed. The National Comparative Audit of Blood Transfusion is a collaborative initiative between the Royal College of Physicians and NHS Blood and Transplant with active participation in several audits from hospitals across the country [23].

Patient information and consent

The last Better Blood Transfusion health service circular [6] recommends that timely information should be made available to patients, informing them of the indication for transfusion, the risks and benefits of blood transfusion and any alternatives available. There is also a need to increase patient awareness regarding the importance of correct identification.

In October 2011, the SaBTO in the UK re-enforced the recommendation that valid consent for blood transfusion should be obtained and documented in the patient's clinical record by the healthcare professional. A standardized information resource for clinicians indicating the key issues to be discussed by the healthcare professional when obtaining valid consent from a patient for a blood transfusion is now available at http://www.transfusion-guidelines.org.uk/index.asp?Publication=BBT&Section=22&pageid=7691.

Patient information leaflets are available from the UK Blood Transfusion Services. There should be a modified form of consent for long-term multi-transfused patients. Patients who have received a blood transfusion and who were not able to give valid consent prior to the transfusion should be provided with information retrospectively. A *good practice guidance* document to help identify the most effective way of providing information retrospectively has been developed by the SaBTO and is available at http://www.transfusionguidelines.org.uk/index.asp?Publication=BBT&Section=22&pageid=7691.

References

1 UK Blood Transfusion & Tissue Transplantation Services. European Blood Safety Directives/Blood Safety and Quality Regulations (BSQR). http://www.transfusionguidelines.org.uk/index.aspx?Publication=REGS (accessed on November 16, 2013).

2 UK Blood Transfusion and Tissue Transplantation Services. Guidelines for the Blood Transfusion Services in the UK (Red Book). 7th edition. London: HMSO; 2005. Also available at: http://www.transfusionguidelines.org.uk/index.aspx?Publication=RB (accessed on November 16, 2013).

3 Health Protection Agency. www.hpa.org.uk/Topics/InfectiousDiseases/InfectionsAZ/BIBD (accessed on November 16, 2013).

4 The Advisory Committee on the Safety of Blood, Tissues and Organs (SaBTO). Cytomegalovirus tested blood components – position Statement. https://www.gov.uk/government/uploads/system/uploads/attachment_data/file/215125/dh_133086.pdf (accessed on December 2, 2013).

5 The Medicines and Healthcare products Regulatory Agency. How we regulate blood. http://www.mhra.gov.uk/Howweregulate/Blood/index.htm (accessed on November 29, 2013).

6 McLelland DBL, ed. Handbook of Transfusion Medicine. 4th edition. Norwich: The Stationery Office; 2007.

7 Department of Health. Better blood transfusion – safe and appropriate use of blood. HSC2007/001. London: HMSO; 2007. http://webarchive.nationalarchives.gov.uk/20130107105354/http://www.dh.gov.uk/prod_consum_dh/groups/dh_digitalassets/documents/digitalasset/dh_080803.pdf.

8 Goodnough LT, Shander A. Patient blood management. Anesthesiology 2012;116(6):1367–76.

9 National Patient Safety Agency. Right patient, right blood: advice for safer blood transfusions. London: HMSO; 2007. http://www.nrls.npsa.nhs.uk/resources/?entryid45=59805 (accessed on November 29, 2013).

10 British Committee for Standards in Haematology (BCSH). Milkins C, Berryman J, Cantwell, C et al. Guidelines for pre-transfusion compatibility procedures in blood transfusion laboratories. Transfus Med 2013;23(1):3–35.

11 Serious Hazards of Transfusion (SHOT). http://www.shotuk.org (accessed on November 29, 2013).

12 British Committee for Standards in Haematology (BCSH). Guideline on the administration of blood components 2009. http://www.bcshguidelines.com (accessed on November 16, 2013).

13 Murphy MF, Waters JH, Wood EM, Yazer MH. Transfusing blood safely and appropriately. BMJ 2013;347:f4303.

14 Tinegate H, Birchall J, Gray A et al. Guideline on the investigation and management of acute transfusion reactions. Prepared by the BCSH Blood Transfusion Task Force. Br J Haematol 2012;159(2):143–53.

15 Retter A, Wyncoll D, Pearse R et al. Guidelines on the management of anaemia and red cell transfusion in adult critically ill patients. Br J Haematol 2013;160(4):445–64.

16 BCSH. Guidelines for the use of platelet transfusions. Br J Haematol 2003;122:10–23.

17 BCSH. Guidelines for the use of prophylactic anti-D immunoglobulin. http://www.bcshguidelines.com/documents/Anti-D_bcsh_07062006.pdf (accessed on November 16, 2013).

18 O'Shaughnessy DF, Atterbury C, Bolton Maggs P et al. BCSH guidelines for the use of fresh frozen plasma, cryoprecipitate and cryosupernatant. Br J Haematol 2004;126:11–28.

19 Goodnough LT, Levy JH, Murphy MF. Concepts of blood transfusion in adults Lancet 2013;381(9880):1845–54.

20 Dzik W, Blajchman MA, Fergusson D et al. Clinical review: Canadian National Advisory Committee on Blood and Blood Products – massive transfusion consensus conference 2011: Report of the panel. Crit Care 2011;15(6):242.

21 Keeling D, Baglin T, Tait C et al. Guidelines on oral anticoagulation with warfarin – fourth edition. Br J Haematol 2011;154(3):311–24.

22 Stanworth SJ, Walsh TS, Prescott RJ et al. A national study of plasma use in critical care: clinical indications, dose and effect on prothrombin time. Crit Care. 2011;15(2):R108.

23 Hospitals & Science. The national comparative audit of blood transfusion. http://hospital.blood.co.uk/safe_use/clinical_audit/National_Comparative/ (accessed on November 16, 2013).

CHAPTER 14

Transfusion Reactions

Therese A. Callaghan
NHS Blood and Transplant, Liverpool, UK
Medical Department, Royal Liverpool University Hospital, Liverpool, UK

Introduction

The possibility of adverse reaction should always be borne in mind when prescribing blood components. Transfusions should be reserved for situations where the clinical indication is clear and no appropriate alternative is available.

Adverse reactions may be acute or chronic and vary in severity from mild to life-threatening. Recognition of a reaction may be difficult in the critical care setting where the symptoms and signs may be masked by the patient's pre-existing clinical condition. Even when a transfusion reaction is suspected, there may be difficulties in establishing the nature and cause of the reaction because of overlapping clinical features.

All suspected transfusion reactions in the UK should be notified to SHOT (Serious Hazards of Transfusion), the national haemovigilance reporting scheme.

Acute reactions

Acute transfusion reactions are those which occur within the first 24 h of transfusion; a severe acute reaction may occur within the first 15 min.

Acute reactions include:
- Acute haemolytic transfusion reaction (AHTR)
- Transfusion-transmitted bacterial infection

- Febrile non-haemolytic transfusion reaction (FNHTR)
- Allergy/anaphylaxis
- Transfusion-associated overload (TACO)
- Transfusion-related acute lung injury (TRALI)

As prompt recognition of acute reactions is essential for management to be effective, careful monitoring of the transfused patient is key. As a minimum, vital signs (temperature, pulse rate, blood pressure) should be monitored before transfusion of each unit, 15 min after the start of each unit and again not more than 60 min after the end of each transfusion episode. Respiratory rate should be recorded at the start and repeated if any of the other vital signs move significantly from baseline values [1].

An overview of acute reactions and their management is outlined in Figure 14.1.

Acute haemolytic transfusion reaction (AHTR)

An AHTR is defined as increased destruction of red cells within 24 h of transfusion. A fall in haemoglobin and plasma haptoglobin is associated with a rise in bilirubin and lactate dehydrogenase. The cause is usually immunological incompatibility between recipient plasma and transfused red cells.

The symptoms and signs of AHTR include:
- Fever, chills or flushing
- Pain at the infusion site or in the loins, abdomen, chest or head

Haematology in Critical Care: A Practical Handbook, First Edition. Edited by Jecko Thachil and Quentin A. Hill.
© 2014 John Wiley & Sons, Ltd. Published 2014 by John Wiley & Sons, Ltd.

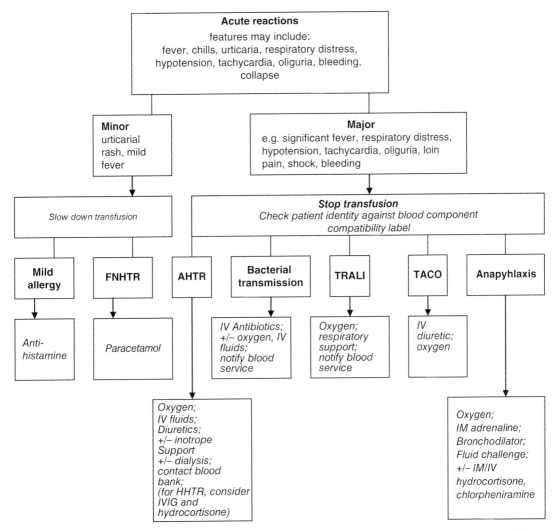

Figure 14.1 Overview of acute reactions and management. FNHTR, febrile non-haemolytic transfusion reaction; AHTR, acute haemolytic transfusion reaction; TRALI, transfusion-related acute lung injury; TACO, transfusion-associated circulatory overload; HHTR, hyperhaemolytic transfusion reaction; IVIG, intravenous immunoglobulin.

• Agitation, nausea/vomiting, dyspnoea, hypotension, hypertension, tachycardia, haemoglobinuria and excessive bleeding

In the unconscious patient, the first sign of an AHTR may be hypotension, uncontrolled bleeding due to disseminated intravascular coagulation (DIC), haemoglobinuria or oliguria.

The main causes of AHTR are:
• Acute immune HTR due to incompatibility of transfused red cells with recipient's antibodies

• Hyperhaemolytic transfusion reaction (HHTR)
Acute haemolysis may also be a feature of reactions due to bacterial contamination; other causes include adverse storage conditions (e.g. excessively high or low temperatures).

Acute immune HTR

An acute immune HTR is most often due to ABO blood group incompatibility where the patient's own naturally occurring anti-A and/or anti-B antibodies react with transfused A or B red cells. Occasionally, other red cell alloantibodies (e.g. anti-Jk^a) may be implicated in the context of a previously transfused and subsequently allo-immunized patient. The direct antiglobulin test (DAT) is usually positive.

Anti-A, anti-B and anti-A,B antibodies are naturally occurring and are regularly present in the plasma of individuals lacking the corresponding antigen. The A and B antigens are strongly immunogenic and often complement binding. ABO incompatibility causes antibody-mediated sequential binding of complement components, leading to intravascular haemolysis, characterized by gross hae-moglobinaemia and haemoglobinuria, and cytokine release progressing to hypotension, DIC and acute tubular necrosis.

The reaction is usually most severe if group A cells are transfused into a group O recipient, and even a few millilitres of blood may be sufficient to cause symptoms in a conscious patient. Less commonly, acute immune haemolytic reactions may occur due to alloantibodies of other blood group specificities or to infusion of incompat-ible high titre donor anti-A or anti-B in plasma-rich com-ponents such as fresh frozen plasma (FFP) or platelets.

Transfusion of the wrong ABO group is inevitably due to an error, which may be related to sampling or labelling, laboratory errors, collection of wrong blood from fridge or failure of the bedside check [2]. When red cells are transfused to an individual other than the intended recip-ient, the chance of ABO incompatibility is about 1 in 3.

It should be borne in mind that an error may involve an identification mix-up between two patients, raising the possibility that another patient may also be at risk. It is therefore essential that the blood transfusion labora-tory is informed immediately so that steps can be taken to prevent another recipient receiving the wrong blood.

Death or serious harm as a result of the inadvertent trans-fusion of ABO incompatible blood components is included in the Department of Health (DH) list of 'never events', defined as 'serious, largely preventable safety incidents that should not occur if the available preventative measures have been implemented by healthcare providers' [3].

Hyperhaemolytic transfusion reaction (HHTR)

Hyperhaemolysis is a rare reaction characterized by a decrease in haemoglobin to a level below the pre-transfusion level, indicating haemolysis of both transfused blood and the patient's own red cells. It is a recognized but uncommon complication of transfusion in patients with sickle cell dis-ease (for more detailed discussion, see Chapter 18) but may also occur in other patient groups. The aetiology of hyper-haemolysis is not well understood as it may occur when no alloantibodies are identified and phenotypically matched units are transfused [4]. Hyperhaemolysis should be sus-pected if the patient develops a more marked anaemia than was present pre-transfusion. Further transfusions may exacerbate the haemolysis and lead to a protracted course or even death. Corticosteroids (hydrocortisone 100 mg 6 hourly) and intravenous immunoglobulin (1 g/kg daily) may be beneficial.

Bacterial transmission

Bacterial septicaemia due to transfusion of an infected blood component should be considered when there is a sustained rise in temperature by 2°C or more or to 39°C or above. Septic shock may develop, and the presenting symptoms and signs may be very similar to an acute immune haemolytic transfusion reaction, with the poten-tial for development of DIC.

Bacterial contamination of red cells is rare but is poten-tially more common with platelet transfusions as platelets are required to be stored at a temperature (22°C) that sup-ports bacterial survival or growth. When bacterial con-tamination does occur, the potential for serious morbidity or death is high, particularly as platelets are often given to immunosuppressed individuals such as those who have received chemotherapy. Organisms which have been implicated include *Staphylococcus epidermidis*, *S. aureus*, *Bacillus cereus*, *E. coli*, *Klebsiella pneumoniae* and *Pseu-domonas* [2]. It is essential that where bacterial transmis-sion is suspected, the supplying Blood Transfusion Service is notified without delay to allow recall of any other prod-ucts from the same donation.

Investigation of suspected AHTR/ bacterial transmission

• Check if patient identity on wristband corresponds to that on the blood pack label and compatibility form.
• Investigations – full blood count, urinary haemoglobin, (visual inspection or dipstick urinalysis), plasma hap-toglobin, bilirubin, DAT, repeat blood group, antibody screening and compatibility testing (pre- and post-transfusion samples), urea and electrolytes and clotting screen, including fibrinogen.
• Blood cultures from patient and blood pack.

Management of suspected AHTR/bacterial transmission

- Stop the transfusion.
- Maintain venous access.
- Resuscitate with crystalloids/colloids.
- Give intravenous broad spectrum antibiotics where bacterial transmission is suspected.
- Monitor urine output.
- Give diuretics (furosemide) to maintain urine output if required.
- Where AHTR confirmed, repeat coagulation and biochemistry screens every 2–4 h.
- Give inotrope support if required.
- Institute haemofiltration or dialysis if required for acute tubular necrosis.
- Where bleeding DIC is present, transfuse blood components as appropriate.
- Where hyperhaemolytic transfusion reaction is suspected, give hydrocortisone and intravenous immunoglobulin.
- Notify the hospital transfusion laboratory.
- Where bacterial transmission is suspected, notify supplying blood service.

Febrile non-haemolytic transfusion reaction (FNHTR)

Febrile non-haemolytic transfusion reactions are relatively common, affecting 0.5–2% of recipients, particularly multi-transfused or previously pregnant individuals. They are caused by anti-leukocyte antibodies in the recipient reacting against white cells in the transfused component or by cytokines in stored platelets. The frequency of FNHTRs has diminished since the introduction of routine pre-storage leukodepletion of cellular blood products. The symptoms and signs of FNHTR include fever of 38°C or above, a rise of 1°C or more from pre-transfusion value, chills/rigours, myalgia and hypotension, occurring during or within 4 h of transfusion without any other identified cause such as AHTR or bacterial contamination or underlying condition.

Management of FNHTR

It is necessary to slow or stop the transfusion. Antipyretics like paracetamol may be helpful. Those patients suffering recurrent or severe FNHTRs, washed red cells may be considered for future transfusions.

Allergy/anaphylaxis

Urticarial and allergic reactions to transfusion of blood components are not uncommon. Platelet and plasma components, particularly FFP, are more frequently implicated than red cells. Most allergic reactions are mild, causing little or no morbidity, but rarely a full-blown life-threatening anaphylactic reaction may occur. The pathogenesis of anaphylaxis is IgE-mediated degranulation of mast cells. Mast cell tryptase (MCT) is typically markedly but transiently raised in severe reactions.

A similar anaphylactoid reaction in transfused patients has been seen in IgA-deficient recipients although the vast majority of IgA-deficient individuals, even those with severe deficiency and anti-IgA antibodies, do not experience adverse reaction to transfusion [5]. The symptoms and signs of allergic reaction include flushing, urticaria, rash, wheeze, bronchospasm, stridor and angiooedema. The clinical features of anaphylaxis are as for allergic reaction, plus severe breathing difficulty, shock, arrhythmias and loss of consciousness

The investigation of moderate or severe allergic or anaphylactic reactions should include serial MCT levels immediately and at 3 and 24 h post reaction [6], serum IgA level and anti-IgA antibody screen (if severe IgA deficiency). The management of mild allergic-type reactions is mainly to slow or stop the transfusion and give antihistamine such as chlorpheniramine but for anaphylactic reaction:
- The transfusion should be stopped.
- Adrenaline 1 in 1000 should be administered (in accordance with the UK Resuscitation Council guidelines) [6].

Washed cellular components should be considered for future transfusions. For IgA-deficient recipients with history of anaphylactoid reaction, consideration should be given to using IgA-deficient blood components (e.g. washed red cells, components from IgA-deficient donors) where time permits. Standard products may be used in emergency situations [5].

Transfusion-associated circulatory overload (TACO)

Transfusion-associated circulatory overload occurs when too much fluid is administered or transfusion is too rapid, resulting in acute left ventricular failure. TACO is under-recognized and under-reported and has an incidence of approximately 6–8% in patients in intensive care [2].

Predisposing factors include cardiac and renal impairment, hypoalbuminaemia and pre-existing fluid overload. Volume overload is a particular risk with 20% albumin solutions. Over-transfusion may result from lack of consideration of the patient's fluid balance and body weight when prescribing red cells and lack of regular monitoring of the patient's haemoglobin after every 2 or 3 U of red cells transfused. Consideration should be given to the administration of diuretics when transfusing red cells to patients with chronic anaemia.

Transfusion-related acute lung injury (TRALI)

Transfusion-related acute lung injury is a severe acute reaction occurring within 6 h of transfusion and characterized by a clinical picture indistinguishable from acute respiratory syndrome (ARDS) and acute lung injury (ALI) [7].

The cause is thought to be preformed antibodies in donor plasma acting against recipient human leukocyte antigen (HLA) or human neutrophil antigen (HNA) on the recipient's white cells. This can lead to pulmonary leukostasis and leukocyte activation with subsequent capillary leak and pulmonary damage. These donor antibodies are formed as a result of previous pregnancy or transfusion.

Blood components with proportionately more plasma, e.g. FFP and platelets, are more likely to cause TRALI, but it may occur even with small amounts of plasma such as is present in concentrated red cells. The introduction of policies to produce plasma components (FFP, cryoprecipitate, plasma for platelet pools) from male donors only has significantly reduced the incidence of TRALI in the UK. Other preventative measures include the screening of female platelet donors for HLA and HNA antibodies and accepting only those who are found to be antibody negative. Rarely, TRALI may result from patient antibodies reacting against donor leukocyte. This is only a possibility where the transfused product is not leukocdepleted, e.g. granulocytes or buffy coats. Transfused HLA and HNA antibodies do not necessarily cause overt lung injury, even if the corresponding antigen is present on the recipient's white cells. It is likely that other predisposing patient factors have to be present suggesting a two-hit mechanism (antibodies, the first hit). Although later testing for donor HLA and HNA antibodies and recipient HLA and HNA typing may provide evidence supporting the diagnosis of

TRALI, the diagnosis in the acute setting is primarily a clinical one. It may be difficult to distinguish TRALI from cardiac failure or non-cardiogenic pulmonary oedema. Chest X-ray typically shows bilateral pulmonary infiltrates. However, in contrast to the findings in TACO, in TRALI, the central venous pressure is normal and the pulmonary wedge pressure is not raised but is low or normal with normal appearances on echocardiography:

• For a diagnosis of TRALI, the presenting features should occur within 6 h of transfusion.

• Donor leukocyte antibody investigations should be considered if high index suspicion of TRALI exists (notify blood service). Recipient HLA/HNA typing is further required if donor antibody screening is positive.

The management of TRALI is primarily to stop the transfusion and provide respiratory support, including ventilation if necessary. Steroids have been used but their value is uncertain. Diuretics should be avoided as loss of circulating volume and hypotension are common and further transfusion should be avoided if possible, but where transfusion is essential, standard products are acceptable.

Delayed reactions

Delayed reactions occur more than 24 h post transfusion and include:

• Delayed haemolytic transfusion reaction (DHTR)
• Post-transfusion purpura (PTP)
• Transfusion-associated graft-versus-host disease (TA-GVHD)

Delayed haemolytic transfusion reaction (DHTR)

Delayed haemolytic transfusion reactions are almost always a consequence of the recipient having been previously sensitized to allogeneic red cell antigens by pregnancy or earlier transfusion. The resulting red cell alloantibody is present at a level too low to cause an acute reaction. But, when the recipient is reexposed to the antigen, there is a secondary immune response resulting in a rapid increase in antibody a few days (typically 5–7 days) after the transfusion. Red cell destruction ensues with fall in haemoglobin and jaundice. Haemolysis is primarily extravascular, and although haemoglobinuria may occur, renal failure is unusual. The DAT becomes positive until the incompatible cells have been removed.

The alloantibodies most commonly implicated are those from the Kidd blood group system (anti-Jk^a, anti-Jk^b) and the Rh system (anti-D, anti-E, anti-e, anti-C, anti-c). The clinical presentation and investigations are similar to ATR.

Management is supportive, but if severe haemolysis occurs with renal compromise, red cell exchange may be required.

Post-transfusion purpura (PTP)

Post-transfusion purpura is a rare complication of transfusion characterized by acute severe thrombocytopenia occurring 5–12 days after transfusion of red cells. Bleeding is common and often severe. The condition affects predominantly middle-aged or elderly females whose platelets are usually negative for human platelet antigen (HPA)-1a and who have been previously alloimmunized by pregnancy with the development of anti-HPA-1a. Reexposure by transfusion leads to a secondary immune response. The reason why the recipient's own platelets are destroyed by the alloantibody is not clearly understood. Other HPA specificities may be implicated, e.g. anti-HPA-5b.

The symptoms and signs of PTP include widespread purpura, bleeding from mucosal membranes, gastrointestinal bleeding and haematuria occurring 5–12 days post transfusion.

Post-transfusion purpura confirmation requires platelet antibody screening and HPA grouping. The management of PTP includes high-dose intravenous immunoglobulin 2 g/kg and high-dose platelets for severe bleeding in acute phase. For future transfusions, use HPA-compatible red cells or platelets if readily available although leukocyte-reduced products are generally regarded as safe.

Transfusion-associated graft-versus-host disease (TA-GVHD)

Transfusion-associated graft-versus-host disease is a rare complication of transfusion, which manifests itself 1–2 weeks post transfusion. It is caused by donor lymphocytes engrafting and proliferating within susceptible recipients. At-risk recipients are those who are profoundly immunosuppressed or who share an HLA haplotype with the donor and include the following patient groups [8]:

- Recipients of peripheral blood stem cell or bone marrow transplants
- Patients with a diagnosis of Hodgkin's disease
- Patients receiving purine antagonists (e.g. fludarabine, cladribine, deoxycoformycin)
- Patients receiving alemtuzumab (anti-CD52) treatment
- Patients receiving anti-thymocyte globulin (ATG) for aplastic anaemia
- Recipients of HLA-matched cellular products
- Recipients of cellular blood products from a family member

In addition, all patients receiving granulocytes or buffy coats are at risk.

The symptoms/signs of TA-GVHD include diarrhoea, fever, maculopapular rash, liver dysfunction and pancytopenia.

Transfusion-associated graft-versus-host disease is almost always fatal, and the mainstay of management is prevention by irradiation of cellular blood products prior to transfusion to at-risk individuals [8].

A total of 13 cases of TA-GVHD were reported to SHOT between 1996 and 2011, all fatal [2]. However, all but one of these cases occurred prior to the introduction of universal leukcodepletion of all cellular blood components (except granulocytes/buffy coats) in late 1999. Two cases in total have been reported in recipients of leukcodepleted products. The last case in the UK reported to SHOT was in 2001.

References

1 British Committee for Standards in Haematology (BCSH). Guideline on the administration of blood components http://www.bcshguidelines.com/documents/Admin_blood_components_bcsh_05012010.pdf (accessed on November 16, 2013).

2 Serious Hazards of Transfusion (SHOT) steering group. SHOT annual reports 1996–2011. http://www.shotuk.org (accessed on November 28, 2013).

3 Department of Health (DH). The 'never events' list 2011/12. Prepared by the Patient Safety Policy Team http://www.dh.gov.uk/prod_consum_dh/groups/dh_digitalassets/documents/digitalasset/dh_124580.pdf (accessed on November 28, 2013); 2011.

4 Garraty G. What do we mean by 'hyperhaemolysis' and what is the cause? Transfus Med 2012;22:77–9.

5 Tinegate H. Investigation and clinical management of suspected reactions to IgA. 2012. http://hospital.blood.co.uk/library/pdf/INF486.pdf (accessed on November 16, 2013).

6 Resuscitation Council (UK). Emergency treatment of anaphylactic reactions. Guidelines for healthcare providers. 2008. http://www.resus.org.uk/pages/reaction.pdf (accessed on November 28, 2013).

7 Popovsky MA, Moore SB. Diagnostic and pathogenetic considerations in transfusion-related acute lung injury. Transfusion 1985;25:573–7.

8 Treleaven J, Gennery A, Marsh J et al. Guidelines on the use of irradiated blood components, prepared by the British Committee for Standards in Haematology blood transfusion task force. Br J Haematol 2010;152:35–51.

CHAPTER 15

The Management of Non-traumatic Massive Haemorrhage

Nicola S. Curry[1,2] and Simon J. Stanworth[2,3]

[1]Oxford Haemophilia and Thrombosis Centre, Oxford University Hospitals, Oxford, UK
[2]Department of Haematology, University of Oxford, Oxford, UK
[3]NHS Blood and Transplant/Oxford University Hospitals NHS Trust, John Radcliffe Hospital, Oxford, UK

Introduction

Massive (or major) bleeding is a life-threatening emergency in hospitalized patients and occurs across most specialities including surgery, medicine (gastrointestinal), obstetrics and neonatology. These patients are not infrequently admitted to intensive care or high dependency units, for continued care and close monitoring. Even if treated outside this setting, they are often managed with input from critical care physicians. Successful haemostatic control in these situations requires the delivery of effective resuscitation, specifically transfusion therapy, in conjunction with surgical and/or radiological interventions.

Traditionally, massive (or major) haemorrhage has been defined as the loss of one blood volume within a 24-h period. Alternative definitions include a loss of 50% blood volume within 3 h or a rate of blood loss of 150 mL/min [1]. These quantitative (and retrospectively applied) definitions are fairly straightforward to understand, but from a practical standpoint are unhelpful. Early identification of severe haemorrhage, or indeed a patient at risk of major haemorrhage, is critical for improving the chances of a successful outcome. Recognition of blood loss ideally needs to be made within minutes rather than at 24 h. However, clinical evidence of blood loss can be difficult to detect, particularly in patients with good cardiovascular reserve, but a high index of suspicion in addition to parameters suggestive of shock, i.e. a systolic blood pressure (SBP) less than 70 mmHg or an SBP less than 90 mmHg after an initial fluid challenge, is a helpful tool.

This chapter will summarize haemostatic changes during major blood loss and how this knowledge has helped to drive changes to transfusion practices; it will focus on general management of major blood loss and apply these to specific clinical settings.

Massive transfusion: An outdated term?

Massive transfusion (MT) is a term that most commonly describes the transfusion of ≥10 U of red blood cells (RBC) within a 24-h period. It is an arbitrary definition and is frequently used synonymously to delineate patients with severe blood loss. However, this would artificially divide patients into different groups, while RBC transfusion should be, in fact, on a continuous spectrum. The phrase also defines a medical condition by its treatment and specifically, treatment by red cell usage rather than haemostatic interventions. Moreover, mortality has not been shown to dramatically increase at any threshold value including greater than 10 U RBC. Furthermore, the CRASH-2 study has demonstrated that tranexamic acid (TXA) when given within 3 h of injury confers mortality benefit to all trauma patients at risk of bleeding. In fact, the largest group to benefit from TXA were those who did not receive *MT* support, i.e. less than 10 U RBC [2].

Red cell transfusions

Patients with major bleeding need red cell transfusions urgently. Maintaining tissue perfusion and oxygenation is key to improving outcomes. Because of the direct link between tissue ischaemia and mortality, RBC transfusions are an early priority in resuscitation. As described later, hospital policies to describe access to emergency-release uncrossmatched RBCs within minutes of identification of major bleeding are essential within major haemorrhage protocols (MHPs). Intra-operative blood salvage, when selectively used for cases involving large volume blood loss such as obstetrics or surgery, may also provide a source of red cell support, but will not be considered further in this chapter.

The coagulopathy of massive haemorrhage

Coagulopathy is frequently identified in patients with life-threatening haemorrhage. Depending on the definition and patient group, it affects between 5% and 30% of patients (e.g. trauma, cardiac surgery patients and acute upper gastrointestinal haemorrhage). Coagulopathic patients, whether or not they are actively bleeding, have a worse overall prognosis. There are several causes of worsening coagulation during major blood loss:

1 *Consumption.* Coagulation factors and platelets are consumed during the formation of clots in an attempt to prevent blood loss through damaged vessels.

2 *Dilution.* This is a consequence of replacement of the whole blood with crystalloid, colloid and red cell transfusions. Replacement of two blood volumes with red cell concentrate alone results in a platelet count in the order of $50 \times 10-9/L$. Furthermore, the volume of fluid administered to a patient has been shown to be proportional to the resultant coagulopathy.

3 *Hypoxia, acidosis and hypothermia.* This triad predisposes to further bleeding. Hypothermia and acidosis

impair the functional ability of both the platelets and the coagulation proteases. Haemostatic defects are most evident once pH values fall below 7.1 and temperatures below 33°C.

4 *Ongoing bleeding.* Anaemia has an effect on primary haemostasis. A low haematocrit reduces axial flow (where all the red cells flow in the middle of the vessel and platelets and plasma are pushed into close proximity to the endothelium) and thus reduces the margination of platelets and platelet–endothelial interaction.

The aforementioned four effects tend to lead to increased bleeding, while the next leads to a prothrombotic phenotype and helps to explain why those patients with severe bleeding are also at increased risk of thrombotic problems including multi-organ failure:

5 *Hormonal and cytokine-induced changes.* Following tissue injury, hormone levels, i.e. adrenaline and vasopressin, rise, and there is an increased generation of cytokines. Vasopressin stimulates both the release of von Willebrand factor (from Weibel–Palade bodies) and expression of P-selectin on the endothelial cell surface. Cytokines, such as TNF and IL-1, as well as thrombin can cause endothelial cell activation and thus effect a slow change in endothelial cell phenotype from antithrombotic to prothrombotic.

Definitions of coagulopathy: Standard laboratory tests or thromboelastography?

There are two reasons for assessing haemostatic function in a patient with major blood loss: the first, to rapidly identify any coagulopathy and/or predict which patients will require early implementation of major haemorrhage therapy and, the second, to guide ongoing therapy and transfusions. The advantages of using standard tests are that every laboratory can provide these results. But there are several disadvantages. The prothrombin time (PT) and activated partial thromboplastin time (APTT) tests were originally designed to evaluate clotting factor deficiencies, not acquired coagulopathy, and have been shown to be poor predictors of bleeding in these circumstances. Furthermore, turnaround times from sampling to obtaining results from the laboratory may be over an hour, a timescale often considered impractical in the setting of ongoing blood loss.

Near-patient testing is therefore often advocated in the setting of major bleeding. The most widely used near-patient testing devices include the thromboelastogram (TEG) or ROTEM. These are whole-blood viscoelastic tests that evaluate the effects of coagulation factors, platelets and red cells on overall clotting potential. Both work along similar principles, whereby progressive clot formation in the presence of an activator is measured. The trace can then be used to determine the activity of separate components of the clotting pathway, including coagulation proteases, platelets and fibrinogen as well as any lytic activity. Advocates for viscoelastic testing argue that the ability to distinguish different haemostatic abnormalities provides a means of individualizing coagulation management and guiding transfusion resuscitation. TEG has been demonstrated to be useful in guiding and reducing transfusion requirements following cardiac and liver transplantation surgery although a validated algorithm to guide blood product use in patients with major blood loss and active bleeding has never been refined and many hospitals use non-validated local policies [3].

Management of massive haemorrhage and its associated coagulopathy in specific clinical settings

Lessons from the trauma literature

Contemporary management of major haemorrhage employs several approaches to combat acidosis, hypothermia, coagulopathy and hypoperfusion simultaneously. In the setting of trauma, this practice is known as damage control resuscitation (DCR). An integral component of DCR is the early and aggressive transfusion of red cells and blood components in high ratio in an attempt to reverse coagulopathy and restore delivery of oxygenated blood to the tissues. Immediate transfusion is not guided by coagulation results.

Although there are reports of case series beginning to appear in the literature where high ratio blood component, RBC transfusion therapy has been used outside the trauma setting, there have been no published data, which compare the underlying coagulopathy profiles or the responses of different patient groups with major haemorrhage to various forms of transfusion therapy.

Patients with non-trauma bleeding have co-morbidities and clinical features very different from trauma patients. This is particularly apparent when the co-morbidities for patients with gastrointestinal bleeding are considered (e.g. older age and the presence of liver disease). Therefore, limitations may exist when considering the direct application of similar transfusion support strategies from trauma to non-trauma patients with major bleeding. Of equal consideration and as described later, the pathophysiology of haemostatic breakdown (including iatrogenic causes for coagulopathy, i.e. anti-platelet agents) in non-trauma patients is different from that observed in trauma.

Critically ill patients with obstetric causes for major bleeding

Major obstetric haemorrhage (MOH) is the leading cause of preventable maternal death worldwide, and 80% of major bleeding episodes occur postpartum. As there is no universally accepted definition for MOH, its incidence varies depending on how it is defined. For Scotland in 2009, the overall rate of MOH – defined as greater than 2500 mL blood loss or greater than or equal to 5 U of RBC within 24 h of giving birth – was 5 per 1000 live births [4].

One critical feature of major haemorrhage in obstetrics is the development of fibrinolysis early on in the haemorrhagic episode. Fibrinogen concentration during the initial period of bleeding may be an informative marker for predicting outcome during MOH. In one study, a fibrinogen concentration of less than 2.9 g/L during labour was associated with an increase in the incidence of postpartum haemorrhage (PPH) (odds ratio = 19.7), and in a second study, the parameter found to correlate best with volume of blood loss ($r = -0.48$; $p = <0.01$) was the maternal fibrinogen concentration [5]. Current guidelines for PPH recommend fibrinogen replacement only when plasma levels fall below 1 g/L, but these recent data provide evidence that a higher trigger, of 2 g/L, for example, is likely more appropriate and may particularly be beneficial if given early during bleeding [6]. Fibrinogen is one of the most important proteins in coagulation, for it is the final point of the coagulation cascade, being converted to insoluble fibrin strands, and is the ligand for platelet aggregation – thereby acting as the bridge for stable clot formation. When levels of fibrinogen fall, patients have a reduced ability to form clots and tend to bleed longer. Indeed, it has been shown that fibrinogen is one of the earliest coagulation proteins to fall in major bleeding.

Although there is no consensus on the optimal use of blood and blood components to treat obstetric patients with severe bleeding, management of MOH has started to mirror treatment of trauma haemorrhage, using high ratio blood component principles [7], with some experts additionally advocating early supplementation by fibrinogen, using either fibrinogen concentrates or cryoprecipitate. Pro-haemostatic drugs have been used in obstetric bleeding, in particular TXA and recombinant factor VIIa (rFVIIa). A systematic review has concluded that TXA reduces postpartum blood loss, but these results were based on two RCTs of questionable quality [8]. The results of a large international RCT – the WOMAN study – to evaluate the effects of TXA in PPH are awaited with interest [9]. WHO currently recommends that TXA is used at a dose of 1 g by slow IV injection, repeated once if bleeding continued. Any beneficial role of rFVIIa is uncertain, as general evidence of effectiveness for this agent does not exist, despite numerous RCTs. A trial has evaluated the efficacy and safety of early versus delayed use of rFVIIa in PPH [10], which is now completed and the results are awaited.

Critically ill patients with cardiac causes for major bleeding

Major bleeding may occur in patients during or after cardiac surgery. Several features of bleeding in cardiac patients may be distinctive. Bleeding in cardiac surgery can be attributed to surgical breach of the vasculature or acquired haemostatic defects or a combination of the two. Haemostatic defects in cardiopulmonary bypass (CPB) surgery are unique, and factors that may contribute to bleeding include platelet dysfunction from the bypass circuit and anti-platelet therapy, reduced thrombin generation due to deranged clotting factor activity, hypofibrinogenaemia and fibrinolysis. Abnormal platelet function, often in combination with thrombocytopenia, is a frequent cause of bleeding in patients undergoing CPB. Increasing the duration of CPB increases the platelet dysfunction, and resolution usually takes 5–24 h. There is also emerging evidence that lower fibrinogen levels in patients both pre-operatively and during CPB procedures are predictive of increased bleeding peri-operatively. Reports from small RCTs support the use of fibrinogen

concentrate in cardiac surgery patients and show reduced bleeding and transfusion need following its use.

Major bleeding in critically ill patients on warfarin

Some patients who present with major or life-threatening haemorrhage will be receiving oral anticoagulant therapy. For these patients, there should be full and rapid reversal of the effect of warfarin. This is most effectively achieved using a prothrombin complex concentrate (PCC), used in combination with intravenous vitamin K. PCCs are plasma-derived coagulation factor concentrates that contain three or four vitamin K-dependent factors at high concentration. Four factor concentrates (widely available in UK) are much preferred and contain factors II, VII, IX and X, as well as variable amounts of anticoagulants and heparin. Studies have shown that PCCs are safe and effective and normalize INR values rapidly when compared to FFP. Outcome data examining the effect of PCCs on bleeding rates and mortality are not yet available.

Critically ill patients with hepatic and gastrointestinal causes for major bleeding

Gastrointestinal bleeding can be divided into causes arising from the upper or lower gastrointestinal tract; upper gastrointestinal bleeding (UGIB) is more common. Non-variceal bleeding accounts for most presentations with major bleeding, and the most common cause is peptic ulcer disease. Patients with gastrointestinal bleeding are often of advancing age and have many co-morbidities such as liver disease or chronic renal failure. The incidence of variceal UGIB in patients with liver cirrhosis is rising, largely driven by alcohol- and obesity-induced liver disease (steatohepatitis). There are no published data on rates of coagulopathy or strategies for resuscitation management in these situations. A recent updated systematic review of TXA in gastrointestinal bleeding indicated that TXA significantly reduced mortality in patients with gastrointestinal bleeding (RR = 0.59, 95% CI 0.42–0.82; $p = 0.002$) [11]. However, the quality of the trials was poor, and most were conducted in an era prior to the widespread availability of therapeutic endoscopy and high dose proton-pump inhibition, and results from a larger trial are awaited.

Coagulopathy and management of bleeding in patients with liver cirrhosis deserve separate mention. Many factors contribute to abnormalities of haemostasis in patients with cirrhosis including anaemia, thrombocytopenia, hypo- and dysfibrinogenaemia, hyperfibrinolysis and deficiencies in both pro- and anticoagulation factors. Again, there is a dearth of data to describe haemostatic changes in bleeding patients. Patients are considered now to have a more balanced deficiency of hypo- and hypercoagulopathic changes in liver disease. As such, there are limitations with regard to the value of standard coagulation tests in monitoring such patients with major bleeding as the PT and APTT really only reflect the levels of procoagulant factors (values are often prolonged due to reduced hepatic synthesis of many of the clotting factors). The PT and APTT provide no information about the balance of haemostasis or the overall capacity for thrombin formation. There is therefore an increasing view that thrombin generation tests provide results that are more representative of the overall pro- versus anticoagulant balance and are more accurately able to predict bleeding risk.

Practical considerations for the management of non-traumatic major haemorrhage

All patients:
• Early recognition of major blood loss is paramount.
• Involve senior physicians, including haematologists for transfusion support and relevant surgical or interventional radiology teams for definitive haemostatic control.
• Activate the MHP (see following texts).
• Take regular full blood counts and coagulation screens, and if available, use viscoelastic tests.

Obstetrics:
• Recognize the potential need for early fibrinogen replacement, with either fibrinogen concentrate or cryoprecipitate (according to local practice).

Cardiac:
• Following CPB, ensure heparin is fully reversed.
• Platelet transfusion may be indicated even in the absence of thrombocytopenia, in light of the acquired platelet dysfunction.
• Consider fibrinogen replacement (according to local practice).

Warfarin and major blood loss:
• Treat with 25–50 IU/kg PCC (according to INR – if known) and according to local hospital policy and administer 5–10 mg intravenous vitamin K. Repeat INR.
• FFP will not reverse warfarin effectively and should not be used for this indication.

GI and hepatic haemorrhage:
• Fluid overload is a concern and those patients with cirrhosis are at highest risk. FFP should be used judiciously and not simply as a volume expander.
• Recognize that standard coagulation tests in patients with liver disease are unreliable.

Major haemorrhage protocols

The delivery of blood and blood components in an emergency presents logistic difficulties. This may be due to the need for immediate transfusion in a highly pressured clinical setting (the majority of severe haemorrhagic deaths occur in the first 6 h) and also due to the large number of people involved. Between October 2006 and September 2010, delays in the emergency provision of blood in UK hospitals led to 11 deaths and 83 incidents of harm being reposted to the National Patient Safety Agency. In light of this, a Rapid Response Report concerning the transfusion of blood in an emergency was produced, which recommended the adoption of MHPs in every hospital [12].

Therefore, a key step in optimizing the support of patients with major bleeding is the development of a local agreed-upon approach to identification and management, which includes plans for regular audit and monitoring of cases, education to key staff and emphasis on the importance of communication between relevant staff. MHPs should provide a structured framework within which emergency red cells and blood components can be accessed rapidly using systems that are adapted to local hospital policies (see Figure 15.1 for an example of a MHP) [13]. Policies must also indicate, where appropriate (i.e. for trauma), the importance of early use of TXA. The initial approach to the care of patients with major bleeding should be in keeping with current principles of resuscitation, such as those detailed in the Advanced Trauma Life Support (ATLS) guidelines, which are regularly updated. Direct control of bleeding by surgery or interventional radiology or therapeutic endoscopy remains the mainstay of initial therapy.

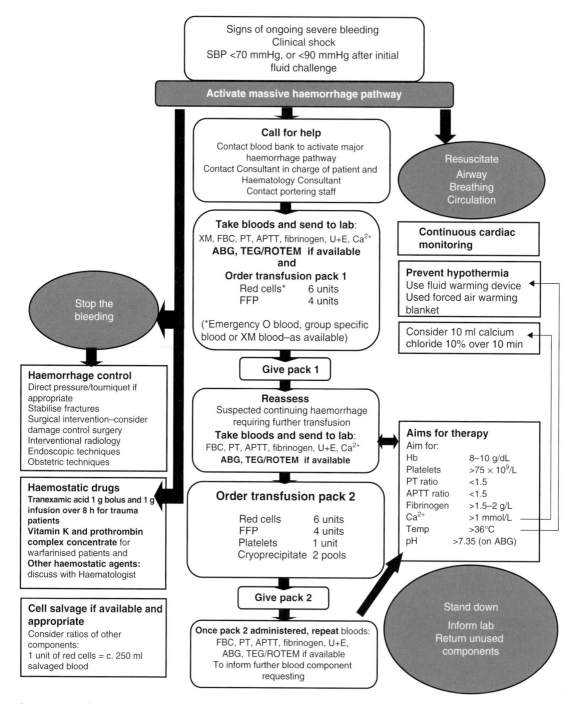

Figure 15.1 Transfusion management of massive haemorrhage. ABG, arterial blood gas; APTT, activated partial thromboplastin time; FBC, full blood count; FFP, fresh frozen plasma; PT, prothrombin time; SBP, systolic blood pressure; TEG/ROTEM, thromboelastography; XM, crossmatch.

References

1 Stainsby D, MacLennan S, Hamilton PJ. Management of massive blood loss: a template guideline. Br J Anaesth 2000;85:487–91.

2 CRASH-2 Collaborators, Roberts I, Shakur H et al. The importance of early treatment with tranexamic acid in bleeding trauma patients: an exploratory analysis of the CRASH-2 randomised controlled trial. Lancet 2011;377:1096–101.

3 Afshari A, Wikkelsø A, Brok J, Møller AM, Wetterslev J. Thrombelastography (TEG) or thromboelastometry (ROTEM) to monitor haemotherapy versus usual care in patients with massive transfusion. Cochrane Database Syst Rev 2011;(3):CD007871.

4 Scottish Confidential Audit of Severe Maternal Morbidity. 7th annual report (data from 2009). 2011. http://www.healthcareimprovementscotland.org (accessed on April 3, 2012).

5 de Lloyd L, Bovington R, Kaye A et al. Standard haemostatic test following major obstetric haemorrhage. Int J Obst Anesth 2011;20:135–41.

6 Solomon C, Collis RE, Collins PW. Haemostatic monitoring during postpartum haemorrhage and implications for management. Br J Anaesth 2012;109:851–63.

7 Saule I, Hawkins N. Transfusion practice in major obstetric haemorrhage: lessons from trauma. Int J Obstet Anesth 2012;21:79–83.

8 Novikova N, Hofmeyr GJ. Tranexamic acid for preventing postpartum haemorrhage. Cochrane Database Syst Rev 2010;(7):CD007872.

9 ISRCTN76912190. The WOMAN trial. London School of Tropical Medicine, London. http://www.thewomantrial.lshtm.ac.uk (accessed on March 21, 2012).

10 NCT 00370877. Recombinant human activated factor VII as salvage therapy in women with severe postpartum hemorrhage. http://clinicaltrials.gov/ct2/show/NCT00370877 (accessed on April 03, 2012).

11 Gluud LL, Klingenburg SL, Langhoz E. Tranexamic acid for upper gastrointestinal bleeding. Cochrane Database Syst Rev 2012;(1):CD006640.

12 National Patient Safety Agency. The transfusion of blood and blood products in an emergency. Rapid response report. NPSA/2010/RRR017. 2010. http://www.nrls.npsa.nhs.uk/alerts/?entryid45=83659 (accessed on March 21, 2012).

13 Dzik WH, Blajchman MA, Fergusson D et al. Clinical review: Canadian National Advisory Committee on Blood and Blood Products – massive transfusion consensus conference 2011: report of the panel. Crit Care 2011;15:242.

CHAPTER 16

Plasma Exchange

Khaled El-Ghariani

Department of Stem Cells and Therapeutic Apheresis Services, NHS Blood and Transplant
and Sheffield Teaching Hospitals NHS Trust, Sheffield, UK, and University of Sheffield, Sheffield, UK

Introduction

Plasma exchange is a therapeutic procedure in which part of the patient's plasma is replaced with an appropriate alternative fluid. The rationale of such a therapy is that plasma removal would also reduce the body content of a substance or substances that are implicated in the pathogenesis of the disorder being treated. Although plasma exchange is mainly used to reduce the immunoglobulin contents of the human body, to ameliorate an immunologically based disease process, the procedure could also deplete other large-molecular-weight substances such as immune complexes; complement components; coagulation factors, particularly fibrinogen and ultralarge von Willebrand factor (vWF) multimers; and low-density lipoprotein. The efficiency of apheresis removal of a substance depends on its density, its rate of synthesis and its predominant presence in the intravascular rather than extravascular compartment, as well as the speed of equilibrium between these two compartments following plasma exchange [1]. IgM and fibrinogen are relatively easily depleted following repeated plasma exchange, followed by IgG and IgA [2]. Given their rate of synthesis and/or extravascular distribution, other smaller molecules are less effectively removed.

The term plasmapheresis (Greek word *aphaeresis*, meaning *to take away*) is sometimes used interchangeably with plasma exchange; however, the term plasmapheresis is best used to describe plasma removal (e.g. plasma donation) without replacement fluid, rather than to describe genuine plasma exchange [3].

Technologies

Plasma exchange can be performed either by centrifugal separation or by membrane filtration. Following carefully adjusted centrifugation, blood separates into layers depending on component density. Red cells, being the most dense, settle on the bottom followed by granulocytes, lymphocytes, platelets and finally plasma on the top [1]. Centrifugal devices often use light sensors to detect the borders of separation between these layers, divert the plasma into discard and infuse the required volume of replacement fluid through the machine's sophisticated tubing system. This technology usually uses citrate as an extracorporeal anticoagulant, and it is popular in haematology practice because it is versatile and can be used to exchange red cells and to collect peripheral blood stem cells. A commonly used centrifugal device is the COBE® Spectra Apheresis System and the next generation called the Spectra Optia® Apheresis System (TERUMO BCT). The advantage with centrifugation technique is that there is no size limit of the molecules being removed.

On the other hand, filtration-based exchange uses membrane separation, usually hollow fibre filtration, and

Haematology in Critical Care: A Practical Handbook, First Edition. Edited by Jecko Thachil and Quentin A. Hill.
© 2014 John Wiley & Sons, Ltd. Published 2014 by John Wiley & Sons, Ltd.

separation is based mainly on particle size. This allows separation of plasma from cellular components. Plasma is removed and replacement fluid is infused into the patient. This system, unlike centrifugation, cannot perform cell collection or exchange [1], and large molecules such as IgM may not pass through the filter and so cannot be efficiently eliminated. This system usually uses heparin as an extracorporeal anticoagulant, and because of its similarities with haemodialysis, it is more commonly used by the renal teams. An example of a filtration device is the HF440 (Infomed blood purification devices). The benefit of filtration method is that a large filter can be easily added to a haemodialysis circuit although the size of the molecules removed is limited by the size of the pore of the filter, which is disadvantageous in thrombotic thrombocytopenic purpura (TTP), where the ultralarge vWF multimers can be very big.

Treatment plan

Prior to embarking on plasma exchange therapy, a physician trained in therapeutic apheresis should draw up a treatment plan for each patient [4, 5]. This should include number of plasma volumes to be exchanged during each procedure, type of replacement fluid to be used, frequency and total number of procedures and type of vascular access most suitable for the patient. Also, the potential impact of both the anticoagulation used and the extracorporeal circulatory volume on the patient must be assessed.

An exchange of a single plasma volume of the patient is expected to reduce the intravascular concentration of a substance by 60%, and exchanging 1.5 plasma volumes will lower the concentration by 75%; however, further increasing of exchange volume is associated with progressively exchanging more infused replacement fluid and is of diminishing clinical value (Figure 16.1). An exchange of 1–1.5 plasma volumes will suit most clinical situations. Plasma volume in the average adult can be calculated using the following formula:

Plasma volume (mL) =
$$(70 \times \text{body weight})(1 - \text{haematocrit})$$

The removed plasma has to be replaced, usually volume for volume, with an appropriate fluid that is able to preserve intravascular oncotic pressure and so maintain the systemic blood pressure. Human albumin solution (HAS,

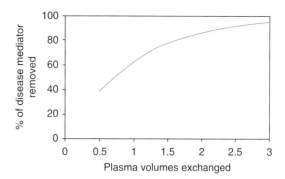

Figure 16.1 Efficiency of plasma exchange. Exchanging more than 1.5 plasma volume is associated with progressively reduced efficiency.

4–5%) is the most commonly used replacement fluid. It is effective and less likely to cause allergic reaction or transmit infection. HAS does not replace clotting factors; hence, following intensive daily exchange, a drop in fibrinogen level may cause deranged laboratory coagulation tests [2] and possibly predispose some at-risk patients to bleeding complications. Fresh frozen plasma (FFP) can also be used as a replacement fluid. FFP replaces clotting factors in patients at high risk of bleeding such as Goodpasture syndrome with pulmonary haemorrhage [2]. In the treatment of TTP, FFP is the recommended replacement fluid [6, 7]. This is because, in addition to the need to remove pathogenic factors, there is a requirement to replace specific missing physiological factors; these are the metalloproteinase enzyme and small vWF polymers. The use of solvent–detergent plasma is associated with less allergic reactions, and because of its safety, it is recommended in the UK for patients who are likely to be infused with large volumes of plasma.

The intensity of a course of plasma exchange should depend on the underlying pathology of the disease being treated. For aggressive disorders such as TTP or Goodpasture syndrome, daily exchange is required until an adequate response is obtained. For clinically less aggressive diseases, a reduction of the total IgG body content by 70–85% can be achieved by 5–6 exchanges. These should be spread over 14 days to allow equilibrium between intravascular and extravascular compartments and hence more effective removal of molecules such as IgG [2]. A successful plasma exchange requires a good blood flow into and out of the apheresis device [1]. Some patients have good antecubital veins to allow this, and others, particularly those who require frequent procedures over a short period of time, may require the insertion of a central venous catheter. This should be rigid enough to prevent lumen collapse under the sucking forces of the apheresis machine [4] and should also have a double lumen to allow the withdrawal and return of blood to and from the patient at the same time. During plasma exchange, the volume of the extracorporeal circulation can be up to 300 mL. The system is usually primed with saline to remove air as well as to ensure isovolaemia. However, at the start of a procedure, the patient will lose red cells, and hence some oxygen-carrying capacity, into the device tubing. Although this is easily tolerated by a haemodynamically stable adult patient, the red cells lost into the extracorporeal circulation at the start of the procedure can be significant in several anaemic or small paediatric patients [1]. In such situations, priming the machine tubing with red cells and saline is required.

Indications

Although for certain disorders, such as TTP, hyperviscosity and myasthenia gravis, the beneficial mechanism of the action of plasma exchange and the subsequent clinical improvement are evident, the complexity of many other pathological processes makes the decision to initiate plasma exchange therapy more challenging. The non-selective nature of plasma exchange, where many useful and harmful plasma factors are removed, and the usual concurrent use of other, possibly potent, therapeutic agents such as corticosteroid make the contribution of plasma exchange to clinical improvement difficult to ascertain, particularly if clinical improvement takes place days or weeks after a course of plasma exchange has been completed.

The American Society for Apheresis (ASFA) produces periodic assessments of clinical evidence to support, or otherwise, the use of therapeutic apheresis, including plasma exchange, in different clinical scenarios [3]. ASFA classifies indications into four categories:

Category I: therapeutic apheresis is considered first-line therapy.

Category II: therapeutic apheresis is considered second-line therapy.

Category III: role of therapeutic apheresis is not established and decision-making should be individualized.

Category IV: evidence suggests that therapeutic apheresis is ineffective or harmful.

American Society for Apheresis guidance is useful and widely used; however, situations will arise, particularly in critical care, where evidence to support the use of plasma exchange is lacking. In such situations, clinicians are encouraged to consider a patient's clinical circumstances on their merits, involve experts from other disciplines, if required, in the discussion to balance risks to patients against expected benefits, ensure informed patient consent and seek to publish their experience to guide others.

Disorders that are more likely than others to require plasma exchange in the critical care setting include TTP, hyperviscosity, severe cryoglobulinaemia, Goodpasture syndrome, catastrophic antiphospholipid syndrome, Wegener's granulomatosis, acute renal failure with myeloma, Guillain–Barre syndrome and myasthenia crisis [7]. There are other disorders for which the evidence for the use of plasma exchange is not very firm. These include overdose [5], venoms and poisoning, sepsis with multi-organ failure and acute liver failure [7]. Decisions to use plasma exchange in these situations should be individualized to a patient's needs.

Thrombotic thrombocytopenic purpura is a haematological emergency characterized by microangiopathic haemolytic anaemia and thrombocytopenia with or without renal or neurological abnormalities and without another aetiology [6, 7]. Daily plasma exchange using FFP as a replacement fluid is thought to remove both the pathogenic antibodies and ultralarge vWF molecules, as well as replace the missing ADAMTS13 and smaller vWF polymers.

High levels of paraprotein, sometimes seen in plasma cell and lymphoproliferative disorders, particularly monoclonal IgM in Waldenström macroglobulinaemia, may significantly increase blood viscosity [7], slow circulation and give rise to neurological signs and symptoms. Paraproteins may also interfere with coagulation factors and platelet function, causing coagulopathy. One to three plasma exchanges using HAS replacement fluid should alleviate patient symptoms and allow time for the primary treatment, usually chemotherapy based, to slow paraprotein production.

Plasma exchange has been shown to expedite recovery in Guillain–Barre syndrome [7], myasthenia gravis and Goodpasture syndrome

Plasma exchange is rarely used to treat poisoning or drug overdose. Theoretically, drugs that bind readily to protein and stay longer in the circulation can be removed effectively with plasma exchange [4]. However, this is not a common practice, and associated clinical evidence is not strong. Such situations should be individually assessed using evidence available at the time.

Complications

Plasma exchange can be associated with a variety of symptoms [4] such as nausea, vomiting, faints, hypotension and palpitation. These could be symptoms of citrate toxicity and associated hypocalcaemia or due to vagal stimulation. They usually respond to skilful symptomatic treatment such as oral or parenteral calcium supplementation or slowing the speed of blood flow into the apheresis device. Unconscious or conscious but ventilated patients should be closely monitored for such symptoms. An important source of morbidity and sometimes mortality in therapeutic apheresis is related to the insertion and care of central venous catheters. These should be inserted and looked after by trained staff [4]. Recirculation of infused and withdrawn fluids at the tip of a dual-lumen catheter can render the procedure of plasma exchange ineffective. This may happen if the lumens are used in reverse or if the catheter is placed in a partially clotted vein.

Using current technologies and in skilful hands, plasma exchange is a relatively safe procedure. Complications are likely to be caused by human errors or staff lacking necessary training. The demand for plasma exchange in the average hospital is sometimes not enough to allow maintenance of staff skills or cost-effective utilization of equipments. A regional model of service delivery, in which services to many hospitals in a region are provided by a single provider, can ensure safer services and may overcome the chronic problem of the lack of robust services in most smaller hospitals or sometimes the lack of out-of-hours services in larger teaching centres.

References

1 Linenberger ML, Price TH. Use of cellular and plasma apheresis in the critically ill patient: part 1: technical and physiological considerations. J Intensive Care Med 2005;20(1):18–27.

2 Brecher ME. Plasma exchange: why we do what we do. J Clin Apher 2002;17:207–11.

3 Szczepiokowski ZM, Winters JL, Bandarenko N et al. Guidelines on the use of therapeutic apheresis in clinical practice-evidence-based approach from the apheresis applications Committee of the American Society for Apheresis. J Clin Apher 2010;25:83–177.

4 Shelat SG. Practical considerations for planning a therapeutic apheresis procedure. Am J Med 2010;123 (9):777–84.

5 Russi G, Marson P. Urgent plasma exchange: how, where and when. Blood Transfus 2011;9:356–61.

6 George JN. How I treat patients with thrombotic thrombocytopenic purpura: 2012. Blood 2010;116:4060–9.

7 Linenberger ML, Price TH. Use of cellular and plasma apheresis in the critically ill patient: part II: clinical indications and applications. J Intensive Care Med 2005;20(2):88–103.

4 SECTION 4

Approach to Red Cell Problems

CHAPTER 17

Appropriate Haemoglobin in Intensive Care

Jonathan Wallis[1] and Stephen Wright[2]

[1] Department of Haematology, Newcastle upon Tyne NHS Acute Hospitals Trust, Newcastle upon Tyne, UK
[2] Department of Perioperative and Critical Care, Freeman Hospital, Newcastle upon Tyne, UK

Introduction

For clinicians working in intensive care unit (ICU), 'what is an appropriate haemoglobin (Hb) concentration for this patient?' is an important and daily question. This chapter will discuss the risks and benefits of anaemia and of transfusion, provide practical advice for those considering blood transfusion in the critically ill, summarize the results of the key transfusion studies and highlight the areas where evidence is lacking.

Background

In the UK, between 8% and 10% of the blood supply is used for patients on the ICU [1]. Some patients are admitted to ICU with anaemia but those who are not commonly develop anaemia during their ICU stay. The aetiology of the anaemia in ICU patients is usually multifactorial (Table 17.1), with ongoing haemorrhage being a relatively uncommon cause. For patients who have a long ICU stay, iatrogenic anaemia from multiple blood sampling can become significant; 40 mL of blood per day is average. Blood transfusion is often used to correct anaemia with around one-third of patients receiving one or more units of red blood cells (RBC) while in the ICU [2, 3].

Anaemia is also common on discharge from ICU – an inevitable consequence of the high prevalence of anaemia

and restrictive transfusion practices in the critically ill. Some patients may recover their Hb concentration before hospital discharge, but in one study, one-third of ICU patients were discharged home with an Hb less than 100 g/L [4]. Little is known about the potential impact of this anaemia on functional recovery, but it is possible that some of the weakness and fatigue common in survivors of critical illness are related to anaemia persisting after discharge from intensive care.

Role of red cells and of transfusion

The primary role of red cells is oxygen delivery to tissues and removal of carbon dioxide. Secondary roles of less certain clinical importance include regulation of haemostasis and microvascular flow through physical flow effects, e.g. endothelial shear stress and forcing platelets to the periphery of small vessels, and through chemical mechanisms such as nitric oxide metabolism and secretion of ATP.

Oxygen delivery to the tissues is mainly controlled by changes in regional and microvascular blood flow. Ischaemia is much more commonly due to hypoperfusion than due to anaemia. However, Hb concentration and oxygen saturation and the HbO_2 dissociation curve are also important, more especially in tissues with higher oxygen demand relative to blood flow. Different tissues extract varying proportions of the oxygen supplied, with (in healthy

Haematology in Critical Care: A Practical Handbook, First Edition. Edited by Jecko Thachil and Quentin A. Hill.
© 2014 John Wiley & Sons, Ltd. Published 2014 by John Wiley & Sons, Ltd.

Table 17.1 Common causes of anaemia in critical illness.

Blood loss	Trauma/surgery
	Occult GI blood loss (e.g. gastric erosions and stress ulceration)
Iatrogenic	Blood tests
	Discarded blood from indwelling venous/arterial catheters
	Clotting of extracorporeal circuits such as continuous haemofiltration
	Haemodilution from intravenous fluid resuscitation
Sepsis and inflammation	Reduced erythropoiesis
	Impaired iron utilization
	Blunted response to erythropoietin
	Reduced red cell survival
Nutritional deficiency	Protein calorie malnutrition/negative nitrogen balance
	Reduced intake of haematinics and micronutrients
Renal impairment	Reduced erythropoietin synthesis

resting subjects) the skin and kidney's extracting less than 10%, the brain about 30% and the heart nearly 60% of delivered oxygen, leaving the heart particularly susceptible to the effects of anaemia. The aim of blood transfusion in the critically ill is largely to maintain adequate oxygen delivery to the tissues and in particular the myocardium.

The efficacy of blood transfusion in reversing the effects of anaemia depends in part on the ability of the transfused cells to bind and release oxygen. During storage, the red cells lose 2,3-DPG with a consequent left shift in the HbO_2 dissociation curve and a lower ability to release oxygen at any given partial pressure of oxygen. This largely recovers by 6 h after transfusion but takes 24 h for full recovery. During storage, the red cells undergo other biochemical, metabolic and structural changes, some of which may never completely recover.

Risks of anaemia and of transfusion

Severe anaemia itself clearly carries some risk, although there are surprisingly few data to tell us how low an Hb concentration is too low. In a cohort of 300 surgical patients who declined blood transfusion for religious reasons, the risk of death was low in patients with post-operative Hb levels of 71–80 g/L, but as post-operative blood counts fell, the morbidity and/or mortality rose and became high with a post-operative Hb below 50 g/L and very high below 30 g/L [5]. The development of anaemia,

as opposed to the anaemia itself, is however likely to be a marker for poor outcome. As transfusion is a widely accepted treatment of anaemia, it is not surprising that there is a great deal of data associating the use of blood transfusion with poor clinical outcomes in the critically ill. In two large cohort studies, the number of RBC units a patient received was independently associated with mortality, and this association remained after allowing for likely confounding variables [2, 3]. A systematic review suggested that RBC transfusions are associated with increased morbidity and mortality in a range of high-risk hospitalized patients, including adult ICU, trauma and surgical patients [6]. In interpreting these studies, two important points need to be remembered: the possibility of residual confounders and bias by indication. Most blood transfusions given in ICU are given for anaemia rather than acute haemorrhage, and whatever the indication, blood transfusion is more likely in sicker patients. Statistical methods can be used to correct for known confounding variables – such as age, APACHE II score or diagnosis – but it is impossible to account for unknown or unmeasured confounding variables. Bias by indication means that the factors that influence the clinical decision to transfuse may also have prognostic importance. This bias can be addressed statistically (using propensity scoring to match patients to a *control*), but the only sure way around these problems is to conduct a prospective randomized trial [7].

The risks associated with RBC transfusion depend on the quality of the product transfused and may vary depending on the age of the red cells and the production method used, including the additive solution used. In the future, we may find a better quality blood product that will change the balance of risks and allow more liberal transfusion. In the meantime, the risks and benefits of transfusion must be considered for each patient bearing in mind the patient's co-morbidities, the degree of anaemia and the clinical condition of the patient.

Transfusion triggers in critical care

Critically ill, non-bleeding patients

In 1999, the TRICC investigators published the results of their multicentre, non-blinded, randomized clinical trial [8]. They found that a restrictive transfusion strategy where Hb concentrations were maintained 70–90 g/L was not inferior to a more liberal strategy of 100–120 g/L.

However, mortality rates were significantly lower in the restrictive transfusion group among patients who were less severely ill (APACHE II score ≤ 20) and among patients who were less than 55 years of age. This study used non-leukcodepleted red cells with significant amounts of plasma, and a harmful effect of transfusion as opposed to a beneficial effect of anaemia seemed probable.

• In stable critically ill patients without ischaemic heart disease, a transfusion trigger of 70 g/L is appropriate for most patients.

Patients with ischaemic heart disease

For patients with stable ischaemic heart disease, the evidence is less clear [9]. A subgroup analysis of the 20% of patients in the TRICC trial with known cardiovascular disease found no difference in outcome between the restrictive and liberal strategies. In particular, there were no significant differences in the rates of cardiac events between groups. The more recent FOCUS study, although in patients with fractured hips rather than the critically ill, provides useful supporting data in this patient group [10]. Using mainly leukcodepleted and plasma-poor red cells, it found no differences in several outcomes between a threshold of 80 and 100 g/L despite only recruiting those with known or likely ischaemic cardiac disease. Together, these studies suggest that moderate anaemia is well tolerated despite cardiac disease, that transfusion may have adverse effects but that the quality of the red cells is important.

• In patients with stable ischaemic heart disease, a transfusion trigger of 70–80 g/L is appropriate.

In patients with an acute coronary syndrome, the risk/benefit may favour a more liberal transfusion to optimize oxygen delivery to the myocardium, although there is no evidence from randomized controlled trials to support this. Observational studies have found anaemia to be associated with mortality after acute myocardial infarction, but these studies are prone to bias as discussed before. As evidence of the lack of certainty, the TRICC investigators urged caution in implementing their restrictive strategy in patients with acute coronary syndromes.

• In patients with an acute coronary syndrome, a transfusion trigger of 80–90 g/L is probably appropriate for most patients.

Critically ill children

The best evidence in children comes from the TRIPICU study, which randomized over 600 critically ill children to either a restrictive (70 g/L) or liberal (95 g/L) transfusion strategy [11]. No differences in the primary end point (new or progressing organs dysfunction) were found.

• In stable, critically ill children, a transfusion trigger of 70 g/L is appropriate.

Resuscitation in severe sepsis and septic shock

In the early resuscitation of a patient with severe sepsis or septic shock, there is some evidence that a more liberal transfusion trigger may be of benefit. A study by Rivers et al. showed improved outcomes in patients resuscitated using an early goal-directed therapy (EGDT) protocol, which included various interventions, such as fluids, inotropes, vasodilators and blood transfusion, aimed at achieving certain physiological goals during the first 6 h of treatment [12]. In the EGDT protocol, patients first received intravenous fluids to restore an adequate circulating volume and inotropic drugs to achieve a mean arterial pressure greater than or equal to 65 mmHg. If the central venous oxygen saturation was then found to be below 70%, patients were transfused to achieve a haematocrit of at least 30%. To be eligible for the study, patients had to have evidence of poor tissue perfusion with either a systolic blood pressure of less than or equal to 90 mmHg or a lactate of greater than or equal to 4 mmol/L; the mean lactate concentration at baseline was actually over 7 mmol/L. While it is difficult to determine which part(s) of the EGDT protocol was most important, it does suggest that blood transfusion to an Hb 90–100 g/L may of benefit in the early resuscitation of patients with severe sepsis or septic shock who have signs of poor tissue perfusion (high lactate or low central venous oxygen saturation) when given alongside fluid resuscitation and inotropic drugs. The results of the single-centre Rivers' study are still to be confirmed by ongoing multicentre randomized controlled trials.

• In patients in the early-phase severe sepsis or septic shock, consider a transfusion trigger of 90 g/L, especially if there are signs of poor tissue perfusion.

Ongoing areas of uncertainty

Since the TRICC trial was published, there have been many changes to the way blood products are processed, most notably the introduction in many countries of universal leukcodepletion. Whether the potentially detrimental effects seen in the TRICC trial would be so apparent now is not clear. Packed red cells can be stored for up to 35 days in the UK (42 days in some countries); during this time, there are marked changes to the RBC including decreased flexibility and loss of shape of the cell membrane and a decrease in 2,3-DPG. There is conflicting observational evidence about the clinical importance of these changes although a large cohort study in cardiac surgical patients showed improved outcomes in patients receiving fresher blood [13]. A prospective, multicentre randomized controlled trial (ABLE study) is currently trying to answer the question whether transfusion of fresh (<1-week-old) RBC compared with standard-issue RBC improves mortality and a range of relevant secondary outcomes.

Erythropoietin has been used in an attempt to improve the Hb level in critically ill patients. The results of a large randomized study showed no significant difference in the need for transfusion or in the number of units of transfused [14]. Treatment with erythropoietin was associated with an increased incidence of thrombosis. Despite this, there was a trend towards a reduced mortality in the treatment group, especially in those with trauma. It is hypothesized that this may be due to the non-erythroid effects of erythropoietin, and while its use in the critically ill will not significantly reduce transfusion requirements, it may find a place for other reasons.

Iron deficiency anaemia and the role of iron supplementation are also an unresolved issue in the critically ill. The interaction between inflammation and the usual

iron indices makes iron deficiency difficult to investigate [15]. The only randomized controlled trial investigating oral iron supplementation in the critically ill showed a reduced transfusion rate in patients receiving iron rather than placebo, but this benefit was only observed in the subgroup with baseline iron deficiency [16]. A small study of intravenous iron replacement found no benefit from intravenous iron in either red cell production (reticulocyte count) or Hb concentration [17].

References

1 Walsh TS, Garrioch M, Maciver C et al. Red cell requirements for intensive care units adhering to evidence-based transfusion guidelines. Transfusion 2004;44:1405–11.
2 Corwin HJ, Gettinger A, Pearl RG et al. The CRIT Study: anemia and blood transfusion in the critically ill – current clinical practice in the United States. Crit Care Med 2004;32:39–52.
3 Vincent JL, Baron JF, Reinhart K et al. Anemia and blood transfusion in critically ill patients. JAMA 2002;288(12):1499–507.
4 Walsh TS, Saleh EE, Lee RJ, MClelland DB. The prevalence and characteristics of anaemia at discharge home after intensive care. Intensive Care Med. 2006;32:1206–13.
5 Carson JL, Noveck H, Berlin JA, Gould SA. Mortality and morbidity in patients with very low postoperative Hb levels who decline blood transfusion. Transfusion. 2002;42:812–8.
6 Marik PE, Corwin HL. Efficacy of red blood cell transfusion in the critically ill: a systematic review of the literature. Crit Care Med. 2008;36:2667–74.
7 Carson JL, Reynolds RC, Klein HG. Bad bad blood? Crit Care Med 2008;36:2707–8.
8 Hébert PC, Wells G, Blajchman MA et al. A multicenter, randomized, controlled clinical trial of transfusion requirements in critical care. Transfusion Requirements in Critical Care Investigators, Canadian Critical Care Trials Group. N Engl J Med. 1999;340:409–17.
9 Geber DR. Transfusion of packed red blood cells in patients with ischemic heart disease. Crit Care Med. 2008;36:1068–74.
10 Carson JL, Terrin ML, Noveck H et al. Liberal or restrictive transfusion in high-risk patients after hip surgery. N Engl J Med. 2011;365:2453–62.
11 Lacroix J, Hébert PC, Hutchison JS. Transfusion strategies for patients in pediatric intensive care units. N Engl J Med. 2007;356:1609–19.
12 Rivers E, Nguyen B, Havstad S et al. Early goal-directed therapy in the treatment of severe sepsis and septic shock. N Engl J Med 2001;345:1368–77.

Box 17.1 Five practical clinical points when considering blood transfusion in ICU

1 Consider the cause of the anaemia, look for signs of bleeding and treat any sign of shock with intravenous fluids initially while waiting for blood.

2 If the Hb is out of keeping with previous results, consider repeating the sample – sampling or labelling errors can lead to false results and unnecessary transfusion.

3 Transfuse 1 U at a time for most top-up transfusions; this should increase the Hb by at least 10 g/L.

4 If unsure of the indication for top-up transfusion, especially when reviewing a stable patient overnight, consider discussion with a senior colleague before prescribing blood.

5 Iatrogenic anaemia is a real problem, particularly for long-stay ICU patients, so consider the need for daily, repeated blood sampling.

13 Koch CG, Li L, Sessler DI et al. Duration of red-cell storage and complications after cardiac surgery. N Engl J Med 2008; 358:1229–39.

14 Corwin HL, Gettinger A, Fabian T et al. Efficacy and safety of epoetin alfa in critically ill patients. N Engl J Med. 2007; 357:965–76.

15 Pieracci FM, Barie PS. Diagnosis and management of iron-related anemias in critical illness. Crit Care Med. 2006;34: 1898–905.

16 Pieracci FM, Henderson P, Rodney JR et al. Randomized, double-blind, placebo-controlled trial of effects of enteral iron supplementation on anemia and risk of infection during surgical critical illness. Surg Infect (Larchmt). 2009;10(1): 9–19.

17 van Iperen CE, Gaillard CA, Kraaijenhagen RJ et al. Response of erythropoiesis and iron metabolism to recombinant human erythropoietin in intensive care unit patients. Crit Care Med. 2000;28:2773–8.

18

CHAPTER 18

Sickle Cell Disease and Thalassaemia in the Critical Care Setting

Andrew Retter[1,2] and Jo Howard[1]

[1] Department of Haematology, Guy's and St Thomas' NHS Foundation Trust, London, UK
[2] Intensive Care Department, Guy's and St Thomas' NHS Foundation Trust, London, UK

Introduction

Sickle cell disease (SCD) and thalassaemia are both inherited disorders of haemoglobin (Hb) associated with considerable morbidity and mortality. Patients with both conditions can present to critical care in a number of different ways. These fall into three distinct categories:

1 An acute complication of their underlying haemoglobinopathy requiring organ support
2 An unplanned admission for an illness unrelated to their underlying haemoglobinopathy
3 A planned admission for post-operative care

This chapter will describe the acute and chronic complications of both conditions that may result in admission or complicate an admission to the critical care unit. The perioperative care of patients with SCD will also be discussed.

Sickle cell disease

Sickle cell disease is the most common inherited disorder worldwide, and there are approximately 12–15,000 affected individuals in the UK. It is an autosomal recessive condition, and patients with homozygous SCD (HbSS) have a severe disease phenotype. The carrier form (sickle trait, HbAS) is in essence an asymptomatic condition. The sickle Hb gene can be also inherited with HbC, β-thalassaemia, HbO-Arab, HbD or HbE, causing the compound heterozygote conditions HbSC, HbS β-thalassaemia and so forth. These tend to be associated with a more moderate phenotype.

The abnormal haemoglobin S (HbS) arises from a point mutation in the β-globin gene. HbS has decreased solubility and increased viscosity compared to HbA, with a tendency to form polymers, which is increased by hypoxia. The formation of Hb polymers irreversibly distorts the cell, disrupting its membrane and producing the classical sickle cell shape on a blood film. These *distorted* cells break down more rapidly, leading to anaemia. They can also become trapped in the microvasculature and cause downstream ischaemia.

Diagnosis of SCD

In the majority of situations, patients will be aware of their diagnosis. Occasionally, the first presentation will be with an acute complication requiring critical care, or a patient may be admitted acutely unwell and unable to inform the medical team of their diagnosis. A suspicion of SCD may arise because of the clinical picture, and patients will usually have an Hb of 60–90 g/dL, although this can be higher in HbSC disease. There is a reticulocytosis, although the reticulocyte count can be low in some situations such as aplastic crisis due to parvovirus B19 infection. The blood film shows marked variation in red

Haematology in Critical Care: A Practical Handbook, First Edition. Edited by Jecko Thachil and Quentin A. Hill.
© 2014 John Wiley & Sons, Ltd. Published 2014 by John Wiley & Sons, Ltd.

cell size with sickle cells and target cells; basophilic stippling is frequently seen in conjunction with Howell–Jolly bodies. A positive sickle solubility test indicates the presence of HbS but cannot differentiate between sickle cell trait and homozygous disease. However, the combination of positive solubility test and a consistent blood film allows a rapid diagnosis to be made. The diagnosis should be confirmed, promptly, with a definitive laboratory test such as high-performance liquid chromatography.

Clinical manifestations of sickle cell anaemia

The dominant clinical feature of SCD is a chronic haemolytic anaemia with repeated episodic acute painful crises due to vaso-occlusion. SCD is also associated with multi-organ acute and chronic complications. The clinical features of SCD are summarized in Table 18.1. Despite our understanding of the precise genetic aberration, there

is profound variability in the clinical severity of SCD. Some patients live an almost normal life, free of significant problems; others develop severe crises from a very young age or have life-threatening disease complications. The life expectancy of patients with SCD is reduced but is increasing due to the improvement in supportive therapies, notably regular antibiotic prophylaxis, primary stroke screening in children, increased use of hydroxy-carbamide or transfusion and improved specialist care.

The complications most likely to require critical care admission are acute chest syndrome (ACS), acute stroke and acute renal injury.

General principles of management of SCD

The management of crises is supportive unless there are specific indications for blood transfusion. The aim of treatment is to interrupt the downward spiral of sickling,

Table 18.1 Clinical features of sickle cell disease (SCD).

Complication	Features
Painful crisis	Occurs in the majority (but not all) of patients with SCD, marked variability in the frequency and severity of symptoms
	May evolve into a chronic pain syndrome
Neurological	Subclinical microvascular occlusion may be seen on MRI in a substantial proportion of patients. May progress to cause cognitive impairment
	Stroke occurs in 10% of children; it is a leading cause of morbidity and mortality
	Can be prevented by regular red cell transfusion
Pulmonary	
Acute chest syndrome	Leading cause of mortality in adults, high risk of acute respiratory failure
Asthma	There is an established association between SCD and increased airway reactivity
Fibrotic lung disease	Difficult and rare complication of SCD, no direct treatment strategies
Gastrointestinal	
Cholelithiasis	The majority of patients have gallstones secondary to the increased haemolysis
Hepatopathy	Rare complication of SCD, which can progress to decompensated liver disease
Renal	Chronic renal failure develops in up to 20% of patients
Urological	Priapism can be devastating in men and lead to long-term sexual dysfunction
Ophthalmology	Proliferative retinopathy is particularly common in patients with HbSC disease
Orthopaedic	
Avascular necrosis	Frequent complication particularly of the hip and shoulders, may require replacement
Osteomyelitis	Salmonella is the most common organism, can be particularly difficult to treat
Haematological	
Haemolytic anaemia	Chronic haemolysis, usual Hb 60–90 g/L, higher in HbSC
Aplastic crisis	Parvovirus B19 infection may trigger red cell aplasia. The combination of impaired red cell production and increased red cell turnover can be fatal
Splenic sequestration	Typically seen in infants with a rapidly enlarging spleen → fluid resuscitation and cautious transfusion

dehydration, hypoxia and acidosis, which precipitates further sickling. Pain is the most common feature. Opiate-naïve patients should be treated as per the World Health Organization analgesic ladder, but subcutaneous morphine or an alternative strong opiate is usually required for the treatment of severe pain. Pethidine should be avoided due to its ability to increase the risk of grand mal seizures. Analgesia should be given within 30 min of presentation, and its efficacy assessed every 15–30 min. Patient-controlled analgesia (PCA) devices are an effective way of achieving good pain control and recommended in national guidelines. Adequate fluid intake is essential.

The acute chest syndrome

Acute chest syndrome is defined as an acute illness with fever and/or respiratory symptoms in the presence of a new pulmonary infiltrate. It is the leading cause of mortality in adults with SCD and the most common cause of critical care admission. ACS requiring mechanical ventilation is reported to have a mortality of 5% [1]. Symptoms include cough, wheeze, shortness of breath and chest pain, which may be pleuritic or affect the ribs and sternum [2]. The differential diagnosis is pneumonia, and while ACS is often associated with an infective aetiology, ACS is unique to SCD and is associated with a more severe course and worse outcome than pneumonia. Hypoxia is not included in the definition but is a useful predictor of severity and may precede clinical or X-ray signs of chest consolidation. Some patients are admitted with the clinical features of ACS, but in the majority of cases, it will develop while in hospital. Untreated ACS can progress rapidly, within hours, to acute respiratory distress syndrome and on occasion to acute multi-organ failure. Therefore, all patients admitted with a painful crisis should be monitored regularly for the development of this complication with frequent pulse oximetry and chest examination.

Any of the features of hypoxia should raise the suspicion of ACS, and treatment with oxygen, intravenous fluids, pain relief and antimicrobials should be commenced. Bronchodilators and steroids should be considered in patients with asthma or evidence of wheeze. Incentive spirometry has been shown to reduce the risk of ACS in children with chest pain [3] and is useful in the management of patients with ACS. Blood transfusion is an effective treatment in ACS and will improve oxygenation. Early top-up transfusion is effective in less severe cases when there is a low Hb (<70 g/L), but an exchange transfusion will be required in deteriorating patients, those with high Hb levels or those with marked hypoxia. Transfusions in this situation should be managed by the haematologists. The target is a final Hb level of 90–100 g/L and percentage of HbS (HbS%) of under 30%.

Worsening hypoxia, severe dyspnoea and increasing hypercarbia causing a respiratory acidosis are indications for initiating advanced respiratory supportive therapies. Risk factors for progression of ACS include a platelet count greater than 200×10^9/L, extensive pulmonary consolidation on chest radiograph and co-existing respiratory disease. Patients with risk factors, or those in whom blood might not be readily available, should be considered for early intervention with advanced respiratory support. Non-invasive ventilation (NIV) may reduce the need for intubation and mechanical ventilation. Increasing mean airway pressure recruits the collapsed lung, improving the functional residual capacity and improving lung compliance. Together, these measures reduce the work of breathing and increase PaO_2. Deteriorating respiratory failure despite maximal NIV support requires endotracheal intubation and ventilation. Standard lung protective ventilation should be adopted. The majority of patients can be managed with conventional ventilation. There are occasional case reports of the use of high-frequency oscillatory ventilation and extracorporeal membrane oxygenation. These measures may be appropriate in centres with sufficient expertise.

Stroke

Ischaemic and haemorrhagic stroke are common in SCD, with a prevalence of greater than 5% [4]. The incidence of stroke in children with SCD has decreased following the introduction of transcranial Doppler screening and primary stroke prevention with transfusion, but it can still occur at any age. A stroke may be precipitated by an intercurrent illness or dehydration. It presents with symptoms and signs similar to patients without SCD. Early imaging is essential to confirm the diagnosis and exclude haemorrhage. MRI is the modality of choice with greatest sensitivity and specificity. If the scan confirms a stroke, the patient should proceed to an immediate exchange transfusion to achieve an HbS less than 30%. If there is strong clinical suspicion and the scan is delayed, the exchange transfusion should commence. In young patients, exchange transfusion rather than thrombolysis is the treatment of choice. In older patients (>50 years), the role of thrombolysis should be discussed with the stroke and haematology teams. Its use will depend on whether stroke aetiology is thought to be primarily due to sickle cell or cerebrovascular disease. Secondary prevention of ischaemic stroke is achieved by long-term exchange transfusion therapy, and there is little evidence for the efficacy of anti-platelet therapy in primary or secondary stroke prevention in SCD.

Sepsis

Patients with SCD are functionally asplenic rendering them at greater risk of infection from encapsulated organisms. Osteomyelitis and Gram-negative sepsis are particular problems. All patients should receive vaccination against *Neisseria meningitidis*, *Haemophilus influenzae* and *Streptococcus pneumoniae*. Daily penicillin V prophylaxis has been shown to be beneficial in preventing pneumococcal infections in children [5] and should be commenced at diagnosis. Adherence to therapy is seldom complete, and therefore, these organisms should always be considered in patients with SCD and acute sepsis.

Other complications of SCD

The kidneys are affected even in children with SCD who have decreased renal concentrating ability and are hence prone to dehydration. Over the longer term, patients can develop proteinuria and chronic renal impairment due to glomerular damage. This leaves patients increasingly vulnerable to acute kidney injury during a crisis, and this may precipitate or complicate critical care admissions. Chronic lung disease is common and manifests as either a restrictive lung defect or an overnight hypoxia and sleep apnoea. Pulmonary hypertension is more common in SCD and can lead to marked hypoxia.

Admission to critical care unit with illness unrelated to the SCD

Patients may be admitted to the ICU with an illness unrelated to their SCD. It is essential that clinicians do not presume that all presentations in patients with SCD are due to their chronic disease and keep an open mind to other co-existing conditions. Patients occasionally present with overwhelming sepsis, fulminant hepatic failure and/or multi-organ failure with unknown aetiology. It may be difficult to ascertain the cause of this acute deterioration, whether it is due to SCD or non-SCD pathology, and urgent transfusion should be discussed with the haematologist as transfusion aiming for an Hb of 90–100 g/L and HbS% of less than 30% will improve tissue oxygenation and perfusion, whatever the underlying aetiology.

Transfusion in SCD patients in ICU

Transfusion should always be undertaken with caution in patients with SCD because of the risk of serious side effects, in particular alloimmunization. The incidence of alloimmunization to red cell antigens is around 20% in SCD [6]. Once a patient has developed alloantibodies, there is a propensity to develop further antibodies with subsequent transfusions. This can make it difficult to provide phenotypically crossmatched blood for future transfusions. An extended red cell phenotype should be determined in all patients with SCD, ideally to the Kell, Duffy, Kid, Lewis, Lutheran, P and MNS groups. Blood should be crossmatch compatible to the ABO, C, D, E and Kell antigens, plus any known antibodies. This has been shown to reduce the incidence of developing alloantibodies.

Alloantibody formation is associated with delayed haemolytic transfusion reactions. These typically occur 7–10 days following a transfusion and are characterized by increasing anaemia, jaundice and haemoglobinuria. They may be associated with severe pain and are often misdiagnosed as vaso-occlusive crises. Usually, the direct antiglobulin test (DAT) is positive, there is a reticulocytosis and a new alloantibody is identified, but sometimes none of these features are present, which makes the diagnosis difficult. Diagnosis is helped by measurement of the HbS and HbA%; after a transfusion, there should be HbA present (amount depending on amount of blood transfused) for up to 3 months, but where there is brisk haemolysis of transfused units, the HbA will decrease and even disappear within a few days. In some cases, the patient's own blood, as well as the transfused blood, can be haemolysed. This is known as hyperhaemolysis and is characterized by the baseline Hb level falling below the pre-transfusion level and, often, reticulocytopenia. This may be exacerbated by further transfusion and should be treated with steroids, intravenous immunoglobulin and erythropoietin [7]. The use of rituximab has been reported in severe cases. Transfusion should be reserved for very severe or life-threatening anaemia and should be given cautiously with simultaneous immunosuppression. These patients will often require treatment in the critical care unit.

When used appropriately, transfusion can be life-saving and prevent progressive organ damage in patients with SCD. Red cells can be given as a simple *top-up* or as an exchange. The target Hb post transfusion should be 90–100 g/L. Higher levels can cause hyperviscosity and risk exacerbating a crisis. Below 60 g/L, a *top-up* transfusion should be used in preference to exchange transfusion. However, when the starting Hb is greater than 90 g/L, an exchange transfusion should be used to alter the HbS%. The abnormal sickle cells are removed and replaced with normal RBCs containing HbA. Approximately 8 U of blood are required to exchange in an adult. The target exchange HbS% after an exchange is less than 30%. The procedure is performed most effectively through a large-calibre central venous line.

Preparation for general anaesthesia and post-operative care

A recent international, multicentre study compared peri-operative complications among patients with SCD (HbSS and HbS β-thalassaemia) undergoing moderate and low-risk surgery. Patients were randomized to receive either best supportive care or pre-operative transfusion with supportive care. In the intervention arm, patients received either a *top-up* if their Hb was less than 90 g/dL or a red cell exchange if Hb was greater than 90 g/dL. There was an increased incidence of serious adverse events in the group randomized not to receive transfusion; 30.3% developed a significant complication compared to 2.9% in the control group [8]. It is now our practice that all patients with HbSS and HbS β-thalassaemia receive

transfusion (as per the study protocol) prior to surgery. The role of pre-operative transfusion in other sickle genotypes is less clear, but patients undergoing moderate and major surgery should probably receive pre-operative transfusion. Patients should have good hydration maintained throughout surgery. It should be remembered that they are at higher risk of infective and thromboembolic complications and will need appropriate prophylaxis.

Patients with thalassaemia in the critical care setting

Patients with β-thalassaemia major are transfusion dependent from an early age but with effective red cell transfusion and iron chelation therapy can be kept free from the majority of complications. If admitted to the critical care unit, they may need additional transfusion support. Their usual transfusion target is 95–100 g/L, which suppresses underlying ineffective erythropoiesis, and this threshold should be used in critical care, not the more common threshold of 70–80 g/L. Patients with thalassaemia may have had a splenectomy to reduce their transfusion requirements. Careful attention should be paid to hyposplenic patients due to the increased risk overwhelming sepsis. *Yersinia* infections may occur in iron-loaded patients, and if a thalassaemic patient is admitted with diarrhoea or gastrointestinal upset, *Yersinia* infection should be actively sought and pre-emptively treated. Other bacteria such as *Klebsiella* species, *E. coli* and *Pseudomonas* also become more pathogenic in an iron-rich environment. Iron overload can be a significant problem in transfusion-dependent patients if compliance with iron chelation has been suboptimal. Cardiac iron overload can lead to cardiac failure and is associated with arrhythmias. Cardiac complications should be treated with standard treatment, but iron overload should be treated aggressively with continuous intravenous desferrioxamine [9]. A raised ferritin level will usually be diagnostic of iron overload but can be falsely high as it is an acute phase reactant or falsely low in someone who has recently started chelating. Cardiac T2* MRI is the gold standard method to determine cardiac iron load.

Patients with thalassaemia intermedia usually run an Hb level of 60–90 g/L and are not transfusion dependent. In a situation requiring critical care, they may be more anaemic than usual and require transfusion.

References

1 Vichinsky EP, Neumayr LD, Earles AN et al. Causes and outcomes of the acute chest syndrome in sickle cell disease. National Acute Chest Syndrome Study Group. N Engl J Med 2000;342(25):1855–65.

2 Ballas SK, Lieff S, Benjamin LJ et al. Definitions of the phenotypic manifestations of sickle cell disease. Am J Hematol 2010;85:6–13.

3 Bellet PS, Kalinyak KA, Shukla R, Gelfand MJ, Rucknagel DL. Incentive spirometry to prevent acute pulmonary complications in sickle cell diseases. N Engl J Med 1995;333: 699–703.

4 Ohene-Frempong K, Weiner SJ, Sleeper LA et al. Cerebrovascular accidents in SCD: rates and risk factors. Blood 1998;91:288–94.

5 Gaston MH, Verter JI. Woods G et al. Prophylaxis with oral penicillin in children with sickle cell anemia. A randomized trial. N Engl J Med 1986;314(25):1593–9.

6 Rosse WF, Gallagher D, Kinney TR et al. Transfusion and alloimmunization in sickle cell disease. The Cooperative Study of Sickle Cell Disease. Blood 1990;76(7):1431–7.

7 de Montalembert M, Dumont MD, Heilbronner C et al. Delayed haemolytic transfusion reactions in children with sickle cell disease. Haematologica 2011;96:801–17.

8 Howard J, Malfroy M, Llewelyn C et al. The Transfusion Alternatives Preoperatively in Sickle Cell Disease (TAPS) study: a randomised, controlled, multicentre clinical trial. Lancet 2013;381:930–8.

9 Davis BA, Porter JB. Long-term outcome of continuous 24-hour deferoxamine infusion via indwelling intravenous catheters in high-risk beta-thalassaemia. Blood 2000;95(4):1229–36.

CHAPTER 19

Management of Patients Who Refuse Blood Transfusion

Derek R. Norfolk[1] and Fran Hartley[2]

[1] NHS Blood and Transplant, Leeds Teaching Hospitals NHS Trust, Leeds, UK
[2] Hospital Transfusion Team, Leeds Teaching Hospitals NHS Trust, Leeds, UK

More than half of all patients admitted to critical care are anaemic (haemoglobin (Hb) <130 g/L), and up to 30% of these have an initial Hb concentration less than 90 g/L [1]. After 1 week, the Hb of 80% of patients is below 90 g/L. Depending on case mix, the typical patient without major haemorrhage receives 2–4 U of red blood cells during their stay in the intensive care unit. Consequently, management of the critically ill patient who refuses potentially life-saving blood component therapy presents significant ethical and clinical challenges to the healthcare team.

Who refuses transfusion and why?

Patients refuse blood transfusion for many reasons, ranging from religious principles to anxiety about potential risks and reactions. The patient, or their family members, may have falsely raised perceptions of the risks of transfusion, such as HIV, hepatitis or variant CJD, based on media reporting or anecdotal experience. In this instance, sympathetic discussion with a well-informed clinician (doctor, nurse or transfusion practitioner) is often successful in allaying concerns (risks of transfusion transmitted infection and their frequency are detailed in Chapter 13). In the UK, the national blood transfusion services provide a range of useful information resources for patients and their families [2], and many hospitals have written policies to support staff in this process. Ultimately, the autonomy of

competent patients must be respected however much the clinician may disagree with their decision.

Jehovah's Witnesses, the most frequent group refusing transfusion, base their decision on strict interpretation of the biblical texts: 'the life of all flesh is the blood thereof: whoever eat it shall be cut off' (Lev. 17:10–16) and 'abstain from the meats offered to idols and from blood' (Acts 15:28–29) (1–3). Most Jehovah's Witnesses refuse the transfusion of *whole blood* and its *primary components* (red cells, platelets, white cells and whole plasma), including preoperative autologous donation, but there are areas of individual choice. *Derivatives* of primary blood components such as cryoprecipitate, coagulation factor concentrates, albumin and intravenous immunoglobulin are acceptable to most Jehovah's Witnesses. There is usually no objection to extracorporeal techniques, such as intra-operative cell salvage (ICS), apheresis, haemodialysis, cardiac bypass or haemodilution, providing equipment is primed with non-blood fluids. Witnesses, like all patients, seek the most effective treatments *within the restrictions of their religious prohibitions* and have no objection to the use of recombinant haemopoietic stimulating agents such as erythropoietin or G-CSF, procoagulants such as recombinant activated factor VII (rFVIIa, NovoSeven™) or other pharmacological supportive therapies such as intravenous iron. Many Jehovah's Witnesses carry a signed and witnessed *Advance Decision Document* (or *living will*) indicating which transfusion modalities they will, or will not, accept, but it is essential, wherever possible, to have a free and frank discussion

Haematology in Critical Care: A Practical Handbook, First Edition. Edited by Jecko Thachil and Quentin A. Hill.

about the risks and benefits of their chosen course of action. Ideally, this should be with the patient alone (if competent) to avoid any possibility of coercion. Where time allows, both the patient and staff may find it helpful to involve the local Hospital Liaison Committee for Jehovah's Witnesses (contact details may be in the hospital's policy document but there is a central UK Coordinating Office – tel 02089062211 (24 h); his@uk.jw.org).

Consent for blood transfusion

Consent is the agreement by a *competent* patient for a health professional to provide care. Helpful guidance has been provided by bodies such as the UK General Medical Council and, in relation to blood transfusion, the Advisory Committee on the Safety of Blood, Tissues and Organs (SaBTO) [3]. Following extensive consultation with professionals and patients, SaBTO endorsed the GMC standards for consent, emphasizing the importance of providing standardized patient information (including alternatives to transfusion), recording the consent process in the clinical record and providing retrospective information about transfusion to patients who were unable to consent at the time urgent transfusion was needed. *Valid* consent implies that the patient has received sufficient information to make an informed decision, including the decision to decline treatment, and is not acting under duress. Patients vary in the extent of information they wish to receive, and clinical judgement is important, but the presumption should be that the patient wishes to be well informed. The discussions and consent, or otherwise, should be clearly documented in the patient record.

A detailed discussion of the legal basis of *consent* and *mental capacity* is outside the scope of this chapter, and it should be noted that the legal position differs slightly in the UK Devolved Authorities. In England and Wales, the Mental Capacity Act (2005) states 'that an adult (aged 16 or over) has full legal capacity to make decisions for themselves (the right to autonomy) unless it can be shown that they lack capacity to make a decision for themselves at the time the decision needs to be made'. Importantly, 'a person is not to be treated as unable to make a decision merely because he makes an unwise decision'. No one can give consent on behalf of an individual with mental capacity. The accompanying Code of Practice [4] details the *decision-specific tests* needed to assess mental capacity

and the individuals and bodies that can become the incapacitated patient's *best interests decision-maker*.

If a patient with mental capacity declines transfusion after appropriate discussion and advice, this decision must be respected. If a patient has a valid signed and witnessed Advance Decision Document, a copy should be lodged in the patient record, clinical staff made aware of this and the specific limitations on treatment made clear to all members of the team.

In the critical care setting, patients often present with *temporary incapacity* due to the severity of their illness, alteration of conscious state or the effects of essential treatment (e.g. sedation for mechanical ventilation). In this situation, the clinician must act in the *best interests* of the patient and give life-saving treatment, including urgent blood transfusion, unless there is unequivocal evidence of refusal such as a valid Advance Decision Document. If family members or friends state that the patient previously expressed a wish to avoid transfusion, they should be invited to provide documentary evidence, but, in the meantime, necessary resuscitation measures should not be withheld. Where doubt exists, it is better to act to save life, but it is essential to record (dated and signed) the discussions and clinical indications for treatment in the medical notes, preferably witnessed by a colleague. If the patient later regains capacity and refuses further transfusion or an Advance Decision Document is produced, then the wishes of the patient (or their legal *best interests representative*) must be followed.

In the case of children under 16 whose parents or legal guardians refuse transfusions (or other interventions) that, in the opinion of the treating clinician, are life-saving or essential for the well-being of the child, a *Specific Issue Order* can be rapidly obtained from a court. All hospitals should have clear policies that describe the mechanism for carrying out this process without delay, 24 h a day. It is important to seek parental consent wherever possible, and the process must be clearly documented in the clinical record.

Strategies to manage anaemia without blood transfusion

The multiple, and interacting, causes of anaemia in critical care patients are listed in Table 17.1, and the major treatment strategies, in the absence of blood transfusion, are shown in Table 19.1. Anaemia at the time of, or soon

| Preventing/reducing haemorrhage | Secure local haemostasis:
   Surgery
   Interventional radiology
Maintain normovolaemia in acute haemorrhage:
   Crystalloid or colloidal plasma expanders
Cell salvage and autologous reinfusion of red cells
Administer high-concentration oxygen
Maintain normothermia and prevent acidosis
Antifibrinolytic drugs (tranexamic acid)
Coagulation factor concentrates
Desmopressin
Recombinant activated factor VII (rFVIIa) |
| Preventing anaemia/ stimulation of haemopoiesis | Reduce *iatrogenic* blood loss:
   Essential diagnostic blood sampling only
   Small volume sample tubes
   Reduce loss of discard blood from indwelling catheters
   Point of care analysis
Ensure adequate haematinics:
   Folic acid +/– B12
   Iron – if on erythropoiesis-stimulating agent
   Enteral/parenteral nutrition and micronutrients
Haemopoietic stimulating agents:
   Erythropoiesis-stimulating agents (such as erythropoietin)
   Recombinant granulocyte colony-stimulating factor (G-CSF) – in
   rare cases where granulocyte transfusion would be considered |

Table 19.1 Strategies to manage anaemia in critical care without blood transfusion.

after, admission to critical care is predominantly due to bleeding, haemodilution and blood sampling, whereas impaired red cell production due to inflammation predominates later in the course. In practice, most transfusions are given for anaemia rather than bleeding. Successful management of the patient refusing transfusion depends on multidisciplinary input from critical care, surgical, haematological, transfusion medicine and laboratory specialists and the development of a clear treatment plan utilizing the blood conservation modalities and transfusion alternatives discussed in the succeeding text. The acceptability of treatments such as cell salvage and derivative blood products should be established as early as possible.

Although the degree of anaemia is a key factor in predicting survival without transfusion, the absolute need for red cell support to ensure adequate oxygen delivery to critical organs varies with age, cardiopulmonary reserve, co-morbidities and the rate and volume of haemorrhage. Current expert consensus, heavily influenced by the North American TRICC trial in adults [5] (later replicated in paediatric and neonatal critical care), favours a restrictive approach to transfusion in most patients with a *transfusion trigger* around 70 g/L (see Chapter 17). An extensive litera-

ture demonstrates the ability of Jehovah's Witness patients to survive severe anaemia associated with surgical or medical conditions and has provided useful information on which to underpin general transfusion guidelines. A review of 4722 medical or surgical patients who refused transfusion with Hb less than 80 g/L [6] found that mortality increased significantly when the Hb fell below 50 g/L (23 of the 50 deaths attributed to anaemia), although 25 patients survived a fall below this concentration, some down to 14 g/L. The experience of *bloodless surgery* institutions has also contributed to our knowledge in this field.

Preventing or reducing haemorrhage

In severe haemorrhage after trauma or surgery, direct control of bleeding by surgery or interventional radiology is a priority [7]. Patients with surgical, obstetric or traumatic blood loss should be offered intra-operative red cell salvage or post-operative reinfusion of blood where appropriate. Ensuring normothermia and preventing acidosis promote normal haemostatic function, and administration of high-concentration inspired oxygen contributes to tissue oxygenation even in severe anaemia. Preventing shock by the administration of crystalloid and/or colloidal plasma expanders helps maintain critical organ function (but accelerates the fall in concentration of circulating red cells, platelets and coagulation factors by dilution).

The CRASH-2 study provides high-level evidence of the survival benefit and safety of the antifibrinolytic drug, tranexamic acid (a synthetic lysine derivative), administered early in the course of major traumatic haemorrhage [8]. This, together with lower-level evidence that tranexamic acid reduces transfusion requirements in cardiac and orthopaedic surgery without increasing thromboembolic complications, suggests a wider role in reducing blood loss in the critical care setting. The dose of tranexamic acid used in CRASH-2 was a loading dose of 1 g over 10 min followed by infusion of 1 g over 8 h, based on evidence that doses of this magnitude are sufficient to inhibit fibrinolysis and larger doses produce no additional haemostatic benefit. There are no high-quality randomized controlled trials of tranexamic acid in critical care patients, but the manufacturer recommends 15 mg/kg by slow intravenous injection every 6–8 h for the treatment of *general fibrinolysis*. The dose must be reduced in patients with renal impairment (see Summary of Product Characteristics on http://www.mhra.gov.uk/home/groups/spcpil/documents/spcpil/con1369117492211.pdf), but no adjustment is required because of hepatic impairment.

Treatment of a coagulopathy will depend on the underlying cause. Anticoagulant drugs should be stopped, and vitamin K +/− prothrombin complex concentrate (PCC) can be given to patients with an elevated prothrombin time secondary to liver disease or vitamin K deficiency. Disseminated intravascular coagulation (DIC) is a common complication of critical illness, especially in the presence of trauma or sepsis. Coagulation factor support is only indicated in the presence of bleeding and should not be used simply to *correct* abnormal laboratory tests. Most Jehovah's Witnesses will accept transfusion of cryoprecipitate (as a source of fibrinogen), fibrinogen concentrate or PCC but not fresh frozen plasma.

Treatment with desmopressin (a vasopressin analogue) or rFVIIa (NovoSeven™) is not recommended for routine use. Desmopressin releases factor VIIIc and von Willebrand factor from endothelial cells and may reduce bleeding in patients with renal failure and platelet dysfunction. However, these coagulation factors are *acute phase reactants*, levels are already high in most critical care patients and there are no studies showing benefit in the critical care setting. rFVIIa generates thrombin at the sites of tissue factor exposure and is widely used *off-licence* for major haemorrhage, often as a *last ditch* therapy, and may be considered for massive, nonsurgical bleeding (see Chapter 28). However, numerous studies show no evidence that it reduces mortality; it is very expensive and carries a significant risk of thromboembolic complications [9]. The widespread tissue/vascular damage or DIC commonly seen in critical care patients may increase the risk of thrombotic problems.

Preventing anaemia

Diagnostic blood sampling is a significant factor in most patients, typically 30–70 mL a day [1]. This can be reduced by limiting blood tests to an essential minimum, the use of small volume (paediatric) sample tubes by arrangement with the laboratory and reducing losses from *discard* blood when sampling from indwelling vascular catheters. Closed systems for sampling from venous or arterial lines, with reinfusion of sterile blood, are available and have been shown to reduce the need for red cell transfusion in small studies. Appropriate point-of-care testing, using low volume or *capillary* samples, will also reduce iatrogenic losses.

Although the *anaemia of critical care* is largely due to inflammatory suppression of normal erythropoiesis, it is important to ensure an adequate supply of haematinics, such as folate and vitamin B12, and micronutrients as part of general nutritional support. Iron administration alone does not improve the anaemia, because of impaired utilization, and may be associated with increased susceptibility to infection. In the absence of unequivocal evidence of iron deficiency, its use should probably be confined to co-administration with erythropoiesis stimulating agents (ESA). Patients who refuse blood transfusion may have been electively treated with ESA and iron pre-operatively for surgical procedures with a high risk of peri-operative anaemia. Critical care patients have a subnormal erythropoietin response to anaemia, and studies suggest that the combination of an ESA, such as recombinant human erythropoietin (rHuEpo), and iron supplements can modestly reduce transfusion requirements in the critical care setting, albeit with a possible increase in thromboembolic complications and no reduction in mortality. The large randomized placebo-controlled trial of 1460 critical care patients reported by Corwin et al. [10] used rHuEpo alfa 40,000 IU once weekly and showed a significant improvement in Hb at day 29 but with no reduction in transfusion using a restrictive transfusion trigger. Reports of ESA treatment in patients refusing transfusion are anecdotal, and they are not licensed for this indication. However, many experts recommend their use in this setting as the risk/benefit ratio is likely to be more favourable. Reported regimens vary considerably and tend to be based on those licensed for treatment of anaemia in renal dialysis patients or to support pre-operative autologous blood donation for surgery. In the absence of evidence-based guidelines, the selection and dose of an ESA should be determined in conjunction with a haematologist, and treatment should be carefully monitored with a *target* of no more than Hb 100 g/L (haematocrit 30%) to reduce the risk of thromboembolic complications. Evidence from patients with chronic kidney disease suggests that co-administration of iron with an ESA is essential to prevent *functional iron deficiency* and accommodates the stimulus to rapid erythropoiesis. Oral iron is poorly effective in this setting, and modern intravenous iron preparations with a low risk of serious allergic reactions, such as iron sucrose, are appropriate and convenient. The optimum dose and frequency of administration of intravenous iron is unknown, but recommended doses include 100 mg elemental iron once to three times weekly during ESA therapy.

Potential future options

Red cell substitutes, such as cell-free Hb solutions or perfluorocarbons, have so far failed to translate from research into clinical practice. Problems include short intravascular half-life and, in the case of Hb solutions, increased risk of myocardial infarction and stroke related to their ability to scavenge nitric oxide and reduce microvascular flow. In the UK, there are currently no compounds licensed for this indication.

Jehovah's Witnesses developing severe bone marrow failure or acute leukaemia have a high risk of early death from thrombocytopenia or anaemia following intensive chemotherapy. First-generation recombinant human thrombopoietic growth factors (rHuTPO) failed to shorten the time to platelet recovery following chemotherapy, but the second-generation TPO-mimetic eltrombopag has a different mechanism of action and further trials are needed.

Conclusion

Successful management of the critical care patient who declines transfusion is challenging to the clinical team, but the decisions of a patient with mental capacity must

be respected. Although mortality is higher, patients can survive severe anaemia, and supportive care is focused on the management and prevention of haemorrhage, reduction of iatrogenic blood loss and stimulation of erythropoiesis.

References

1 Walsh TS, Lee RJ, McIver CR et al. Anaemia during and at discharge from intensive care: the impact of restrictive blood transfusion practice. Intensive Care Med 2006;32:100–9.

2 NHS Blood and Transplant: *Will I need a blood transfusion?* Updated July 2011 (available in 6 languages). http://hospital. blood.co.uk/library/pdf/2011_Will_I_Need_English_v3.pdf (accessed on November 21, 2013). Scottish National Blood Transfusion Service: *Receiving a transfusion: Information for patients and relatives.* Version 6, November 2010. http://www. scotblood.co.uk/media/11442/receiving_a_transfusion_ v2_9738_15.12.10_lr_rgb_2_.pdf (accessed on November 21, 2013).

3 Advisory Committee on the Safety of Blood, Tissues and Organs. Consent for blood transfusion. October 2011. http:// www.dh.gov.uk/prod_consum_dh/groups/dh_digitalas-sets/@dh/@ab/documents/digitalasset/dh_130715.pdf (accessed on November 21, 2013).

4 Mental Capacity Act. Code of Practice (issued 2007). 2005. http://webarchive.nationalarchives.gov.uk/; http://www.dca. gov.uk/legal-policy/mental-capacity/mca-cp.pdf (accessed on November 21, 2013).

5 Hebert PC, Wells G, Blajchmann MA et al. A multicentre, randomized, controlled clinical trial of transfusion requirements in critical care. Transfusion Requirements in Critical Care Investigators, Canadian Critical Care Trials Group. New Engl J Med 1999;340:409–17.

6 Viele MK, Weiskopf RB. What can we learn about the need for transfusion from patients who refuse blood? The experience with Jehovah's Witnesses. Transfusion 1994;34:396–401.

7 Rossaint R, Bouillon B, Cerny V et al. Management of bleeding following major trauma: an updated European Guideline. Crit Care 2010;14:R52.

8 The CRASH-2 Collaborators. Effects of tranexamic acid on death, vascular occlusive events, and blood transfusion in trauma patients with significant haemorrhage (CRASH-2): a randomised placebo-controlled trial. Lancet 2010;376: 23–32.

9 Lipworth W, Kerridge I, Little M, Day R. Evidence and desperation in off-label prescribing: recombinant factor VIIa. BMJ 2012;344:d7926.

10 Corwin HL, Gettinger A, Fabian TC et al. Efficacy and safety of epoetin alfa in critically ill patients. N Engl J Med 2007; 357:965–76.

5

SECTION 5
Approach to White Cell Problems

CHAPTER 20

Infectious Complications in the Immunosuppressed Patient

Tim Collyns¹ and Elankumaran Paramasivam²

¹Leeds Teaching Hospitals Trust, St James's University Hospital, Leeds, UK
²St James's University Hospital, Leeds, UK

Introduction

Patients with many haematological disorders have an increased susceptibility to infections. This may be due to disruption of the patient's host defences by the underlying condition and/or the subsequent haematological treatment. Some examples are listed in Table 20.1; however, the spectrum of infectious diseases which may be involved varies with the type and severity of the haematological condition and the associated therapy [1–3]. It is also related to the infectious agents which are circulating in the patient's surrounding environment and community and to which they have been exposed to.

Depending on the haematological disease, patients may present with more than one infectious complication, either concurrently or consecutively. Patients may require critical care level support due to the systemic sequelae of an infection, or they may acquire certain infections while in the critical care environment. This chapter outlines some of the more common scenarios in the critical care setting and approaches to their diagnosis and successful management. Infectious complications contribute significantly to the overall morbidity and mortality of haematological diseases; hence, there will usually be local guidelines in place which should be consulted as required.

Neutropenic fever

This is the archetype of an infectious complication in the setting of haematological diseases. Standard, internationally applied definitions are available (Table 20.2), but there may be local variation in interpretation of both *neutropenia* and *fever* [1, 2, 4]. Diagnostic criteria for assessing sepsis severity are also outlined in Table 20.2 [5, 6]. The National Institute for Health and Clinical Excellence (NICE) in the UK has recently issued guidance for the *prevention and management of neutropenic sepsis* – in which the criteria for a diagnosis of *sepsis* includes a fever greater than 38°C alone, while neutropenia is defined as the patient's neutrophil count being equal to, or less than, 0.5×10^9/L [4].

Neutropenic fever often arises in those with haematological malignancy undergoing chemotherapy. The absence of neutrophils, coupled with disruption of skin and mucosal barriers, predispose the patient to infection. The risk is inversely proportional to the absolute count, and 10–20% of patients with a neutrophil count less than 0.1×10^9/L will have a bloodstream infection. Fever is an early, albeit non-specific, sign of infection, although classic symptoms and signs may be reduced or absent [1, 2]. Only 20–30% of neutropenic fevers are due to clinically identified infection [2].

The aetiology of likely infecting organisms varies with length of neutropenia, previous or current antimicrobial

Haematology in Critical Care: A Practical Handbook, First Edition. Edited by Jecko Thachil and Quentin A. Hill.
© 2014 John Wiley & Sons, Ltd. Published 2014 by John Wiley & Sons, Ltd.

Table 20.1 Some specific infections associated with, and/or more severe in, specific conditions [1–3].

Neutropenia	Viral infections
	  HSV reactivation
	Bacterial infections (see also Table 20.3)
	  Gut translocation: Enterobacteriaceae (coliforms)
	  Line associated: staphylococci
	Fungal infections
	  Candida species
	  Aspergillus species, most common Aspergillus fumigatus (other moulds)

Hypogammaglobulinaemia/impaired humoral immunity	Encapsulated bacteria: principally Streptococcus pneumoniae, also Haemophilus influenzae, Neisseria meningitidis Sinopulmonary infections, +/− septicaemia
Lymphopenia/impaired cellular immunity	Herpesviruses, respiratory viruses Listeria monocytogenes, Nocardia species Mycobacteria: Mycobacterium tuberculosis and non-tuberculous Cryptococcus species, P. jirovecii Toxoplasma gondii reactivation
Asplenic/functionally hyposplenic	Encapsulated bacteria, principally S. pneumoniae, also H. influenzae, Capnocytophaga spp.; parasite infections, malaria, babesiosis
Acute leukaemias	If neutropenic, see preceding text. Patients with acute myeloid leukaemia (AML) or myelodysplastic syndrome (MDS) may be functionally neutropenic, i.e. detectable but ineffective neutrophils Acute lymphocytic leukaemia (ALL): Pneumocystis
Chronic lymphocytic leukaemia (CLL)	Hypogammaglobulinaemic – see preceding text CLL treatment (e.g. alemtuzumab, MabCampath®): wide range, including Pneumocystis, CMV reactivation
Multiple myeloma	Functionally hypogammaglobulinaemic – see preceding text If neutropenic – see preceding text
Sickle cell disease	Functionally hyposplenic – see preceding text Salmonella osteomyelitis
Iron overload (e.g. thalassaemias) and/or iron chelator therapy such as desferrioxamine	Yersinia spp.; other bacteria may have increased pathogenicity in presence of iron-rich milieu fungal infection (Zygomycetes)

Haemopoietic stem cell transplant (HSCT) recipients

Relative risks vary considerably with source/type of transplant and conditioning regime, as well as underlying disease and previous treatment. Allogeneic recipients are more likely to have infectious complications, and be at risk for longer, than autologous recipients. In the former, the presence of significant GVHD notably increases the probability of certain infectious complications

Conventionally for allogeneic recipients: 3 phases post HSCT

Pre-engraftment (day 0 usually to < day 30)

Neutropenic: see preceding text (also present post autologous HSCT though usually less prolonged)

Early post-engraftment (up to day 100)

Lymphopenic – see preceding text

Specific risks include CMV reactivation (seropositive recipient and/or donor)

Respiratory viruses, including adenovirus

BK virus (haemorrhagic cystitis)

Aspergillus species and other moulds

Pneumocystis

T. gondii (seropositive recipient)

Late post-engraftment (day 100 to reconstitution of immune function – usually around 18 months post allogeneic HSCT but delayed in presence of GVHD/associated treatment)

Sinopulmonary infections: *S. pneumoniae, H. influenzae, Pneumocystis, Aspergillus* species and other moulds

Varicella zoster virus (VZV) (seropositive recipient)

Table 20.2 Diagnostic criteria.

Neutropenic fever	Absolute neutrophil count <0.5 × 10⁹/L blood or <1 and expected to fall to <0.5 within the next 48 h
	Single temperature ≥38.3°C (i.e. 101°F) or ≥38°C for 1 h or more
	(NB NICE definitions: ANC < 0.5, temperature > 38°C [4])
Sepsis	Infection (suspected or proven) coupled with deranged parameters indicative of systemic response, including:
	Pyrexia (>38.3°C) or hypothermia (<36°C)
	Tachycardia (>90 beats/min)
	Tachypnoea (>30 breaths/min)
	Significant oedema or positive fluid balance (>20 mL/kg/24 h)
	Abnormal blood tests:
	Leukocytosis* (>12 × 10⁹/L) or leukopenia* (<4)
	Thrombocytopenia* (platelet count <100 × 10⁹/L)
	(*NB often not applicable in haematology patient setting)
	Significantly elevated CRP (or PCT)
	Hyperglycaemia (plasma glucose >7.7 mM/L) without diabetes
	Arterial hypotension (see also severe sepsis)
	Organ dysfunction or tissue perfusion markers (see also severe sepsis)
Severe sepsis	Sepsis with dysfunction or hypoperfusion of organs not primarily infected, e.g. lactic acidosis, oliguria (<30 mL/h or <0.5 mL/kg/h), altered mental state and/or hypotension (systolic pressure < 90 mmHg, mean arterial pressure <70 mmHg or drop of > 40 mmHg from baseline) – which is correctable with fluid resuscitation
	Organ dysfunction can be recorded/monitored using validated scoring systems, such as Multiple Organ Dysfunction (MOD) or Sequential Organ Failure Assessment (SOFA) scores
Septic shock	Sepsis-induced persistent arterial hypotension which requires pressor therapy to correct
Refractory septic shock	Septic shock that lasts >1 h despite the use of pressor therapy

Adapted from [1, 2, 4–6].

therapy, as well as with clinical source. It is also influenced by the patient's setting – whether in the community or in hospital and, if in the hospital, the particular unit's microflora. Some attributes of the more common bacterial isolates are detailed in Table 20.3.

Diagnostic assessment

History: Document the nature of the underlying disorder and what therapy has been received. Note any previous infections and antimicrobials received – either as prophylaxis or treatment. Aim to identify a possible focus of infection on systemic enquiry.

Examination: Full examination including assessment of intravascular access device(s) if present; skin; sinuses; chest; digestive tract, including mouth and perianal area; and presence of mucositis. Assess for evidence of concomitant sepsis/its severity (see Table 20.2).

Tests: Full blood count (FBC) (including differential leukocyte count) and urea, creatinine and electrolytes (U&Es) and liver function tests. Lactate, C-reactive protein (CRP), +/– other markers for infection, such as procalcitonin (PCT) if locally available. Consider chest X-ray (CXR) – notably if respiratory symptoms or signs [1, 2, 4].

Microbiology
• Blood cultures: preferably taken pre-starting or changing antimicrobials – ideally concurrent luminal and peripheral sets [2, 5].
• Urine should be sent if patient catheterized, localizing symptoms present or abnormal urinalysis [1, 2].
• Other suitable site-specific samples as clinically indicated [1, 2].

Antimicrobial therapy
Timing
Start early – i.e. empirically (*best guess*) – don't wait for positive microbiological results. If neutropenia suspected post chemotherapy and the blood count is awaited, manage as if neutropenic until result is available.

In the critical care setting, first dose(s) of suitable regimen should be administered as soon as possible (though ideally still after blood cultures collected) – certainly within 1 h of presentation if septic [2, 4–6].

Choice
There is a plethora of comparative trials of agents – both alone and in combination – and associated systematic reviews [1, 2, 4, 7, 8]. The complication of infection in

Table 20.3 Some common bacterial pathogens [1–3, 6].

Gram-negative bacilli

Enterobacteriaceae (*coliforms*)

e.g. *Escherichia coli*, *Klebsiella pneumoniae*, *Enterobacter* spp., other genera such as *Citrobacter* spp., *Serratia* spp.

Likely sources: gut translocation; urinary tract, respiratory tract (vascular catheter)

Treatment: usually susceptible *in vitro* to suitable broad-spectrum β-lactams such as piperacillin–tazobactam, carbapenems (imipenem/meropenem) and ceftazidime, although resistance is increasing. Carbapenems most reliable against antibiotic-resistant isolates, such as extended-spectrum β-lactamase (ESBL) producers or those with derepressed chromosomal AmpC gene – though carbapenemase-producing isolates are also emerging. Aminoglycosides usually also active and synergistic with a suitable β-lactam

Non-lactose-fermenting Gram-negative bacilli

e.g. *Pseudomonas aeruginosa*, other *Pseudomonas* spp., *Acinetobacter* spp., *Stenotrophomonas maltophilia*

Likely sources: vascular catheter, respiratory tract (gut translocation of *P. aeruginosa*)

Treatment: less predictable sensitivity patterns than Enterobacteriaceae. Suitable empirical febrile neutropenia regimes need effective anti-*P. aeruginosa* activity

S. maltophilia intrinsically resistant to the carbapenems. Antimicrobial of choice for this organism is usually co-trimoxazole (at *mid*-dose: e.g. 1.44g twice daily for 75kg patient)

Gram-positive bacilli

Staphylococci

e.g. *Staphylococcus aureus*, coagulase-negative staphylococci (including *Staphylococcus epidermidis*)

Likely sources: vascular catheter, skin and soft tissue infection (*S. aureus*), skin flora contaminant (coagulase-negative staphylococci)

Treatment: If meticillin susceptible, suitable β-lactam such as flucloxacillin. Carbapenems also active. If meticillin resistant, glycopeptide, linezolid, daptomycin

Streptococci

e.g. *Streptococcus pneumoniae*

Likely sources: respiratory tract, head (sinuses, ear, meninges)

Treatment: piperacillin–tazobactam, aforementioned carbapenems usually active (consider *de-escalation* to benzylpenicillin or amoxicillin), certain fluoroquinolones (e.g. levofloxacin or moxifloxacin, not ciprofloxacin), macrolide (e.g. clarithromycin), linezolid, glycopeptides

β-Haemolytic streptococci: Lancefield groups A, B, C, G

Likely sources: skin/soft tissue infection, gut translocation (Group B streptococcus)

Treatment: as for *S. pneumoniae*

Viridans streptococci

Likely sources: translocation in patients with mucositis, respiratory tract (consider endocarditis)

Treatment: as for *S. pneumoniae* – though these streptococci more commonly resistant to penicillins and other antimicrobial classes. Most reliably active: glycopeptides, linezolid

Enterococci

e.g. *Enterococcus faecalis*, *Enterococcus faecium*

Likely sources: gut translocation, vascular catheter (notably if femoral site) (urinary tract)

Treatment: *E. faecalis* – piperacillin–tazobactam, imipenem usually active (consider *de-escalation* to amoxicillin), glycopeptides, linezolid, daptomycin

E. faecium: resistant to β-lactams – therefore glycopeptides, linezolid, daptomycin

Corynebacteria (Gram-positive bacilli – *diphtheroids*)

Likely sources: vascular catheter, skin flora contaminant

Treatment: similar to that for *viridans* streptococci in the preceding text

---

neutropenia is not a homogenous monolith – stratification strategies have been developed, which include assessing the risk of significant sequelae [1, 2, 4]. In the critical care setting, intravenous antibiotics, at least initially, are appropriate. The specific choice is influenced by patient factors (e.g. clinical condition/any identified focus, previous microbiological results, drug allergy history) and institutional factors (e.g. individual agent availability, organism susceptibility patterns). A β-lactam with antipseudomonal activity, e.g. piperacillin–tazobactam or a suitable carbapenem such as meropenem or imipenem, is the most common first choice, either alone or with an aminoglycoside such as gentamicin or amikacin. There is a consistent lack of evidence that the routine addition of an aminoglycoside is of benefit; however, such combination therapy may still be appropriate in the initial management of a patient with severe sepsis or septic shock [1, 2, 4, 5, 8]. Piperacillin–tazobactam has been associated with overall lower all-cause mortality than other single agents; however, in the critical care setting, the carbapenems are appealing due to their greater spectrum of activity against antibiotic-resistant bacteria [2, 5, 7]. An *inappropriate* empirical regimen, i.e. one which is not active against the relevant infecting organism(s), has been associated with increased mortality from sepsis [5, 6, 9]. The routine addition of a glycopeptide such as vancomycin or teicoplanin is not appropriate – it should be reserved for specific cases such as when significant catheter-related infection is clinically suspected or microbiologically confirmed or in setting of current or previous isolation of a β-lactam-resistant Gram-positive pathogen [1, 2, 4].

If clinical and/or radiological suspicion of lower respiratory tract infection (RTI) – notably if community acquired – anti-atypical pneumonia pathogen cover should be considered in addition, e.g. a macrolide such as clarithromycin or azithromycin, or fluoroquinolone such as levofloxacin or ciprofloxacin [1].

Allergy

For patients who are reported to be *allergic to penicillin*, try to find out the nature of the reaction and which antimicrobials the patient has received previously without adverse effect.

For cases with a reported immediate hypersensitivity type I reaction or other severe adverse event, the combination of a glycopeptide and either aztreonam (unless previous reaction specifically to aztreonam or ceftazidime) or ciprofloxacin (unless on fluoroquinolone prophylaxis) is usually reasonable, whereas for less marked reactions to a previous penicillin, a carbapenem may be considered [2].

Other supportive therapy

Depending on the overall clinical condition of the patient, other early goal-directed interventions are important in improving survival [5, 6]. In the setting of severe sepsis or septic shock, these include:
• Fluid resuscitation to restore cardiovascular function (aiming for central venous pressure 8–12 mmHg, mean arterial pressure ≥ 65 mmHg, urine output ≥ 0.5 mL/kg/h and either central venous oxygen saturation ≥70% or mixed venous ≥ 65%) [5, 6].

• Respiratory support: Almost half of these patients will suffer acute lung injury/acute respiratory distress syndrome [6].
• Renal function support: For actual replacement therapy, continuous venovenous haemofiltration (CVVH) may be easier to manage in haemodynamically unstable patients than intermittent haemodialysis, although this has not been shown to improve overall survival [5, 6].

Follow-on

Review the empirical therapy, agents and length, in light of clinical response and latest microbiological results. An appropriate empirical regimen does not need to be altered on the basis of persistent fever alone if the patient is clinically stable or otherwise improving [1, 4].

If no aetiology identified, and the patient has been afebrile for 48 h or more, consider stopping the empirical agents [4]. If a causative organism is identified, therapy should be modified as required, and for bacteraemias with a Gram-negative organism, a minimum of 1-week effective therapy is normally appropriate, while for *Staphylococcus aureus* or *Candida* species, a minimum of 2 weeks is recommended [1].

If the fever persists, or recurs, despite 4–7 days of appropriate antibacterials, empirical antifungal therapy may also be warranted [1, 2].

Respiratory tract infection (RTI)

The respiratory tract may be the focus of infection precipitating the need for critical care level support, or the haematology patient may acquire an RTI while receiving such support – notably if mechanically ventilated, with a *ventilator-associated pneumonia* (VAP).

The likely aetiologies of a precipitating infection, as for all patients, vary as to whether the infection was acquired in the community or while in the hospital. Some of the more common causes are in Tables 20.1 and 20.3; however, the range of potential pathogens is extensive, and the comparative risk varies with the nature and degree of the immune compromise.

If ventilator associated, the most likely culprits are those that cause such infections in any critical care patient – though remember that some haematology patients will have received extensive prior antimicrobial exposure, either as treatment or prophylaxis.

Certain invasive fungal infections (IFI), notably those due to moulds such as *Aspergillus* species, may present with respiratory tract symptoms. These infections are more frequently found (and suspected) in patients with certain underlying haematological conditions. Patients at highest risk of IFI include those with prolonged neutropenia (>10 days) and allogeneic haemopoietic stem cell transplant (HSCT) recipients, notably those with significant graft-versus-host disease (GVHD) on high-dose steroid therapy [1]. Confirming this diagnosis can be challenging, and hence, patients at risk are often treated with a suitable antifungal, either empirically (as in the preceding text) or *pre-emptively* – in which there is some suggestive evidence of an invasive fungal aetiology such as suspicious lesion(s) on a chest high-resolution CT (HRCT) scan or positive blood test(s) for fungal material, such as *Aspergillus* galactomannan antigen or the broader range 1,3-β-D-glucan assay, and/or nucleic acid by PCR [2].

Some haematological disorders/associated therapy also predisposes to pulmonary disease due to *Pneumocystis jirovecii* – basonym *P. carinii*, i.e. *Pneumocystis* pneumonia (*PcP*). Some of these are listed in Table 20.1.

Viral infections, e.g. with respiratory syncytial virus (RSV), parainfluenza or human metapneumovirus (hMPV), may present with lower respiratory tract manifestations – notably in high-risk hosts such as lymphopenic allogeneic HSCT recipients – as well as influenza and adenovirus [1, 3]. Pneumonia is also the commonest presentation of end-organ CMV disease in allogeneic HSCT recipients.

Diagnostic assessment
History
Symptoms suggestive of fungal aetiology include *pleuritic-type* chest pain and haemoptysis. Patients with PcP may have marked dyspnoea, coupled with non-productive cough and fever. Ascertain if the patient is currently prescribed with (and taking) any prophylaxis, as the likelihood of PcP is much less in patients, otherwise at risk, who are on effective PcP preventative therapy; similarly, the likely aetiology of an invasive mould infection will vary with preceding prophylaxis.

Examination
The findings vary widely in accordance with degree of lung involvement and nature of infection.

Tests
FBC, U&Es, arterial blood gases, and CRP (+/− PCT)
CXR: presence and pattern of any infiltrate(s)
HRCT: can detect abnormalities not identified on CXR – notably those suggestive of IFI [1]

Microbiology
Infections may present with unusual clinical features, concurrently or consecutively. Investigate with:
- Blood cultures.
- Urine for *Legionella* (primarily *Legionella pneumophila*, serogroup 1) and *Streptococcus pneumoniae* antigens.
- Blood serology for *atypical* pneumonia pathogens (e.g. for *Mycoplasma pneumoniae* IgM antibodies). Also consider a sample for nucleic acid detection (e.g. by PCR) of certain viruses, e.g. CMV and adenovirus.
- Suitable respiratory tract samples: if the patient is intubated, a bronchoalveolar lavage (BAL), either bronchoscopically directed or collected *blind*, is very useful. Such fluid, depending on laboratory provision, can be tested for:
  ○ Bacterial pathogens (preferably including semi-quantitative count – if querying VAP, $\geq 10^4$ colony-forming units (cfu) of a pathogenic bacterial species per mL of fluid suggest lower RTI as opposed to upper respiratory tract (URT) colonization)
  ○ Fungi (microscopy with calcofluor white, culture and testing for fungal products such as *Aspergillus* antigen and/or by PCR, as well as for *Pneumocystis*, e.g. by PCR or immunofluorescence)
  ○ Respiratory viruses such as RSV, parainfluenza (types 1–4), hMPV, along with influenza A and B, adenovirus, HSV and CMV
  ○ Acid-fast bacilli (AFBs)

However, intubation and mechanical ventilation should be avoided unless indicated due to respiratory insufficiency; and in the non-intubated patient, a bronchoscopic-directed BAL may itself trigger sufficient deterioration for a patient to require ventilatory support [6]. In this setting, sputum, if available, should be sent for bacterial and fungal (+/− AFB) investigations and suitable URT samples (e.g. nose and throat swabs or a nasopharyngeal aspirate (NPA)) for respiratory viral studies [1, 2].

Antimicrobial therapy
Neutropenic patients should be managed in accordance with the principles in the preceding text. Piperacillin–tazobactam and the carbapenems have good activity

against common community bacterial pathogens such as *S. pneumoniae* or *Haemophilus influenzae*. These antibiotics are also suitable for the initial management of non-neutropenic patients who are severely unwell with an RTI. The carbapenems are more reliable against meticillin-sensitive *S. aureus* than piperacillin–tazobactam. If a meticillin-resistant *S. aureus* (MRSA) is suspected, then a specific additional agent may need to be added, such as linezolid or vancomycin [1, 2].

Patients with community-acquired RTI should usually have specific cover for *atypical* pneumonia pathogens, such as *Legionella*, *Mycoplasma* and *Chlamydophila* – usually with a macrolide or fluoroquinolone [1].

If *Pneumocystis* is clinically and/or radiologically suspected, then co-trimoxazole at *high dose* (i.e. 100–120 mg/kg/day if adequate renal function) is warranted. Remember that co-trimoxazole is potentially active against many other common pneumonic pathogens – including *atypical* ones and MRSA – with the notable exceptions of *Pseudomonas aeruginosa* and *Mycoplasma*; therefore, if co-trimoxazole is being used, other *additional* agents such as linezolid or a macrolide are often not required.

If IFI is suspected, then an appropriate antifungal should also be included in the therapeutic regimen (i.e. an amphotericin B formulation, an echinocandin such as caspofungin or an appropriate triazole [1, 2]). Consider using a different class to that of any recent anti-mould prophylaxis.

Specific antiviral treatment, such as nebulized ribavirin, is normally only instituted on the basis of positive microbiological results. An exception is during the annual influenza season, when empirical therapy with neuraminidase inhibitor (oseltamivir or zanamivir) in patients presenting within 48 h of suggestive symptoms (e.g. high fever, myalgia, coryza, dry cough) may be added to standard antimicrobials [1, 2].

Modify empirical therapy as appropriate on the basis of microbiological results/clinical response.

Catheter-related infections

Patients with haematological conditions may have a *long-term* intravenous catheter *in situ* (i.e. planned to be present for >14 days) – to allow the administration of certain chemotherapy agents and blood products and facilitate blood sampling [10]. These catheters, such as Hickman

or Groshong lines, are surgically implanted with a portion in a subcutaneous tunnel. A patient requiring critical care level support may also have *short-term* central venous and/or arterial lines inserted. Venous catheters are a significant source of bloodstream infections in the haematology setting [2]. The frequency of infection is affected by a number of factors, including the catheter type and site, and the standards of asepsis applied when inserting and using the catheter [10]. The hub/lumen is the primary route of organism acquisition by long lines, and hence, these catheter-related bloodstream infections (CRBSIs) are predominantly caused by Gram-positive organisms which colonize the skin, such as coagulase-negative staphylococci, *S. aureus* and corynebacteria (see Table 20.3) [2, 10]. Other organisms include *Candida* species, enterococci, Gram-negative bacilli and rapidly growing mycobacteria [2, 10].

Diagnosis
History/examination
Localizing symptoms/signs may be mild or absent. There may be visible purulence or inflammation of skin at the exit site +/− that overlying the subcutaneous tunnel if present. Fever +/− rigors may be temporally associated with accessing the line.

Microbiology
• If line being preserved at the time, blood cultures should be taken concurrently from a peripheral vein and via each lumen of the catheter(s) – with similar volume of blood inoculated per bottle. If one or more luminal blood cultures flag with positive growth on an automated blood culture machine 2 h or more faster than the peripheral set, this *differential time to positivity* (DTP) is considered significant and is strongly suggestive of the catheter being the source of infection [2, 5, 10]. Quantitative blood cultures are not performed in most routine microbiology laboratories [10]. Note that blood cultures positive for *S. aureus*, coagulase-negative staphylococci or *Candida* raise the suspicion per se of CRBSI if no alternative clinically apparent source [10].
• Exit site swab if exudate present [10].
• If catheter is removed and cultured, the growth of greater than or equal to15 cfu from the tip rolled on an agar plate indicates the catheter was (at least) colonized – although this technique doesn't detect intra-luminal growth [10].

Management

Decide whether to attempt catheter salvage – i.e. treating the infection with the catheter remaining in place. Whether this should be attempted is influenced by a range of factors, including:

Catheter type: Salvage may be appropriate for *long-term* catheters – infected short-term catheters should normally be removed forthwith [10].

Clinical condition: If patient is systemically severely unwell; remove catheter(s) if potentially infected; or in the presence of tunnel infection, suppurative thrombophlebitis or associated endocarditis [5, 10].

Pathogen involved: Some organisms are more virulent and/or difficult to eradicate successfully without removal of infected line. Organisms in which line removal is usually *mandatory* include *S. aureus*, *P. aeruginosa*, fungi and mycobacteria [10].

If line salvage is being attempted, then for a CRBSI, this normally involves *locking* the lumen(s) of the line with an antimicrobial solution – as this is usually the primary source of the infection, combined with systemic antimicrobials – the latter at least until the patient is clinically stable. The antimicrobial lock concentration in the small volume of the line lumen (~2 mL for a standard Hickman line) is much greater than can be achieved in the overall circulation. Line lock agents need to be sufficiently stable, such as a glycopeptide for a Gram-positive organism (e.g. vancomycin at concentration 5 mg/mL) or an aminoglycoside for a Gram-negative isolate [10]. Other potential agents include some not used systemically, such as taurolidine or ethanol. The lock dwell time should be as long as practical, usually up to 1 week, with 8 h as a suggested minimum. If the line has two lumens and some line access is required, consider alternating the locked lumen every 24 h. Seven to fourteen days in total is normally appropriate, with subsequent luminal blood cultures to assess microbiological efficacy.

Prevention

Trying to avoid infectious complications involves a number of different strategies, for example, universal asepsis for vascular catheter insertion and access, and techniques shown to reduce VAP rates. Granulocyte colony-stimulating factor (G-CSF) may be used after chemotherapy to shorten the duration of neutropenia and reduce the risk of febrile neutropenia in high-risk patients, although there is a lack of evidence against its routine use [4, 11]. It may also be used in patients with febrile neutropenia at high risk of poor clinical outcome [11].

Specific antimicrobial prophylaxis may be appropriate. This may include antiviral, antibacterial and antifungal agents.

Antiviral

Aciclovir: during period(s) of neutropenia, primarily to prevent HSV reactivation

CMV infections are normally managed *pre-emptively*. This is done by monitoring for viral reactivation in patients adjudged at sufficiently high risk by regular (e.g. 1–2 times per week) blood testing for viral DNA. Such patients include certain allogeneic HSCT recipients early post transplant (see Table 20.1). Patients at highest risk of reactivation are those who are CMV seropositive pre-HSCT, receiving cells from a seronegative donor. At less risk are recipients (positive or negative) with CMV-seropositive donor. If *significant* viral reactivation is detected – the trigger threshold varies with method used – antiviral therapy (usually initially with ganciclovir) is instituted before progression to end-organ disease.

Antibacterial

Fluoroquinolone (levofloxacin or ciprofloxacin) prophylaxis during expected period(s) of neutropenia post chemotherapy [1, 2, 4].

Anti-pneumococcal: penicillin (or macrolide if penicillin allergic) in asplenic or functionally hyposplenic patients.

Antifungal

This may be anti-yeast (fluconazole) or also anti-mould, e.g. a broader-spectrum azole (currently itraconazole, posaconazole or voriconazole), an echinocandin or amphotericin B formulation [1, 2]. For longer-term prophylaxis, the azoles are appealing as they are available orally.

Anti-*Pneumocystis*

For patients at risk (see Table 20.1 for some examples), co-trimoxazole is the first choice and effective – reducing PcP rate to less than 1% of allogeneic HSCT recipients [3]. It is also active against many bacterial species, as well as other organisms – such as preventing *Toxoplasma gondii* reactivation.

If co-trimoxazole is contraindicated (e.g. due to allergy), consider dapsone (NB this agent is *not* active vs. bacteria such as *S. pneumoniae*).

Immunosuppressed haematological patients should also be offered appropriate vaccinations, in accordance with national +/− local guidelines.

Conclusions

Haematological patients are at risk of a wide gamut of infectious complications, both in aetiology and severity. It is often appropriate to manage these complications aggressively at the outset, aiming to *get it right first time* and then de-escalating therapy when possible on the basis of test results and clinical response.

References

1 National Comprehensive Cancer Network. Clinical Practice Guidelines in Oncology: Prevention and treatment of cancer-related infections, Version 1. 2013. National Comprehensive Cancer Network, Jenkintown, PA, USA. www.NCCN.org (accessed on November 21, 2013).

2 Freifeld AG, Bow EJ, Sepkowitz KA et al. Clinical Practice Guideline for the use of antimicrobial agents in neutropenic patients with cancer: 2010 update by the Infectious Diseases Society of America. Clin Infect Dis 2011;52:e56–e93.

3 Young JH, Weisdorf DJ. Infections in recipients of hematopoietic cell transplantation. In Mandell GL, Bennett JE, Dolin R (eds), Mandell, Douglas and Bennett's Principles and Practice of Infectious Diseases, 7thedition. Philadelphia: Churchill Livingstone Elsevier, 2010. p. 3821–37.

4 National Institute for Health and Clinical Excellence. Neutropenic sepsis: prevention and management of neutropenic sepsis in cancer patients. NICE clinical guideline 151. 2012. www.nice.org.uk (accessed on November 21, 2013).

5 Dellinger RP, Levy MM, Rhodes A et al. Surviving Sepsis Campaign: international guidelines for management of severe sepsis and septic shock: 2012. Crit Care Med 2013; 41:580–637.

6 Penack O, Buchheidt D, Christopeit M et al. Management of sepsis in neutropenic patients: guidelines from the infectious diseases working party of the German Society of Hematology and Oncology. Ann Oncol 2011; 22:1019–29.

7 Paul M, Yahav D, Bivas A, Fraser A, Leibovici L. Antipseudomonal beta-lactams for the initial, empirical, treatment of febrile neutropenia: comparison of beta-lactams. Cochrane Database Syst Rev 2010;(issue 11). Art. No.:CD005197.

8 Drgona L, Paul M, Bucaneve G, Calandra T, Menichetti F. The need for aminoglycosides in combination with β-lactams for high-risk, febrile neutropaenic patients with leukaemia. Eur J Cancer 2007;Supplement 5;13–22.

9 Paul M, Shani V, Muchtar E. Systematic review and meta-analysis of the efficacy of appropriate empiric antibiotic therapy for sepsis. Antimicrob Agents Chemother 2010; 54:4851–63.

10 Mermel LA, Allon M, Bouza E et al. Clinical Practice Guidelines for the diagnosis and management of intravascular catheter-related infection: 2009 update by the Infectious Diseases Society of America. Clin Infect Dis 2009;49:1–45.

11 Smith TJ, Khatcheressian J, Lyman LA et al. 2006 Update of recommendations for the use of white blood cell growth factors: evidence based Clinical Practice Guideline. J Clin Oncol 2006;24:3187–205.

CHAPTER 21

Haematopoietic Stem Cell Transplantation (HSCT)

John Snowden[1,2] and Stephen Webber[3]

[1]Department of Haematology, Sheffield Teaching Hospitals NHS Foundation Trust, South Yorkshire, UK
[2]Department of Oncology, University of Sheffield, Sheffield, UK
[3]Department of Anaesthesia and Critical Care, Sheffield Teaching Hospitals NHS Foundation Trust, South Yorkshire, UK

Introduction

Haematopoietic stem cell transplantation (HSCT) is a complex and toxic procedure [1], with a high risk of procedural mortality and serious morbidity reflected by 11–40% of patients subsequently requiring intensive care support [2]. The necessity for a close working relationship between the HSCT and critical care teams is highlighted by the fact that unhindered access to critical care support is now a mandatory accreditation requirement for HSCT programmes [3]. Intensive care specialists and their medical, nursing, pharmacy and allied health professional colleagues need to be familiar with the process of HSCT (Figure 21.1), the rationale for performing such procedures (Table 21.1) and the justification for exposing patients to a high risk of treatment-related complications. A working knowledge is not only essential for optimizing clinical outcomes in critically ill HSCT patients but also for effective communication with colleagues and families who are supporting the patient.

The aim of this chapter is to familiarize the critical care reader with the process of HSCT and focus on specific complications that may lead to admission to critical care or otherwise feature in the clinical picture and require ongoing collaborative management. Inevitably, all types of HSCT render patients pancytopenic and at risk of neutropenic infection, septic shock, bleeding and a need for various transfused blood products. These aspects are considered in Chapters 20 (infection), 25 (shock), 3 and 15 (bleeding) and 13, 14 and 17 (transfusion).

Definitions and rationale for HSCT

The practice of HSCT has grown massively since the first clinical bone marrow transplantation (BMT) procedures in the late 1960s. With the increasing use of other sources of haematopoietic stem cells (HSC), particularly peripheral blood stem cells (PBSC) and umbilical cord blood (UCB), the term HSCT is now more appropriate, although BMT persists in common parlance.

Haematopoietic stem cell transplantation is an umbrella term referring to the reconstitution of the blood, bone marrow and immune systems by an infusion of HSC following the administration of intensive myelo- and/or lympho-ablative cytotoxic therapy (see Figure 21.1). HSCT may be from a donor, i.e. allogeneic HSCT, either within the family or unrelated, or from the patients themselves, termed autologous HSCT. Rarely, identical twins may be used (syngeneic HSCT). Various sources of HSC may be used, including the most *traditional* source of bone marrow harvested by direct

Haematology in Critical Care: A Practical Handbook, First Edition. Edited by Jecko Thachil and Quentin A. Hill.
© 2014 John Wiley & Sons, Ltd. Published 2014 by John Wiley & Sons, Ltd.

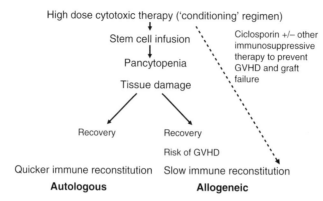

Figure 21.1 Phases of haematopoietic stem cell transplantation (HSCT). HSCT is initiated by administration of the *conditioning regimen*, which consists of intensive cytotoxic chemotherapy +/– total body irradiation (TBI) and anti-lymphocyte antibodies (such as ATG or alemtuzumab). In autologous HSCT, the main aim is to dose intensify cytotoxic treatment to increase cancer cell killing and to use autologous cell infusion to hasten haematological recovery, which may not otherwise occur for months or years. Despite neutrophil recovery, patients may remain immunosuppressed due to the treatment or their underlying disease (myeloma, lymphoma). In allogeneic HSCT, the conditioning therapy has the dual purpose of destroying the underlying disease process and creating immunological *space* for the transplanted graft. Allogeneic HSCT also routinely requires the administration of additional immunosuppressant medication (such as ciclosporin) to prevent graft rejection and graft-versus-host disease (GVHD). GVHD may result in varying degrees of acute and chronic multi-organ dysfunction, which usually require immunosuppressive treatment. In addition, there is slow reconstitution of the transplanted immune system in the allogeneic HSCT recipient, potentially perturbed by GVHD and its treatments, and a long-term risk of infection susceptibility frequently persists. On the positive side, GVHD provides the additional dimension of an ongoing graft-versus-leukaemia/lymphoma (GVL) effect, which may contribute to long-term cure by elimination of low-level residual disease. This forms the principle of donor lymphocyte infusions (DLI), sometimes given post HSCT to maximize the GVL effect.

aspiration under general anaesthetic, but now, the vast majority of HSC are PBSC mobilized with granulocyte colony-stimulating factor (+/– chemotherapy) and collected by apheresis, which have the advantage of quicker engraftment. The use of UCB, banked or as directed donations, is also on the increase, particularly in paediatric practice.

The long-term risks of treatment-related mortality (TRM) and morbidity are substantially higher for allogeneic HSCT compared with autologous HSCT. Although individualized in practice, typical estimates of 1-year TRM given during the consent process are up to 3% for autologous HSCT but up to 20% for fully matched allogeneic HSCT and potentially higher for mismatched and UCB transplantation. Age and co-morbidities are also important considerations, although in recent years reduced intensity conditioning (RIC) regimens and better supportive care have extended the application of HSCT to older and less fit patients, including patients in their 70s.

In every patient, the risks of TRM, serious morbidity and impact on quality of life have to be justified by clear potential for incremental survival over and above the alternative management options. This process should take place initially within the multidisciplinary team (MDT) meeting and then explained to the patient and their family during the consent process for HSCT. For example, provided the TRM risks are recognized, autologous HSCT can achieve cure in the majority of patients with aggressive non-Hodgkin's lymphoma or Hodgkin's disease in chemosensitive relapse, whereas the probability is much lower (at around 10%) with less intensive chemotherapy. By the same logic, the chances of long-term cure in many patients with poor-risk acute leukaemia are boosted by over 30% by allogeneic HSCT, although TRM risks are more substantial. Although the alternative treatment options may offer only remote chances of long-term disease control, this should not be a reason alone for offering HSCT. In addition, patients selected for autologous or allogeneic HSCT must be psychologically motivated and of sufficient physical fitness for an intensive and often complicated and protracted phase of treatment.

Table 21.1 Indications for allogeneic and autologous HSCT in adults and paediatrics (with relative frequencies).

Allogeneic HSCT		Autologous HSCT	
Acute myeloid leukaemia	31%	Myeloma and other plasma cell disorders	44%
Myelodysplastic syndrome/ myeloproliferative diseases	16%	Non-Hodgkin's lymphoma	31%
Acute lymphoblastic leukaemia	15%	Hodgkin's disease	12%
Non-Hodgkin's lymphoma	9%	Leukaemias	4%
Hodgkin's disease	3%	Neuroblastoma	3%
Aplastic anaemia and other bone marrow failure syndromes	6%	Germinal tumours	2%
Myeloma and other plasma cell disorders	5%	Other solid tumours	3%
Chronic myeloid leukaemia	3%	Autoimmune diseases	1%
Chronic lymphocytic leukaemia	3%		
Haemoglobinopathies (thalassaemia, sickle cell disease)	3%		
Paediatric immunodeficiency diseases	3%		
Others (including metabolic diseases, solid tumours, autoimmune diseases)	3%		

Source: Passweg [4]. Copyright Nature. Reproduced with permission of Nature Publishing Group.

Complications generating or featuring in a referral to critical care

Complications of HSCT may be categorized in a number of ways and depend on the type of HSCT. In both autologous and allogeneic HSCT, they include cytotoxic damage induced by the *conditioning regimen* to many tissues. The generation of pancytopenia leads to potential infective and bleeding complications and a dependency on transfused products. Other complications common to all intensive cytotoxic therapy, such as oropharyngeal and gastrointestinal (GI) mucositis, are frequently more pronounced in HSCT patients due to the higher intensity of cytotoxic regimen.

Some complications are relatively unique or largely restricted to HSCT practice, particularly after allogeneic

HSCT. Despite apparent haematological recovery, deficits in cell-mediated immunity typically persist for many months and potentially years following allogeneic HSCT, resulting in increased risk of acquisition or reactivation of a range of opportunistic viral and fungal infections. Allogeneic HSCT may also be associated with acute and chronic graft-versus-host disease (GVHD), a unique and broad spectrum of pathology requiring additional immunosuppressive treatment, which, in turn, adds to the state of infection susceptibility. Some HSCT patients therefore walk a fragile *tightrope* between infection and GVHD. Even after many years post transplant (and cure of their underlying disease), patients may destabilize with infection or other complications and require specialist critical care referral.

While the *mainstream* complications of cytotoxic therapy are considered in Chapter 30, the following will cover those specific complications that directly result in or otherwise feature in the referral to critical care. Needless to say, there are frequently overlapping pathologies, and each patient is relatively unique, depending on their underlying condition, co-morbidities and degree of pre-HSCT treatment, type of transplant, donor source and compatibility and pre-existing parameters such as co-morbidities and viral status (Table 21.2).

Respiratory complications

As in other haematological settings, the most common reason for critical care referral in the HSCT patient is the onset of respiratory failure. In the HSCT setting, the range of infective and noninfective pathology is substantially greater than with chemotherapy alone. The more complex differential diagnosis in HSCT, along with the tempo of deterioration, and frequently narrower window for reversibility all highlight the need for vigilant baseline monitoring for respiratory failure in HSCT, with routine monitoring of oxygen saturation alongside other standard observations.

Respiratory failure, usually detected by falling oxygen saturation, should be addressed by urgent attention to identify the cause. If not rapidly corrected by simple measures, e.g. by diuretic administration, a rapid diagnostic workup should be part of a standard protocol agreed between haematologists, radiologists, microbiologists, respiratory and critical care specialists within an HSCT programme, which facilitates early HRCT scanning and fibre-optic bronchoalveolar lavage

Table 21.2 Early and late complications of HSCT. Side effects of drugs may feature at any stage.

		Early (<3 months)	Late (>3 months)
Infection		Bacterial	Bacterial
		Gram negative	Encapsulated bacteria
		Gram positive (from central lines)	
		Viral	Viral
		Reactivation (HSV, CMV, HHV-6, VZV, adenovirus, EBV)	Reactivation (HSV, VZV, EBV)
		Acquired (RSV, influenza A and B, parainfluenza, norovirus)	Acquired (RSV, influenza A and B, parainfluenza, norovirus)
		Fungal	Fungal
		Aspergillus	*Aspergillus*
		Candida	*P. carinii*
		Pneumocystis carinii	
		Protozoal	
		Toxoplasma gondii	
GVHD		Acute GVHD	Chronic GVHD
			Cutaneous (sclerodermatous)
		Cutaneous (inflammatory)	Mucosal and eyes
		Gastrointestinal (GI)	Liver and GI
		Liver	Lung
			Muscle, fascia, joints
			Immunodeficiency
Other noninfective		Respiratory/cardiovascular	Respiratory/cardiovascular
		Diffuse alveolar haemorrhage	Obliterative bronchiolitis (OB)
		Idiopathic pneumonia syndrome	Bronchiolitis obliterans with organizing pneumonia (BOOP)
		Fluid overload	Obstructive airways disease
		Capillary leak	Arterial disease
		Liver	Cardiomyopathy
		Veno-occlusive disease (VOD)	
		Drugs	Endocrine
			Hypothyroidism
		Renal/Urogenital	Metabolic
			Hypogonadism
		Thrombotic microangiopathy (TMA)	Hypoadrenalism
		Drugs	Metabolic syndrome
		Haemorrhagic cystitis	Transfusion-related iron overload

(FOBAL). An example is provided in Figure 21.2. Specialized microbiological input is key to directing therapy of infective causes. In addition, a range of potential noninfective causes may account for respiratory failure following HSCT. These are usually diagnosed by the exclusion of infective causes supplemented with other more specific investigations, where available. As noninfective lung damage may require corticosteroid or other immunomodulatory treatment, there is a need for confident exclusion of infections, and, in this respect, negative microbiology results following FOBAL and other investigations can sometimes be very valuable.

In the absence of a rapid diagnostic pathway, there is a risk of missing the window of opportunity to perform FOBAL safely without destabilizing the patient. Targeted antimicrobial therapy is highly desirable, as a failure to rapidly confirm a diagnosis often results in blind broad-spectrum anti-infective treatment with potentially unnecessary toxicity and costs. The routine use of FOBAL compared with non-invasive tests is frequently challenging in the acute clinical situation and, arguably, controversial as its precise impact on survival and mortality outcomes remains to be proven. The potential benefits of early diagnosis and modification of therapy are counterbalanced by the risk of precipitating a respiratory

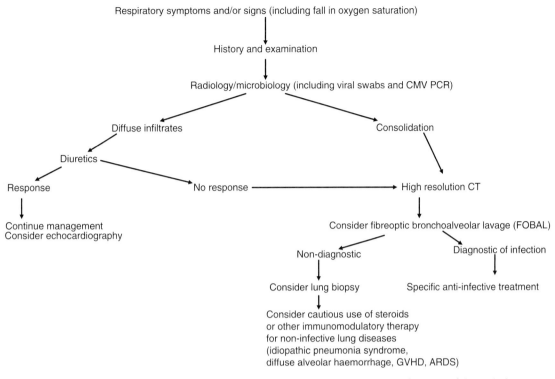

Figure 21.2 Example of a protocol for evaluation of respiratory failure in the HSCT patient. The degree of respiratory failure and other organ compromise determines the tempo of referral to critical care and the feasibility of bronchoalveolar lavage and radiology. A low threshold for evaluation, investigation and referral for critical care review is essential in the hypoxaemic patient.

deterioration. The overall diagnostic yield of FOBAL is 42–65% and is greatest when the procedure is performed early from onset of symptoms (<4 days) and prior to the initiation of empirical antimicrobials. Conversely, yields are lower when performed late or in patients with neutropenia, GVHD or diffuse lung infiltrates on radiological imaging. Non-intubated patients requiring a high inspired oxygen concentration or those receiving noninvasive ventilation are particularly at risk of a respiratory deterioration following FOBAL. Early critical care referral is therefore valuable to familiarize the critical care team with a patient who may destabilize, especially if FOBAL is being considered. There may be an advantage of transfer to critical care prior to FOBAL. Although invasive ventilation is never desirable, if it is necessary, FOBAL should be attempted in the ventilated state [5–8].

The infective pathogen may influence the presentation, e.g. acute bacterial or emergence of fungal infections is often associated with focal consolidation, and viral infections typically present with a more diffuse pneumonitis, but there are no absolute rules and microbiological sampling is key. Noninfective pathologies may present as focal or diffuse radiological changes. The most common is pulmonary oedema, which may respond to simple diuretic therapy, but in the HSCT setting, non-cardiogenic pulmonary oedema (and fluid retention generally) may arise in the context of drug- and engraftment-related capillary leak phenomena and nutritional hypoalbuminaemia. Other noninfective lung pathologies unique to HSCT include diffuse alveolar damage and idiopathic pneumonia syndrome. As with any severe septic or life-threatening process, ARDS may supervene. Acute GVHD rarely affects the lung. All of these noninfective pathologies potentially respond to corticosteroid and other immunomodulatory therapy and highlight the need for early microbiological sampling to exclude or at least adequately identify treatable infection before immunosuppressive treatment is introduced.

In the longer term, chronic lung complications of HSCT may result in referral to critical care for respiratory support. Infective problems may arise many months to years post HSCT, but, in addition, varying degrees of chronic lung damage may limit respiratory reserve. Noninfective pulmonary complications include obliterative bronchiolitis (OB) and bronchiolitis obliterans with organizing pneumonia (BOOP). Some are progressive and may require immunosuppressive treatments, which add to the infection susceptibility. The broad differential of infective and noninfective diagnoses warrants a systematic multidisciplinary approach.

Gastrointestinal (GI) and hepatic complications, with nutritional support

The nutritional status of HSCT patients is invariably compromised, both by GI factors (e.g. mucositis, infections or GVHD) and non-GI factors, such as poor oral intake or catabolic processes. Active measures are routinely employed from the start of HSCT, and the involvement of a specialized dietician in an HSCT programme is an accreditation requirement. Maintenance of nutritional support becomes acutely important when the patient develops complications that warrant transfer to critical care for any cause but especially with GI complications that may reduce absorption or require rest of the gut.

Mucositis is probably the most common and usually self-limiting GI complication of HSCT. While acutely distressing for the patient, it also both predisposes to infections through increased gut permeability and impacts significantly on nutritional status. Management is usually supportive (particularly pain relief, antidiarrhoeals and nutrition). Recombinant keratinocyte growth factor (palifermin) may be administered before cytotoxic therapy to reduce severity but has no role in established mucositis. Rarely, measures need to be taken to protect the upper airway.

Infectious processes may also affect the GI tract, from common bacterial infections such as *Clostridium difficile* to more specialized infections such as viral colitis due to CMV and adenovirus. Common viruses, such as norovirus, which are normally self-limiting, may have a protracted and sometimes fatal course in the HSCT patient.

In the allogeneic HSCT setting, both acute and chronic GVHD may affect the gut and the liver. The onset of acute GVHD typically presents shortly after engraftment with a number of GI symptoms, including poor appetite, nausea and vomiting, as well as varying degrees of diarrhoea, ranging from loose stools to frank blood loss and acute abdominal emergencies. Liver function tests may progressively rise, typically with an obstructive picture (principally affecting alkaline phosphatase and bilirubin). In addition to exclusion of other pathologies, such as infections, it is usually desirable to obtain biopsies of affected sites, particularly as treatment of GVHD involves intensifying immunosuppression. Chronic GVHD may also affect the gut, including the mouth, and the liver and requires long-term immunosuppressive and supportive treatments.

Hepatic veno-occlusive disease (VOD), also known as sinusoidal obstruction syndrome (SOS), is caused by intensive cytotoxic therapy and most commonly presents in the first month following HSCT with a triad of jaundice, tender hepatomegaly and weight gain due to fluid retention and ascites. Diagnosis is primarily clinical, although ultrasound may be useful to confirm the hepatomegaly, ascites and reversed portal flow. Liver biopsy may be undertaken but is usually too hazardous in the midst of thrombocytopenia and deranged coagulation. Management is usually supportive with tightly controlled fluid balance, maintenance of intravascular volume and prevention of hepatorenal syndrome. The anticoagulant defibrotide has been used successfully to help reverse the picture. Some patients make a full recovery, but others develop progressive hepatic failure or chronic liver disease and require specialist management.

Renal and genitourinary complications

Renal complications may arise in any patient undergoing HSCT, particularly if they have underlying renal compromise due to co-morbidities. Occasional patients (e.g. with myeloma kidney disease) may already be maintained on various forms of renal support prior to HSCT. Before proceeding to HSCT, any compromise of GFR should be fully investigated and renal advice sought where appropriate. Renal compromise arising during HSCT is usually temporary and part of a multi-organ compromise requiring critical care support. Permanent and isolated injury requires collaborative working with specialist renal teams.

The most commonly encountered renal complications during HSCT include sepsis and drugs. The calcineurin inhibitors, ciclosporin and tacrolimus, have well-recognized renal toxicity in allogeneic HSCT. Renal toxicity may be minimized by tight control of blood levels.

However, in a complex HSCT setting, drug levels may be challenging to control, or patients suffer other renal insults (especially sepsis, dehydration and other renal toxic drugs). Some patients are also sensitive to thrombotic microangiopathy (TMA) syndrome with calcineurin inhibitors and develop renal failure, haemolytic anaemia and neurological complications. Unlike classic TMA, which requires plasma exchange, management is to withdraw the ciclosporin or tacrolimus and supportive measures.

Haemorrhagic cystitis may be caused by chemotherapy, particularly if high-dose cyclophosphamide is not given with sufficient hydration and mesna (Uromitexan®), which protects against urothelial damage by the metabolite acrolein. The other principal cause is infection, which, in addition to typical bacterial urinary sepsis, may be caused by specific viral pathogens, including polyoma BK virus and subtypes of adenovirus. Severity may range from presence of mild positivity on dipstick testing to massive blood loss, clot retention and obstructive uropathy. Management includes antiviral therapy where appropriate, withdrawal of immunosuppression and supportive measures, including correction of thrombocytopenia and bladder irrigation. Specialist urological input is necessary in severe cases where cystoscopic clot evacuation and other surgical interventions are required.

Neurological complications

Neurological complications account for approximately 10% of indications for referral to critical care [9]. Like any thrombocytopenic patient, HSCT patients are at increased risk of intracranial bleeding, but with good general prophylactic platelet transfusions and correction of clotting abnormalities, such events are rare. Intracranial bleeding may be a feature of an infective process, especially fungal infections.

One of the most common causes of reduced conscious level in the HSCT patient is drug related, including opiates used for control of oropharyngeal mucositis and the neurotoxic effects of ciclosporin and tacrolimus, which may cause a range of symptoms from reduced conscious level to fitting, even at levels in the monitored therapeutic range. Sometimes, neurological features are part of calcineurin inhibitor-related TMA.

Infections of the CNS may occur following HSCT and are occasional causes for referral to critical care. They may arise from a variety of viral, bacterial, fungal and protozoal pathogens and present as encephalitis, cerebritis, meningitis or focal ring-enhancing lesion. In the longer term, EBV-related post-transplant lymphoproliferative disorder (PTLD) and progressive multifocal leukoencephalopathy (due to JC virus) also present with neurological deterioration. Brain biopsy and culture may be necessary and result in critical care involvement. GVHD manifests itself in the CNS very rarely, if at all, although its treatments such as high-dose corticosteroids and ciclosporin may have neuropsychological side effects.

Skin

Although cutaneous complications rarely warrant critical care support in their own right, the skin is affected by a variety of processes that complicate the HSCT patient while on critical care. These include drug eruptions, infections and pressure sores, all of which are commonly encountered in routine critical care practice. In the case of allogeneic HSCT, the skin is a primary target organ for acute and chronic GVHD. Without treatment of the underlying cause and other supportive care measures, the skin may be a source of infection as well as distressing symptoms that compromise the patient overall.

Acute GVHD is frequently the first sign of engraftment and may present as an acute inflammatory macular erythema, affecting any part of the skin, including the palms and soles. Although the diagnosis may be made clinically, it should be confirmed with rapid skin biopsy. Most patients respond to corticosteroids and other immunosuppressive therapies, but more aggressive forms may evolve with desquamation, painful blistering, ulceration, disturbed thermoregulation and fluid shifts, resembling burns. Chronic skin GVHD often overlaps with earlier acute GVHD but is a different disease process, more akin to scleroderma. Chronic skin GVHD may be localized, but in severe cases, mobility may limited from the *hidebound* skin, as well as involvement of the subcutaneous fascia and tendons. Other vital organs are often compromised in such patients, who may not only have significant disability but also a limited prognosis. Extensive chronic GVHD requires prolonged immunosuppressive treatment with attendant risks of infection that may require critical care support.

Relapse of underlying disease

Patients who have undergone HSCT have by definition a disease with a high risk of relapse, which was the justification for accepting the risks of HSCT, and persistence or relapse of malignancy or other disease processes remains a significant undesired outcome. The majority of relapses occur in the first 2 years post HSCT but can potentially occur at any stage (even over a decade). Remission status should therefore always be a consideration in an acutely deteriorating patient. In the acute situation, where major decisions may have to be made regarding escalation of critical care support, urgent bone marrow examinations or imaging may be useful in establishing the remission status. It is important to emphasize that relapse is not necessarily a reason to deny escalation of critical care support, as, in some diseases, effective means of salvage of relapse are increasingly available. In these situations, close liaison between senior specialists in critical care and HSCT is essential.

Late effects of HSCT and other cytotoxic treatments

There is increasing recognition of a range of pathology in long-term survivors of cancer and HSCT arising from exposure to cytotoxic treatments, including endocrine, metabolic and cardiovascular problems and also new secondary malignancies. Most *late effects* are insidious in onset and largely managed in the outpatient setting, but some will feature in referrals to critical care and may require involvement of other disease specialists. Occasionally, *late effects* may impact on prognosis and quality of life in patients in the critical care unit and thereby feature in decision-making in relation to escalation of care.

Prognosis of HSCT patients requiring critical care

Recent data suggest that the hospital mortality for HSCT patients admitted to critical care in the UK is 65% [10]. Short-term mortality of the HSCT patient admitted to critical care is related to the severity of the acute illness, with more severely unwell patients being less likely to survive to discharge from either critical care or hospital [2,10]. However, longer-term outcomes (beyond 6 months) are more related to the underlying haematological condition, i.e. remission status or presence of GVHD. HSCT itself increases the odds ratio for hospital mortality by 1.81 when compared to non-transplanted patients with haematological malignancy [10]. Admission to critical care during the engraftment period is associated with better outcomes than admission in the post-

engraftment period [11]. While the evidence is conflicting, pooled data supports a poorer prognosis following critical care admission for allogeneic HSCT compared with autologous HSCT [9].

Patients requiring mechanical ventilation post HSCT have a poor prognosis, with reported mortality rates exceeding 80% in most studies [9]. The combination of mechanical ventilation plus additional organ failures carries a particularly poor prognosis [11,12]. The 1-year mortality for HSCT patients requiring critical care is approximately 80% but is substantially higher in patients requiring invasive procedures such as mechanical ventilation or haemodialysis [13]. However, as not all HSCT patients with multi-organ failure will die, absolute prognostication is not possible.

The outcomes of HSCT patients admitted to critical care may be improving with time and experience [9, 14]. Agarwal et al. found an ICU mortality of 39% in a cohort of HSCT patients admitted to critical care between 1998 and 2008 compared with mortality rate of 72% in the preceding 10 years. This was in spite of higher APACHE scores in the more recent group [14].

In summary, the decision to admit an HSCT patient to critical care, or escalate the level of support after admission, can be difficult and should be made jointly by HSCT and critical care specialists considering the degree of physiological derangement, the level of organ support required, the potential for reversibility, the longer-term prognosis of the underlying haematological condition and the patient's expressed wishes.

Conclusion

Haematopoietic stem cell transplantation is now a relatively common medical procedure in most tertiary adult and paediatric centres. Despite refinements and better supportive care, there remains a substantial level of risk intrinsic to HSCT procedures. Understanding the process of HSCT, its potential outcomes and intrinsic toxicities, along with the justification for taking risks, should help to optimize clinical management of HSCT patients and support of their families. HSCT teams should work closely with critical care colleagues not only in the acute day-to-day management of shared patients but also in the educational and training programmes, production of policies and protocols and audit of outcomes of HSCT patients admitted to critical care.

References

1 Apperley J, Carreras E, Gluckman E, Masszi T. Haematopoietic Stem Cell Transplantation. The EBMT Handbook. 6th edition. Paris: European School of Haematology/Forum service editoire; 2011.

2 McDowall KL, Hart AJ, Cadamy AJ. The outcomes of adult patients with haematological malignancy requiring admission to the intensive care unit. JICS 2011;12:112–25. http://journal.ics.ac.uk/pdf/1202112.pdf (accessed on November 1, 2013).

3 FACT-JACIE international standards for cellular therapy product collection, processing and administration. 5th edition. Omaha: Foundation for Cellular Therapy, 2012. Available at http://www.jacie.org (accessed on November 21, 2013).

4 Passweg JR, Baldomero H, Gratwohl A et al. The EBMT activity survey: 1990–2010. Bone Marrow Transplant 2012; 47(7):906–23.

5 Burger CD. Utility of positive bronchoalveolar lavage in predicting respiratory failure after hematopoietic stem cell transplantation: a retrospective analysis. Transplant Proc 2007; 39(5):1623–5.

6 Harris B, Lowy FD, Stover DE, Arcasoy SM. Diagnostic bronchoscopy in solid-organ and hematopoietic stem cell transplantation. Ann Am Thorac Soc 2013;10(1):39–49.

7 Shannon VR, Andersson BS, Lei X, Champlin RE, Kontoyiannis DP. Utility of early versus late fiberoptic bronchoscopy in the evaluation of new pulmonary infiltrates following hematopoietic stem cell transplantation. Bone Marrow Transplant 2010;45(4):647–55. Epub 2009 Aug 17.

8 Azoulay E, Mokart D, Rabbat A et al. Indicative bronchoscopy in hematology and oncology patients with acute respiratory failure: prospective multicenter data. Crit Care Med. 2008;36(1):100–7.

9 Afessa B, Azoulay E. Critical care of the hematopoietic stem cell transplant recipient. Crit Care Clin 2010;26(1): 133–50.

10 Hampshire PA, Welch CA, McCrossan LA, Francis K, Harrison DA. Admission factors associated with hospital mortality in patients with haematological malignancy admitted to UK adult, general critical care units: a secondary analysis of the ICNARC Case Mix Programme Database. Crit Care 2009;13(4):R137. Epub 2009 Aug 25.

11 Pène F, Aubron C, Azoulay E et al. Outcome of critically ill allogeneic hematopoietic stem-cell transplantation recipients: A reappraisal of indications for organ failure supports. J Clin Oncol 2006;24:643–49.

12 Bach PB, Schrag D, Nierman DM et al. Identification of poor prognostic features among patients requiring mechanical ventilation after hematopoietic stem cell transplantation. Blood 2001;98:3234–240.

13 Scales DC, Thiruchelvam D, Kiss A, Sibbald WJ, Redelmeier DA. Intensive care outcomes in bone marrow transplant recipients: a population-based cohort analysis. Crit Care. 2008;12(3):R77. Epub 2008 Jun 11.

14 Agarwal S, O'Donoghue S, Gowardman J, Kennedy G, Bandeshe H, Boots R. Intensive care unit experience of haemopoietic stem cell transplant patients. Intern Med J. 2012;42(7):748–54.

CHAPTER 22

Multiple Myeloma and Hyperviscosity Syndrome

Amin Rahemtulla[1] and Joydeep Chakrabartty[2]

[1] Department of Haematology, Imperial College Healthcare NHS Trust, Hammersmith Hospital, London, UK
[2] MIOT Hospital, Chennai, India

Myeloma

Multiple myeloma (MM) (myeloma) is a clonal B-cell disorder characterized by uncontrolled proliferation of plasma cells secreting immunoglobulins or light chains which can be detected in urine, serum or both [1]. Very rarely, the plasma cells may be nonsecretory. Plasma cells are mainly centred in the bone marrow but can also accumulate to form localized soft tissue or bone *plasmacytomas*. These can result in fractures or cause local compressive symptoms.

Myeloma accounts for approximately 1% of all cancers and 10% of haematological cancers. The annual incidence in the UK is approximately 4–5 per 100,000. Myeloma occurs in all races though the incidence is higher in Africans and African Americans. It is slightly more common in men. Myeloma is a disease of older adults. The median age at diagnosis is 66 years, and only 10% and 2% of patients are younger than 50 and 40 years, respectively.

In some studies, over 10% of myeloma patients required intensive care support for indications such as sepsis, acute renal failure and metabolic complications. Hospital mortality appears to be falling with time for myeloma patients admitted to intensive care, and admission to intensive care earlier after hospital admission has also been associated with lower mortality [2].

Clinical features and presentation:
• May vary from asymptomatic disease to increased tiredness, fatigue, bony pain and pathological fractures.

• Spinal cord compression.
• Symptoms of bone marrow infiltration causing anaemia, thrombocytopenia and recurrent infections because of low white cell count.
• Recurrent infections due to immune paresis.
• Renal failure secondary to cast nephropathy (myeloma kidney), amyloidosis, drugs, radiological contrasts, hypercalcaemia, etc.
• Hypercalcaemia causing confusion, pain and constipation.
• Hyperviscosity syndrome (HVS).
• Peripheral neuropathy is uncommon in myeloma at the time of initial diagnosis and, when present, is usually due to amyloidosis. An exception to this general rule occurs in the infrequent subset of patients with POEMS syndrome (osteosclerotic myeloma) in which neuropathy occurs in almost all patients.
• CNS involvement – Spinal cord compression from plasmacytomas is common, but leptomeningeal involvement is rare. When the latter is present, the prognosis is poor with survival measured in months. Rare cases of encephalopathy due to hyperviscosity or high blood levels of ammonia, in the absence of liver involvement, have been reported.

All myeloma cases have a prophase where a paraprotein can be found in the blood but without other features of myeloma. These plasma cell dyscrasias are monoclonal gammopathy of uncertain significance (MGUS) and the more advanced *smouldering myeloma*. Diagnostic criteria are explained in the following text [3].

Diagnostic criteria for multiple myeloma and related disorders
Multiple myeloma (all three criteria must be met)
- Presence of a serum or urinary monoclonal protein
- Presence of clonal plasma cells in the bone marrow or plasmacytoma
- Presence of end-organ damage related to the plasma cell dyscrasia, such as:
    ◦ Increased calcium concentration
    ◦ Lytic bone lesions
    ◦ Anaemia
    ◦ Renal failure

Smouldering (asymptomatic) multiple myeloma (both criteria must be met)
- Serum monoclonal protein greater than or equal to 30 g/L and/or greater than or equal to 10% clonal bone marrow plasma cells
- No end-organ damage related to plasma cell dyscrasia

Monoclonal gammopathy of undetermined significance (MGUS) (all three criteria must be met)
- Serum monoclonal protein less than 30 g/L
- Bone marrow plasma cells greater than 10%
- No end-organ damage related to plasma cell dyscrasia

Prognosis and staging: Serum β2 microglobulin and albumin at presentation can be combined to predict survival. Additionally, the cytogenetic markers $t(4;14)$, $t(14;16)$, deletion17p, deletion 13q and hypoploidy predict more aggressive disease.

Typical treatment strategies are discussed in Chapter 24.

Common medical emergencies in myeloma
Infections
Early infection is common in myeloma with up to 10% of patients dying of infective causes within 60 days of diagnosis. Atypical or opportunistic infections such as *Pneumocystis* pneumonia may occur after starting chemotherapy or stem cell transplantation, and viral infections such as *varicella zoster* reactivation (shingles) are frequently encountered. Most patients now receive prophylaxis when treatment is started. Chemotherapy may result in neutropenia and result in further Immunodeficiency.

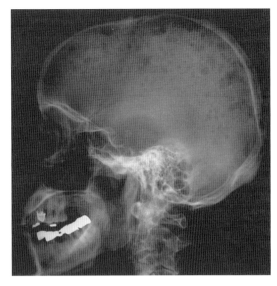

Figure 22.1 Skull x-ray of a patient with myeloma showing multiple lytic lesions.

Steroid doses are reduced in elderly patients to minimize toxicity and death due to infection. When treating bacterial infection, aminoglycosides or other nephrotoxic antibiotics should be used cautiously.

Myeloma bone disease
This can be localized, presenting with a fracture or more diffusely with osteopenia or multiple lytic lesions (Figure 22.1). Although a skeletal survey has been used traditionally (x-rays of the axial skeleton), magnetic resonance imaging (MRI) is a more sensitive imaging modality. Bone fractures and impending fractures might need orthopaedic intervention, and a single fraction of radiotherapy (8–10 gy) helps to reduce pain as well as improve healing. Bisphosphonate therapy should be instituted in all patients.

Vertebral fractures and collapse can be treated with pain killers, rest, thromboprophylaxis when immobile, palliative radiotherapy and procedures such as vertebroplasty or kyphoplasty.

Spinal cord compression
This is manifested by weakness, sphincter disturbance, sensory loss and paraesthesia. This occurs in around 5% of patients during the course of their disease. If there is a clinical suspicion of spinal cord compression, then the patient should be commenced on steroids (dexamethasone 40 mg daily for 4 days) and investigated urgently

with an MRI scan or a CT scan if MRI is unavailable. Structural compression or spinal instability requires surgery. Otherwise, urgent radiotherapy is the treatment of choice. If compression is the presenting feature of myeloma, a full diagnostic workup is required with systemic therapy started as quickly as possible.

Hypercalcaemia

Approximately 10% of patients have hypercalcaemia at diagnosis, which is attributed to increased osteoclast activity. This may be asymptomatic or present with anorexia, nausea, vomiting, polyuria, polydipsia, constipation, weakness, pancreatitis, confusion or stupor. By inhibiting antidiuretic hormone secretion, hypercalcaemia can dehydrate and contribute to renal impairment. Older patients may have more pronounced neurological symptoms at lower concentrations of serum calcium. Bisphosphonates are important agents for the treatment of hypercalcaemia in myeloma. They inhibit osteoclast activation and thereby inhibit bone resorption. These drugs can themselves cause renal impairment and require dose reduction in renal failure. A self-limiting acute-phase reaction of fever, arthralgia and headache can occur in up to 30% of first infusions of a nitrogen-containing bisphosphonate. Osteonecrosis of the jaw is another complication, and when started for bone disease, dental review and any necessary extractions should be carried out prior to the commencement of intravenous (IV) bisphosphonates. This is seldom possible in the acute setting of hypercalcaemia.

Management of hypercalcaemia
• Consider alternative causes, e.g. hyperparathyroidism, thiazide diuretics, excess vitamin D intake, thyrotoxicosis or a calcium-binding paraprotein.
• If mild (corrected calcium 2.6–2.9 mmol/L), oral or IV fluids.
• If moderate or severe (corrected calcium >2.9 mmol/L), prescribe IV fluids (normal saline) and a bisphosphonate. Consider a loop diuretic (improves urinary calcium excretion) if not hypovolaemic.
  ○ Zoledronic acid is recommended as a first-line bisphosphonate if renal function is normal and can be repeated after 72 h if hypercalcaemia persists [3].
  ○ In severe renal impairment (creatinine clearance <30 mL/min), consider pamidronate at a reduced dose of 30 mg over 2–4 h [3].

• In refractory cases, consider steroids or calcitonin.
• In renal or cardiac failure, dialysis may be required.
• Myeloma-driven hypercalcaemia is also an indication for anti-myeloma therapy.

Renal failure

Renal impairment affects up to 50% of patients during the course of their disease, and although reversible in most cases, 2–12% will require renal replacement therapy. There are multiple reasons for renal failure in MM, and although renal biopsy is sometimes helpful to distinguish the cause, the majority of cases are due to light-chain damage to the renal tubules as a result of cast nephropathy (myeloma kidney).

 Management of acute renal failure
• Stop nephrotoxic drugs (e.g. nonsteroidal anti-inflammatory drugs, aminoglycosides, radiological contrasts).
• Treat hypercalcaemia , hyperuricaemia and sepsis.
• Rehydrate with IV fluids (central venous pressure monitoring and consider early nephrology input).
• Dexamethasone (typically 40 mg daily for 4 days) is effective at reducing serum-free light chains (SFLC) and should be started while investigations are being carried out. Definitive therapy should be started without delay. Bortezomib with dexamethasone would usually be considered as first-line therapy in renal impairment due to their rapid reduction of SFLC. SFLC should be monitored during treatment.
• Haemodialysis may be required for severe renal impairment. The successful use of plasma exchange or large-pore haemofiltration to remove SFLC and enable dialysis withdrawal has been reported, and further studies are underway.

Bleeding and thrombosis

Though bleeding is not commonly seen at presentation, troublesome bleeding can occur as a result of disease progression, thrombocytopenia (immune mediated or due to marrow infiltration), renal failure, infection and treatment toxicity. Additionally, the paraprotein in myeloma has, in some cases, been reported to cause bleeding due to acquired von Willebrand disease (VWD), platelet dysfunction, fibrin polymerization defects, hyperfibrinolysis or circulating heparin-like anticoagulant. Patients with secondary AL amyloidosis may develop factor X deficiency. A careful clinical and laboratory evaluation is therefore required. Though there is no consensus in treatment of bleeding, plasma exchange, IV immuno-globulins, desmopressin, prothrombin complex concen-trates, recombinant factor VIIa and splenectomy have all been used, depending on the causative factor.

Myeloma and other plasma cell disorders have a well-established association with venous thromboembolism (VTE). Drugs such as thalidomide and lenalidomide fur-ther increase the risk of thrombosis such that outpatients receiving these agents also receive risk-assessed primary thromboprophylaxis with aspirin, low-molecular-weight heparin or warfarin. Steroids, immobilization, active can-cer and hyperviscosity all contribute to the risk of throm-bosis. Adequate thromboprophylaxis should be ensued during an intensive care admission, and a very low threshold should be maintained for treatment and inves-tigations relating to possible thromboembolism.

Hyperviscosity syndrome (HVS)

This is a clinical condition resulting from increased blood viscosity [4]. This can be either due to proteins such as immunoglobulins as seen most commonly in Waldenström's macroglobulinaemia (WM) and myeloma or due to cellular elements such as a high white cell count in acute leukaemia (leukostasis) or high red cell count in polycythaemia. The management of leukostasis and polycythaemia is discussed in Chapter 4.

Pathophysiology

In normal subjects, fibrinogen is the major determinant of blood viscosity. In paraproteinaemias, such as WM and myeloma, excessive amounts of circulating immuno-globulins are produced. IgM is the largest immunoglobu-lin (molecular weight, 900,000) and is predominantly intravascular. It is therefore the most likely paraprotein to cause hyperviscosity, but HVS has also been documented in cases of myeloma with other types of paraprotein, most commonly IgA.

Clinical features: The classic triad of neurological abnormalities, bleeding and visual disturbances is not always seen.
• Neurological symptoms include confusion, somnolence, vertigo, ataxia, headaches, seizures, stroke and coma.
• Retinal changes include sausage-like beading in the retinal veins, retinal haemorrhage, exudates and papil-loedema.

• Mucosal haemorrhage arises from the circulating para-protein interfering with platelet function. Bleeding time may be prolonged.
• Cardiac and pulmonary symptoms include shortness of breath, acute respiratory failure and hypotension.
• Without prompt treatment, patients may develop con-gestive heart failure, acute tubular necrosis, pulmonary oedema with multi-organ failure and death.

Diagnosis

Though the diagnosis is mainly clinical, confirmation can be achieved by measuring the plasma viscosity. Though it is not always proportional to symptoms, values between 2 and 4 are only rarely symptomatic, while symptoms occur in most patients with values between 5 and 8. Values above 10 are invariably associated with symptoms.

Treatment: Patients with HVS due to paraproteinae-mias, presenting with severe neurological impairment, such as stupor or coma, should be treated urgently with plasmapheresis which can reverse most clinical manifes-tations. Visual disturbance is another urgent indication for treatment due to the risk of retinal haemorrhage or detachment leading to permanent visual loss. Initial one plasma volume exchange, replaced with albumin and saline, is repeated daily until symptoms subside and then at intervals to keep viscosity below the symptomatic threshold. Cascade filtration, with on-line separation of the large-molecular-weight polymers with a *secondary* filter, can be used in patients in whom excessive volume is problematic such as those in heart failure. Plasma exchange by itself does not affect the disease process; therefore, chemotherapy should be started immediately to treat the cause.

References

1 Palumbo A, Anderson K. Multiple myeloma. N Engl J Med 2011;364(11):1046–60.
2 Peigne V, Rusinova K, Karlin L et al. Continued survival gains in recent years among critically ill myeloma patients. Intensive Care Med 2009;35(3):512–8.
3 Bird JM, Owen RG, D'Sa S et al. Guidelines for the diagnosis and management of multiple myeloma 2011. Br J Haematol 2011;154(1):32–75.
4 Stone MJ, Bogen SA. Evidence-based focused review of management of hyperviscosity syndrome. Blood 2012; 119(10):2205–8.

CHAPTER 23

Palliative Care for the Patient with Haematological Malignancy in Intensive Care

Suzanne Kite

Palliative Care Team, St James's University Hospital, Leeds, UK

Introduction

Nearly one-fifth of patients dying from haematological malignancy will do so on ICU [1]. The majority of haematology patients who require ICU will do so as the consequence of prolonged and highly intensive hospital treatment. Therefore, there will usually have been opportunities to clarify the patient's preferences and priorities regarding intensity of treatment, location of care and life goals, all of which underpin medical decision-making and informed consent. Clear communication with patients and families is vital to prevent patients being cared for and dying in circumstances that they might not otherwise have chosen. This is particularly true for patients receiving treatments of uncertain benefit and known toxicity offered late in life. Identifying such patients early is crucial for providing best possible end-of-life care and support for their family and healthcare team. However, crisis management is sometimes inevitable, and the transition from stability and good response to critical illness and death can be very brief. Such a rapid transition in the goals of care, and the aspirations of patient and family, is an added source of stress at an already sad and distressing time, and this can have a major impact on all, including the healthcare team.

There is benefit in applying a palliative care approach to all ICU patients for whom recovery is uncertain as the core palliative care principles are those of good multiprofessional healthcare. Given the high mortality within ICUs, embedding high-quality end-of-life care in a systematic way within routine ICU practice offers the most reliable and effective way of meeting patients' palliative care needs. Most major centres have access to specialist palliative care (SPC) services for additional support.

Palliative care needs of haematology patients

The palliation of haematological malignancy can be challenging, requiring complex skills and experience:

• *Decision-making*: The relative benefits and harms of intensive medical treatments, including palliative measures, can be finely balanced, and a delay in diagnosing dying can have serious consequences for the patient and family. Difficult choices regarding location and intensity of care need to be informed by the skilful eliciting of patient preferences and priorities while maintaining realistic hope.

• *Communication*: Negotiating intent of treatment and communicating poor response and a change in direction requires excellence in communication skills, with patients, families and the healthcare team.

Haematology in Critical Care: A Practical Handbook, First Edition. Edited by Jecko Thachil and Quentin A. Hill.
© 2014 John Wiley & Sons, Ltd. Published 2014 by John Wiley & Sons, Ltd.

• *Symptom management*: Debilitating symptoms are common and require a multifaceted approach which can be adapted as the intention of treatment evolves.
• *Psychological support*: The need for psychological and emotional support of patients and carers can be considerable.
• *Care planning*: Coherent, prioritization of present and anticipated needs into a realistic care plan, with review.

Models of palliative care provision

Patients with haematological malignancies are far less likely to receive SPC services than those with other cancer diagnoses [2] and are twice as likely to die in hospital [3]. In a retrospective review, 18% of patients dying from haematological malignancy died in ICU, with none receiving SPC [1]. Possible causes for this include a late diagnosis of dying, an ongoing management by the haematology and ICU team, an uncertain transition to a palliative approach and a highly technological palliation [2]. Prolonged hospitalization may also weaken relationships with primary and community care services, particularly for patients travelling a distance to a regional cancer centre.

Different models of palliative care provision to ICUs have evolved in response to local service provision. The two main models are as follows:

1 SPC team inreach, by physician, specialist nurse or multiprofessional team to see all patients requiring palliative care
2 Embedding palliative care in routine ICU practice via:
   a Staff training in palliative care skills
   b The introduction of tools and documentation to support best possible end-of-life care
   c SPC team support for patients and families with complex, unresolved needs

The latter is the preferred model in the UK [4, 5], as a workforce trained and skilled in end-of-life care offers the most consistent approach around the clock. There are particular advantages in this approach for clinical areas with a high mortality, such as ICUs. A systematic approach to support best possible end-of-life care decision-making, care planning, symptom management, psychosocial care and documentation is in keeping with the drive to improve the reliability, consistency and

quality of healthcare. An example is the development of a care bundle for those with limited prognosis for whom recovery from acute illness is uncertain [6]. Hospital-based SPC teams are available in most acute hospitals in the UK. SPC teams offer telephone advice and/or full patient assessment for symptom management, psychosocial support, support for carers and links with community-based SPC services and hospices, and SPC services are usually resourced to advise on those patients with complex, unresolved palliative care needs.

Palliative care assessment

Multidisciplinary assessment encompasses physical symptoms, psychosocial concerns and an understanding of the patient and family's insight and expectations, priorities and preferences. The assessment informs the overall care plan and the prioritization of symptom management and defines information and communication needs. A full assessment includes:

• What the patient and their family understand about their illness, prognosis and goals of care
• The patient's main concerns – physical, psychological, social, spiritual and financial
• The family's main concerns
• The patient's priorities and preferences regarding intensity of treatment approach, goals and location of care
• The impact of the illness and treatment on the patient and those close to them and their coping strategies
• What is important to the patient regarding their faith, beliefs and values

Such a holistic assessment is a process which underpins care from the time of diagnosis and which can be added to and reviewed as relationships with the treating team develop and transitions in care are reached.

Symptom management

Physical symptoms such as dyspnoea, fever, pain, haemorrhage and infection are common and frequently compounded by emotional distress, psychological concerns and insomnia. Cognitive disturbances due to direct disease involvement or delirium and drowsiness may be distressing and add to the complexity of symptom management. Treatment toxicities including mucositis, vomiting and diarrhoea or constipation also need to be addressed.

Particular care should be taken with patients unable to self-report pain, and an approach based upon the observation of behaviours and physiological variables, including the adoption of standardized scoring systems, may prevent undertreatment of distressing symptoms [7].

A systematic, stepwise approach to symptom management can be helpful (see Box 23.1).

Advance care planning

Illness or sedation prevents up to 95% of patients on the ICU from making their own healthcare decisions [8]. Where possible, opportunities should be sought to establish patient treatment goals and preferences earlier on in the course of the illness [5]. There is then the opportunity to plan accordingly and to obtain true patient consent to treatment. In particular, patients with advanced disease may not appreciate that in choosing hospital-based treatment, they may also be opting for hospital-based end-of-life care.

When patients lack the capacity to make medical decisions on their own behalf, the relevant legislation of the jurisdiction will apply, such as the Mental Capacity Act 2005 of England and Wales [9]. Steps should be taken to maximize the capacity of the patient to make necessary decisions wherever possible. In the ICU, it may be possible to stop sedative medication for individual patients in order to involve them directly in decision-making; however, this will be rarely appropriate or effective where the underlying illness is too severe or significant pain and suffering would ensue [7].

A clear plan regarding escalation of treatment, including CPR status, needs to be made, communicated and documented.

Withholding or withdrawing treatment

In the UK, professional guidance on withholding or withdrawing treatment is available [5]. For many haemato-oncology patients, the decision to withdraw intensive treatment will coincide with a rapid transition from

Box 23.1 An approach to symptom management.

1 Seek to elicit all the patient's physical and psychological symptoms and the interrelationship between them.

2 Assess each symptom for potential causes and evaluate the impact on the patient. Causes may be due to malignancy, noncancer causes (pre-existing, e.g. pain from arthritis, or new, such as pain from pressure areas) and treatment effects.

3 Correct the correctable where appropriate, i.e. where the burden of doing so is outweighed by the potential gain in patient comfort.

4 Agree a symptom management plan with the patient or with their family if the patient lacks capacity:
   • Based on a shared understanding of patient priorities and treatment intent.
   • Clarify expectations, particularly when symptoms may prove hard to control while maintaining realistic hope.
   • Setting interim goals can be encouraging.
   • Communicate plan to the whole team and document.

5 Review regularly and adjust treatment accordingly:
   • The timeline for review depends upon treatment severity. For severe, distressing symptoms such as pain, breathlessness and anxiety, this would be within the hour initially, with lengthening review as symptoms subside.
   • Persistent symptoms need regular, background control, with additional medication to be available p.r.n.

6 Update the patient, family and team regularly.

7 Consider non-pharmacological approaches, for example:
   • Repositioning may help pain and noisy oropharyngeal secretions.
   • TENS machines may help localized musculoskeletal pain.
   • Some patients find complementary therapies comforting.

8 Plan ahead and try to pre-empt problems if possible, or prepare patient and family for these if not.

9 Seek help:
   • Local symptom management guidelines may be available.
   • SPC team may be contacted for advice or for patient referral.
   • Professional guidelines may help to clarify the expectations of doctors in end-of-life care, e.g. 'Treatment and care towards the end of life: good practice in decision making' [5].

restorative to palliative care [7]. Patients and families will be faced with having to adapt to this sudden change at a highly stressful and emotional time when they are also called upon to inform decision-making. Clear communication of the situation, carer support and clarity of the purpose of a decision-making discussion, and the role of patient and family, are vital. Experienced clinicians will usually aim to:

• Establish and communicate the intended benefit, likely success, and associated timescales of the intervention at the outset, within the context of stage of disease and overall plan of care.

• Listen to the patient and carers, eliciting their understanding, values and wishes and acknowledging and addressing their emotions.

• Assess the patient's mental capacity for any specific decisions they need to make at any stage in the decision-making process and adhere to mental capacity legislation and to relevant professional guidelines.

• Participate in multidisciplinary assessment of the clinical benefit or otherwise of the intervention.

• Clarify the purpose of discussion regarding potential withdrawal of treatment:
  ○ To ascertain a patient/carers' view on the advisability of continuing a potentially beneficial intervention, i.e. participating in decision-making
  ○ To communicate a decision that treatment has not achieved its intended purpose and withdrawal of treatment is advised

• Offer assurance that the patient will continue to be cared for, will not suffer and will not be abandoned.

• Be aware of the potential for conflict between clinical team and patient/caregiver, how to manage this and the process to follow if it remains unresolved. Conflict may arise due to differing interpretations of the intended benefits of treatment. Clarifying expectations and seeking to achieve consensus is the first step, before discussion can progress to whether treatment received can achieve this:
  ○ Doctors are not obliged to offer physiologically futile interventions, but care must be taken to ensure that it is the futility of the treatment (i.e. it cannot achieve what it was intended to do) that is communicated rather than the impression that the patient's life itself is futile.
  ○ A second opinion may be needed and can be supportive for all concerned.

• Thoroughly review the efficacy and appropriateness of all medical treatments being received, in the context of the therapeutic goal. Regarding terminal care:
  ○ The focus is on comfort.

  ○ All interventions, monitoring and treatments that do not directly contribute to comfort can be discontinued.
  ○ More intensive treatment, such as non-invasive ventilation, may be indicated for the palliation of distressing symptoms in particular individuals.

• Clarify as necessary the distinction between euthanasia and the withdrawal of life-sustaining treatment that cannot achieve the therapeutic goals for which it was intended.

• Consider organ or tissue donation where appropriate.

Family members and those close to the patient have a particularly important role to play in the ICU setting where the majority of patients lack capacity. In the UK, the role of relatives and significant others in decision-making for the patient will be clearly laid out in the mental capacity legislation of the relevant jurisdiction.

Managing symptoms around the time of treatment withdrawal

Exacerbation of symptoms on withdrawal of intensive treatment needs to be considered and managed to prevent or minimize any suffering to the patient. Symptoms may be related directly to withdrawal of invasive treatment, such as dyspnoea, abnormal breathing patterns, increased airway secretions and agitation, or be a consequence of reducing sedative and analgesic infusions, with the resurgence of pain and convulsions.

The withdrawal of some interventions, such as dialysis, will not cause immediate distress, whereas cessation of mechanical ventilation needs careful planning. The evidence base regarding the technical aspects of withdrawing intensive treatment, including the indications and contraindications of weaning treatments and of neuromuscular blocking agents, is lacking, and clinicians need to draw on theoretical considerations and clinical experience [7]. Ventilatory support may be stopped abruptly with the administration of opioids and/or benzodiazepines at a dose to prevent dyspnoea, or it may be weaned down with concomitant titration of medications to manage symptoms. Ethically, there is no difference between these approaches, and the practicalities of patient experience should govern decisions [7].

Table 23.1 Approach to managing patients on intravenous sedatives and opioids.

Reassess delivery of sedation and analgesia	Route: will receiving wards be confident with the intravenous route if the patient is transferred from ICU?
	If an opioid or sedative infusion continues to be required, consider changing to a continuous subcutaneous infusion, with p.r.n. subcutaneous medication at a dose appropriate to the background dose prescribed
	Dose: are the doses prescribed to support intensive therapy still necessary?
For the individual consider	Analgesic and anxiolytic requirements prior to admission to ICU
	Current opioid and sedative infusion rates
	Plans to titrate intravenous infusions downwards
	Need for anticonvulsants
	Renal function
Background considerations	Conversion ratios between opioids vary, due to wide interindividual variation in opioid handling, and there is no national or international consensus. Therefore, local organizational guidelines should be consulted
	The first-line opioid for analgesia is usually morphine, but an alternative (e.g. alfentanil) may be required in the presence of severe renal impairment
	The SPC team can advise on the choice of opioid, probable doses and dose conversion ranges
	Opioid and sedative doses used to manage symptoms in palliative care can be significantly lower than those required for anaesthetic sedative purposes
	Pathophysiology and pharmacological site of action. For example, consideration of whether an intact neurocortex is required for optimal drug efficacy (e.g. for benzodiazepines) might influence the choice of drug and dose in patients in vegetative states
	Check and document dose calculations

During the transition from intravenous to subcutaneous infusions, the patient should be closely monitored and should only be transferred from ICU once symptoms are relatively stable with a management plan in place, including documentation of the rationale for the chosen drug regime

Pharmacological approach needs to be tailored to the individual patient, based on previous drug history, response to p.r.n. medications for symptom relief, current ICU treatment and likely physiological impact on treatment withdrawal:

• Considerations regarding intravenous sedatives and opioids are summarized in Table 23.1.
• Consider the pre-emptive use of intravenous methyl-prednisolone to reduce postextubation stridor [10]: a dose of 100 mg methylprednisolone at least 6 h before extubation has been suggested [11].
• Anticipate likelihood of excessive airway secretions after withdrawal of prolonged ventilation: look for iatrogenic overhydration and treat as appropriate with diuretics [11]. Consider the administration of hyoscine (e.g. 20 mg hyoscine butylbromide or 400 µg hyoscine hydrobromide) stat subcutaneously before extubation [11].
• Neuromuscular blocking agents may have been used therapeutically, and the decision on whether or not to continue or stop these after withdrawal of ventilation will need careful consideration on an individual basis, applying the principles of best practice in withdrawing

treatment (preceding text). The expectation is that neuromuscular agents would only be continued in very rare and exceptional clinical circumstances [7, 12], with clear documentation of the clinical objective for this management plan. There is no justification for starting paralytic agents de novo at the time of withdrawal of life support, and the intention of doing so would be seen to be deliberate termination of life [7, 12].

Technological palliation of symptoms, such as non-invasive ventilation, may be required as an interim or ongoing measure. Clear and coherent decision-making regarding the overall continuation and discontinuation of intensive treatments is essential to minimize patient burden and misunderstandings regarding goals of care.

Terminal care

Once a decision has been made to withdraw intensive treatment, the patient's terminal care needs must be assessed, and support for those close to the patient should be provided. An individualized care plan for terminal care should encompass assessment of information needs, symptom management, psychospiritual care, ongoing review, carer support and care after death. Symptom management for intensive care patients has been shown to be improved by regular, frequent and standardized assessment [11]. The following prompts may be useful:

Communication

For patients dying following treatment withdrawal in the ICU setting, there will usually be a shared understanding that death is now imminent. For other critically ill patients, the risk or likelihood of dying may need to be communicated. Patients and/or their families should be offered the opportunity to discuss:
• What to expect regarding symptoms and signs, and time course, including how this may vary between individuals
• What care and support will be provided and where
• How those close to the patient can be contacted and when
• Any other concerns they may have

Those close to the dying patient often ask whether or not their loved one can hear them. Dying patients can appear responsive to the human voice, and it is a good professional practice to communicate with and around dying patients as if they can hear, even if they are apparently asleep or comatose, and to avoid potentially distressing conversations for them in their earshot. Relatives can be encouraged to offer words of comfort to the patient.

Most ICUs will already have arrangements in place to contact relatives and to meet their needs such as for car parking, overnight accommodation and availability of meals.

Place of care

The decision on whether the patient should remain on ICU or be transferred back to the referring ward is an individual one. Family members can find such a move unsettling at a time when familiarity and confidence in healthcare staff is so important, and care should be taken to provide reassurance on continuity of care, to explore expectations and to ensure that their comfort and personal needs are considered.

Most people would prefer not to die in hospital, and it may sometimes be possible to arrange discharge home or to hospice for terminal care if this is the patient's wish and the necessary services can be arranged. A key consideration is the extent of technical symptom management support required, e.g. high-flow oxygen, or the management of indwelling drains and whether facilities exist to continue this support outside hospital. An individual's need for home nursing must be assessed, and the availability of round-the-clock nursing cannot be assumed. Discussion with community services at the earliest opportunity is strongly advised. Such discharges can be complex to arrange, but the benefit for patient and family can be huge.

Psychosocial and spiritual care

The patient, where possible, and their family should be given the opportunity to discuss what is important to them at this time, including their wishes, feelings, faith, beliefs and values. Familiar photographs or music may be comforting, and certain religious needs may need to be met. Chaplaincy staff can support both spiritual and religious needs and have the time to explore the patient's needs in greater depth.

Food and fluids

Patients should be assessed individually for their nutritional and hydration needs. Patients should be supported to take food and fluids by mouth for as long as tolerated. Symptoms of thirst or a dry mouth are often due to mouth breathing or medication/oxygen therapy and good mouth care is essential. The use of clinically assisted hydration needs to be considered on an individual basis, taking into account the pathophysiology of the patient's underlying medical conditions, their preferences and current symptoms.

If clinically assisted hydration or nutritional support is in place, review the rate, volume and route according to individual need. Possible benefits of withdrawing or reducing clinically assisted hydration/nutrition include reduced vomiting and incontinence and reduced painful venepuncture.

Symptom management

Please see Box 23.1 for an overall approach to symptom management and Table 23.1 for guidance on the use of sedative and opioid infusions. A plan needs to be in place to manage existing symptoms and to pre-empt other problems which may arise:

• Review the ongoing need for all interventions and medications and discontinue those no longer offering clear patient benefit. This includes review of routine blood tests, antibiotics, routine recording of vital signs, intravenous vasoactive medications and dialysis.

• Appropriate as needed medication should be prescribed p.r.n. for symptoms common in the last hours or days of life, particularly for pain, agitation, dyspnoea, nausea and retained oropharyngeal secretions. Consult local symptom algorithms as appropriate. As a minimum, p.r.n. medication to be prescribed subcutaneously should include opioid analgesic, sedative/anxiolytic/anticonvulsant, broad-spectrum antiemetic and antisecretory agent to treat retained oropharyngeal secretions (e.g. hyoscine or glycopyrronium).

• Respiratory tract secretions. Retained oropharyngeal secretions in those too weak to swallow or expectorate effectively may pool in the upper airways causing a rattling noise that may be unfamiliar and distressing for those close to them:

  ◦ Reassurance should be given that it is unlikely to be distressing the patient.

  ◦ Repositioning of the patient may help.

  ◦ Antisecretory drugs should be used promptly, followed by continuous subcutaneous infusion.

  ◦ For resistant secretions, consider other causes such as gastric or chest secretions and manage accordingly.

  ◦ Occasionally, suctioning may be required but should only be used after careful consideration of the particular benefits and burdens for the individual patient.

• Comfort care:

  ◦ Good regular mouth care (minimum hourly).

  ◦ Pressure area care.

  ◦ Positioning.

  ◦ Continence – consider catheter, convene or pads and monitor for signs of retention.

  ◦ Bowel care – assess for bowel problems that may cause discomfort, such as constipation or diarrhoea.

• Those close to the patient should be prepared for the symptoms and signs of the dying process, particularly if these are likely to be difficult to manage or potentially distressing. Tracheal obstruction, haemorrhage and fits are rare and can usually be anticipated and planned for with the nursing team, with appropriate p.r.n. medication available to relieve distress, and sedation is sometimes necessary. Family may well be unfamiliar with the possibility of noisy breathing, and the abnormal breathing pattern that may precede death, characterized by gasping, laboured breathing and sometimes myoclonus. The term *agonal respiration*, while correct, is best avoided as it may imply *agony* to family members [7]. Reassurance that the patient will not be suffering as a result of these should be provided.

• If symptoms prove difficult to control, explanation on the reasons for this should be given, along with the proposed management plan including timescales for review.

Care after death

Assistance with practicalities will be appreciated, not least with the timely issuing of the death certificate and thoughtful return of property. High-quality terminal care, considerate care of the body after death and the comfort and support offered to the bereaved can have a lasting impact on the memories of those left behind. Conversely, poor care at the end of life can be an enduring source of distress, eclipsing excellent care earlier on in the illness.

References

1 Ansell P, Howell D, Garry A et al. What determines referral of UK patients with haematological malignancies to palliative care services? Palliat Med 2007;21:487–92.

2 Howell D, Shellens R, Roman E, Garry AC, Patmore R, Howard MR. Haematological malignancy: are patients appropriately referred for palliative and hospice care? Palliat Med 2011;25(6):630–41.

3 Howell D, Roman E, Cox H et al. Destined to die in hospital? Systematic review and meta-analysis of place of death in haematological malignancy. BMC Palliat Care 2010;9(9).

4 Department of Health. End of Life Care Strategy. London: DH; 2008.

5 GMC. Treatment and Care Towards the End of Life: Good Practice in Decision Making. General Medical Council; 2010. www.gmc-uk.org (accessed on November 21, 2013).

6 Morris M, Briant L, Chidgey-Clark J et al. Bringing in care planning conversations for patients whose recovery is uncertain: learning from the Amber Care Bundle. BMJ Support Palliat Care 2011;1:72.

7 Truog RD, Campbell ML, Curtis R et al. Recommendations for end-of-life care in the intensive care unit: a consensus statement by the American College of Critical Medicine. Crit Care Med 2008;36(3):953–63.

8 Luce JM. Is the concept of informed consent applicable to clinical research involving critically ill patients? Crit Care Med 2003;31(3 Suppl.):S153–60.

9 Mental Capacity Act. 2005; www.opsi.gov.uk/acts/acts (accessed on November 21, 2013).

10 Cheng K-C, Hou C-C, Huang H-C, Lin SC, Zhang H. Intravenous injection of methylprednisolone reduces the incidence of postextubation stridor in intensive care unit patients. Crit Care Med 2006;34(5):1345–50.

11 Gay EB, Weiss SP, Nelson JE. Integrating palliative care with intensive care for critically ill patients with lung cancer. Ann Intensive Care 2012;2:3.

12 Kompanje EJO, Van der Hoven B, Bakker J. Anticipation of distress after discontinuation of mechanical ventilation in the ICU at the end of life. Intensive Care Med 2008;34: 1593–99.

SECTION 6

Admission to Intensive Care

CHAPTER 24

Haematological Malignancy Outside Intensive Care: Current Practice and Outcomes

Charlotte Kallmeyer

Department of Haematology, St James's University Hospital, Leeds Teaching Hospitals NHS Trust, Leeds, UK

Significant progress has been made over the last two decades in the treatment and prognosis of most haematological malignancies. The improvements in outlook have resulted in part from intensification in treatment, e.g. increased use of allogeneic stem cell transplant due to the introduction of reduced intensity regimens. However, most of the progress has been due to the introduction of novel agents with more targeted mechanisms of action than traditional DNA-damaging chemotherapy. In parallel, there have been improvements in supportive care, particularly regarding prophylaxis and treatment of infectious complications.

Despite the overall increase in survival for patients with haematological cancers, some patient groups have benefitted relatively little. These include in particular patients older than 65 years, whose outlook remains very poor for some diseases and generally inferior to younger patients. It is also worth noting that outcomes reported in trials tend to be better than in population-based analysis. This is due to the frequent exclusion of patients with poor performance status or short survival time from interventional trials. For a population-based summary of epidemiology and relative overall survival (OS) for different haematological malignancies, see Table 24.1.

Acute leukaemia

Acute myeloid leukaemia (AML)

This is the most common acute leukaemia in adults and represents a heterogeneous disease with the outcome heavily influenced by acquired genomic abnormalities. Median age at diagnosis is 66 years.

In younger patients (<60 years) and selected older patients without adverse disease features or significant co-morbidities, intensive therapy is given with curative intent. Therapy is generally divided into a remission induction and a consolidation phase. The mainstay of induction therapy for the last 40 years has been intravenous chemotherapy with cytosine arabinoside (Ara-C) in combination with an anthracycline, usually given for two cycles. The consolidation phase generally consists of regimens containing high-dose Ara-C for one to three cycles and/or, in patients with adverse disease factors, allogeneic stem cell transplantation. With current treatments, remission induction is successful in greater than 80% of patients [2]. A 5-year OS is 42% but varies considerably by disease risk status. For example, acute myeloid leukaemia (AML) with core binding factor translocations or isolated nucleophosmin-1 (NPM1) mutations has a 5-year survival greater than 60%, whereas corresponding survival for patients with adverse chromosome abnormalities is less

Haematology in Critical Care: A Practical Handbook, First Edition. Edited by Jecko Thachil and Quentin A. Hill.
© 2014 John Wiley & Sons, Ltd. Published 2014 by John Wiley & Sons, Ltd.

Table 24.1 Epidemiology of different haematological malignancies according to the National Cancer Institute based on the US population data 2005–2009.

	Median age at diagnosis (years)	Annual incidence (per 100,000)	5-year relative OS (%)
Acute lymphoblastic leukaemia (ALL)	14	1.6	65.2
Acute myeloid leukaemia (AML)	66	3.6	23.4
Chronic lymphocytic leukaemia (CLL)	72	4.2	78.8
Chronic myeloid leukaemia (CML)	64	1.6	59.1
B-cell non-Hodgkin's lymphoma (NHL)	66	19.6	68.2
Hodgkin's lymphoma (HL)	38	2.8	84.7
Multiple myeloma	69	5.8	41.1

Source: National Cancer Institute [1].
UK survival rates are on average 2–3% lower. Relative overall survival (OS relative to an age- and sex-matched normal population).

than 20%. The main complications of treatment are infections due to the prolonged period of severe neutropenia. Infections are usually bacterial and less commonly fungal in origin.

In older patients (>60 years), survival remains less satisfactory with cure rates of less than 10% and a disappointing median survival of less than 1 year overall. Swedish registry data indicate that for most patients up to 79 years of age, intensive therapy produces a better outcome with remission rates around 50% and a 2-year survival of 20% [3]. The relatively poorer outcome in older patients is not strongly influenced by age per se [4] but is due both to patient-related factors, i.e. co-morbidities, and disease-related factors, i.e. higher rate of adverse cytogenetic abnormalities. For frailer patients, low-intensity treatment, for example, with subcutaneous Ara-C or oral hydroxycarbamide, can achieve disease control for a period of weeks or months.

An important subtype of AML (10%) is acute promyelocytic leukaemia (APL), which enjoys a markedly superior long-term OS of greater than 80%. Treatment is based on chemotherapy with an anthracycline in combination with all-*trans*-retinoic acid (ATRA), which induces terminal differentiation of the abnormal promyelocytes. Recent data suggests that combination treatment of ATRA with arsenic trioxide can achieve similar outcomes and may allow cure without cytotoxic chemotherapy. Early death rate is still greater than 10%, mainly due to coagulopathy (fibrinolysis) and thrombocytopenia leading to haemorrhage. Aggressive management of such early complications is essential as patients surviving these will have an excellent long-term prognosis (see Chapter 4 for acute management of suspected APL).

Acute lymphoblastic leukaemia (ALL)

In contrast to children and adolescents, acute lymphoblastic leukaemia (ALL) is uncommon in adults. Similar to AML, the outcome for ALL patients differs significantly between patients less than 60 years and older patients. Treatment with curative intent consists of an induction phase usually containing dexamethasone, vincristine, asparaginase and daunorubicin, followed by exposure to cyclophosphamide and Ara-C. The consolidation phase generally contains agents to prevent central nervous system (CNS) relapse, e.g. intravenous methotrexate, and may include periods of intensification using similar agents as during induction phase. Treatment is completed by a long maintenance phase of oral mercaptopurine and methotrexate in addition to intermittent intravenous vincristine and intrathecal chemotherapy. Overall, in patients not undergoing allogeneic stem cell transplant, total treatment duration is around 24–30 months. Remission can be achieved in 80–95% of patients. However, the majority will relapse. Despite recent improvements, outcome in adults remains strikingly inferior to paediatric results, and long-term survival, even with intensive treatment, can only be achieved in around 30–40% of patients. Allogeneic stem cell transplantation instead of maintenance is considered for eligible patients with high-risk and standard-risk disease and results in long-term survival of around 50%.

Philadelphia chromosome-positive ALL (25%) previously resulted in very poor outcome. However, the addition of tyrosine kinase inhibitors (TKIs), primarily imatinib, to standard chemotherapy has led to dramatic improvements with achievement of remission in 90–100% of patients. The outlook in patients able to undergo post-induction allogeneic stem cell transplantation is now comparable to Philadelphia chromosome-negative ALL with a 4-year OS of around 40%.

The outlook for older ALL patients (>60 years) remains poor with a median survival of less than 1 year and long-term survival in less than 10%.

Treatment-related complications consist primarily of infections during the induction phase, with a particular risk of fungal as well as bacterial infections.

Chronic leukaemia

Chronic myeloid leukaemia (CML)

This was the first haematological malignancy in which the treatment and prognosis were revolutionized by the introduction of targeted treatment. The inhibition of the disease-specific Bcr–Abl gene translocation by the TKI imatinib has led to a 5-year OS of around 85% [5] and estimated median survival of greater than 20 years in patients with chronic-phase chronic myeloid leukaemia (CML). The response and outcome are comparable in older and younger patients.

Conventional chemotherapy treatment upfront is now obsolete for patients in chronic phase. Intensive AML-type chemotherapy and allogeneic stem cell transplant, however, are still recommended for patients with accelerated phase or blast crisis, as well as for patients developing resistance to TKIs.

Chronic lymphocytic leukaemia (CLL)

Chronic lymphocytic leukaemia (CLL) is unusual in its extreme heterogeneity of aggressiveness ranging from the indolent forms not requiring treatment for several decades to aggressive chemotherapy-resistant forms. The majority of patients (70%) are now diagnosed with stage A disease, often incidentally found on routine blood tests. Although treatment is not recommended in asymptomatic patients, there is increasing evidence that these patients have inferior survival compared to the general population.

Symptomatic disease can generally be controlled for several years with intermittent immuno-chemotherapy using rituximab, a monoclonal B-cell-specific anti-CD20 antibody, in combination with fludarabine, cyclophosphamide or bendamustine. Progression-free survival is around 6 years for initial treatment and 30 months for relapse treatment. Intensification of treatment with autologous stem cell transplant (ASCT) has not been shown to improve survival and is no longer routinely performed. Chlorambucil, the mainstay of treatment for several decades, is still a useful option in patients too frail for more intensive treatment.

Despite the generally indolent nature of CLL, a small group of patients (7% at diagnosis) has aggressive disease identifiable in particular by p53 deletion conveying a high degree of chemotherapy resistance. Treatment in these patients usually takes the form of high-dose steroids and/or alemtuzumab, a monoclonal antibody against CD52 expressed on lymphocytes and macrophages. However, long-term survival in these patients can only be achieved with allogeneic stem cell transplantation.

Chronic lymphocytic leukaemia-specific complications include infections, primarily bacterial and herpes virus infections, due to reduced immunoglobulin levels in almost all patients, and autoimmune phenomena like autoimmune haemolytic anaemia and immune thrombocytopenia due to dysregulation of the immune system. The introduction of highly immunosuppressive treatments, e.g. fludarabine and alemtuzumab, has led to an increased frequency of unusual or opportunistic infections like CMV and *Pneumocystis carinii*.

Lymphoma

Hodgkin's lymphoma (HL)

Hodgkin's lymphoma (HL) remains the most frequently cured lymphoma. Standard treatment for the last 25 years has consisted of chemotherapy with Adriamycin, bleomycin, vinblastine and dacarbazine (ABVD), resulting in a 5-year OS of around 85–90%. Radiotherapy to residual masses or areas of bulky disease remains part of standard treatment. Recent advances and trials have concentrated on intensification of treatment in patients with adverse features, e.g. identified by the early use of PET/CT scans, and de-escalation of chemotherapy/radiotherapy in good prognosis patients to avoid long-term side effects.

In contrast to most other haematological cancers, marked advances have been made in the cure rate of patients with poor-risk disease identified by a high International Prognostic Index (IPI) score, who can now achieve a 5-year OS of 70–75%.

Older patients greater than 60 years have a significantly lower response rate to treatment but can achieve a 5-year OS of around 50–65%.

Thirty to forty per cent of patients with advanced disease will eventually relapse. However, with the use of salvage chemotherapy followed by ASCT, these patients still have a significant chance of cure, resulting in OS of 50–80%.

B-cell non-Hodgkin's lymphoma (NHL)
Aggressive B-cell NHL
The most common subtype is diffuse large B-cell lymphoma (DLBCL) accounting for 30% of all lymphomas. This potentially curable disease has seen recent improvements in survival due to the addition of the monoclonal anti-CD20 antibody rituximab to standard chemotherapy with cyclophosphamide, doxorubicin, vincristine and prednisolone (CHOP). Depending on the risk factors incorporated into the IPI, 5-year OS rates are now between 50% and 90% [6] with average survival of around 65–75%.

Around one-third of patients will suffer from relapse. In relapsed patients able to undergo intensive chemotherapy with ASCT, cure rates of around 40% can be achieved. However, in patients not eligible for this approach due to co-morbidities or chemotherapy-refractory disease, cure is impossible, and treatment is palliative.

The other much less common aggressive non-Hodgkin's lymphoma (NHL) is Burkitt lymphoma, which is among the most proliferative cancers with a proliferation index of greater than 95%. It comprises 30% of paediatric lymphomas but less than 1% of adult NHL. Treatment consists of intensive combination chemotherapy including high doses of alkylating agents and CNS-directed therapy. As the tumour cells express CD20, rituximab now forms part of standard treatment. With this approach, cure rates in adults are around 65–90%. The outcome for patients greater than 40 years is significantly inferior to younger patients with a 2-year OS of 39% compared to 71%.

Due to the rapid cell turnover, there is a risk of tumour lysis syndrome with initial therapy.

Indolent B-cell NHL
This encompasses a diverse group of malignancies with distinct natural histories. Although incurable with standard chemotherapy, OS is excellent, and treatment is aimed at providing maximum quality of life with avoidance of treatment in asymptomatic patients. The exception is patients with localized disease, who have a cure rate of

70% with radiotherapy alone. Multiple treatment regimens are in use providing broadly comparable outcomes. These include chemotherapy with alkylating agents, e.g. cyclophosphamide, or purine analogues, e.g. fludarabine, immunotherapy with or without chemotherapy and local radiotherapy. The choice of treatment depends on patient factors, disease subtype, funding considerations and physicians' preference. In more aggressive forms or in relapsed disease, high-dose chemotherapy with ASCT may form part of standard treatment.

The most common subtype is follicular NHL accounting for 40% of all lymphomas in the USA and Western Europe. Disease aggressiveness and need for treatment can vary greatly, which is reflected in a wide range of 5-year OS rates between 52% and 90% depending on IPI scores [7]. In common with other low-grade lymphoproliferative diseases, it does not require treatment in asymptomatic patients. For patients with symptomatic disease, the introduction of rituximab to standard treatment has resulted in improved median survival of 12–14 years. The first-line treatment often takes the form of cyclophosphamide, vincristine and prednisolone with or without doxorubicin (CVP/CHOP) in combination with rituximab. A 2-year maintenance course of rituximab after initial treatment can improve OS further. For frail patients, treatment with chlorambucil still provides an acceptable balance of efficacy and toxicities.

Treatment options at relapse are similar to first-line treatment. In younger patients, ASCT should be offered, which results in a 4-year OS of around 70%.

Follicular NHL carries an inherent risk of transformation to high-grade disease, usually with a DLBCL phenotype. The risk is estimated at 30% over 10 years. The outcome for these patients is generally poor. However, DLBCL-type chemotherapy, consolidated with ASCT if possible, can lead to a 5-year OS of around 50%.

Marginal zone lymphoma (MZL) accounts for around 10% of B-cell NHL. It is divided into mucosa-associated lymphoid tissue (MALT), splenic and the rare nodal MZL. MALT lymphomas in particular are often initially driven by chronic infection or inflammation, e.g. *Helicobacter pylori* in gastric MALT lymphoma. Other associations include salivary gland involvement in Sjögren's disease, thyroid involvement in Hashimoto thyroiditis and splenic lymphoma in chronic hepatitis C. Gastric MALT lymphoma shows regression in two-thirds after *H. pylori* eradication. In non-responding patients, both low-dose radiotherapy and chemotherapy are appropriate options with excellent 5-year OS. Non-gastric MALT lymphomas, e.g. in salivary glands, thyroid gland and lungs, only show an occasional association with chronic infection. These lymphomas show a very indolent behaviour and can often be controlled with low-dose local radiotherapy, resulting in a 5-year OS of greater than 90%. Splenic MZL can be treated with splenectomy or splenic irradiation to control symptoms. If systemic therapy is required, agents similar to other low-grade lymphomas are used, e.g. rituximab with fludarabine. A 5-year OS for splenic MZL is around 70–80%.

Lymphoplasmacytic lymphoma/Waldenström's macroglobulinaemia accounts for only 1–2% of NHL. It is usually characterized by the presence of a monoclonal IgM paraprotein, which can cause hyperviscosity (see Chapter 22). In this situation, urgent plasma exchange is required. Treatment options in symptomatic patients include alkylating agents, nucleotide analogues and rituximab. Most combination treatments lead to progression-free survival of 3–4 years.

Mantle cell lymphoma (MCL) represents about 6% of NHL and occupies a position between indolent and aggressive lymphomas. It is characterized by generally advanced disease at presentation, frequently with extranodal manifestations, and aggressive course. In contrast to DLBCL, cure with chemotherapy alone is unachievable, and median survival is around 4–6 years. The addition of rituximab and the use of ASCT have improved the outcome for younger patients recently with a 5-year OS of 75–80%. However, the only curative strategy remains allogeneic stem cell transplant. The addition of rituximab should be considered with all chemotherapy regimens, which include similar drugs as DLBCL treatment, with the addition of Ara-C, e.g. the hyper-CVAD regimen.

T-cell NHL

T-cell NHL are much less common than B-cell NHL, accounting for only 10–15% of lymphomas in Western Europe and the USA. They include a number of distinct subtypes of varying aggressiveness. Treatment is similar to B-cell NHL with the exception of rituximab, which has no role in T-cell disease. Apart from very indolent forms like cutaneous T-cell lymphoma, the outcome generally is less good than in B-cell NHL.

Multiple myeloma

The introduction of several novel agents, in particular thalidomide, bortezomib and lenalidomide, over the last 20 years has improved OS significantly [8] such that many patients can now enjoy prolonged treatment-free periods.

For younger patients (<65 years), initial chemotherapy includes either an immunomodulatory drug, i.e. thalidomide or lenalidomide, or a proteasome inhibitor, i.e. bortezomib, with steroids and possibly an alkylating agent like cyclophosphamide. After maximum response, this is followed by high-dose chemotherapy with ASCT, resulting in a median remission duration of 3 years and a 3-year OS of 70–90%. With improvement in relapse treatment, OS for this age group is currently around 5 years.

Older patients follow the same treatment plan apart from omission of the high-dose chemotherapy/ASCT and have an OS of around 3–4 years. The effect of maintenance therapy, e.g. with lenalidomide or bortezomib, is currently undergoing evaluation. In addition, several second- or third-generation novel agents, as well as agents aimed at new targets, are being introduced into clinical practice and are likely to improve OS further.

Bone disease resulting in chronic pain or fractures remains one of the disease manifestations causing significant morbidity. Bone-protective treatment with bisphosphonates now forms part of standard care. Other factors impairing quality of life are side effects of treatment, in particular peripheral neuropathy and thromboembolic complications, as well as a disease-inherent impairment in immunity resulting in increased risk of infection, in particular bacterial. This remains the most frequent cause of death.

References

1 National Cancer Institute. Surveillance epidemiology and end results. http://seer.cancer.gov/statfacts/ (accessed on November 21, 2013).

2 Burnett AK, Hills RK, Milligan D et al. Identification of patients with acute myeloblastic leukemia who benefit from the addition of gemtuzumab ozogamicin: results of the MRC AML15 trial. J Clin Oncol 2011;29:369–77.

3 Juliusson G, Antunovic P, Derolf A et al. Age and acute myeloid leukemia: real world data on decision to treat and

outcomes from the Swedish Acute Leukemia Registry. Blood 2009;113:4179–87.

4 Walter RB, Othus M, Borthakur G et al. Prediction of early death after induction therapy for newly diagnosed acute myeloid leukemia with pretreatment risk scores: a novel paradigm for treatment assignment. J Clin Oncol 2011;29:4417–23.

5 Druker BJ, Guilhot F, O'Brien SG et al. Five-year follow-up of patients receiving imatinib for chronic myeloid leukemia. N Engl J Med 2006;355:2408–17.

6 Ziepert M, Hasenclever D, Kuhnt E et al. Standard International prognostic index remains a valid predictor of outcome for patients with aggressive CD20 + B-cell lymphoma in the rituximab era. J Clin Oncol 2010;28:2373–80.

7 Solal-Céligny P, Roy P, Colombat P et al. Follicular lymphoma international prognostic index. Blood 2004;104:1258–65.

8 Kumar SK, Rajkumar SV, Dispenzieri A et al. Improved survival in multiple myeloma and the impact of novel therapies. Blood 2008;111:2516–20.

CHAPTER 25

Early Care of the Unstable Patient: Preventing Admission to the Intensive Care Unit

Andrew Breen

Adult Critical Care, St James's University Hospital, Leeds, UK

Introduction

A requirement for admission to the intensive care unit (ICU) is associated with increased morbidity and mortality, and strategies to prevent critical illness are based on early recognition and treatment of disease. The aims of admission to the ICU can be to support a patient who has developed organ dysfunction or to try to prevent the development of worsening organ dysfunction in a patient at risk. As such, when caring for the unstable patient, preventing admission to ICU entails preventing early organ dysfunction, recognizing deteriorating organ dysfunction and then responding with organ support in such a way as to minimize the duration and severity of an episode of organ failure.

Although preventing admission to critical care is desirable in terms of limiting the severity of a disease process, a critical care facility may be the most suitable venue in which to intervene when a patient has shown early signs of deterioration. An example of this is a haemodynamically unstable patient who is in need of fluid therapy: although fluid administration can be carried out on a haematology ward, it can be delivered more accurately and judiciously in a critical care facility with the use of cardiac output monitoring.

Finally, one must consider whether the critical care environment has the potential to introduce risk to the patient's care. The risk of hospital-acquired infection may be higher in a critical care facility if the same levels of source isolation found on a haematology ward are not available. As with all areas of medicine, the benefit must outweigh the risk, and a judgement will frequently need to be made regarding whether admission to critical care is likely to be of overall clinical benefit.

The role of the critical care outreach team

Since 1999, critical care outreach teams (CCOT) have proliferated in UK hospitals. Among their many responsibilities and competencies, these teams aim to help in the early recognition and prompt treatment of patients at risk of developing organ failure. The service is ordinarily staffed by nurses and doctors with critical care training, and track and trigger systems are utilized by ward staff to inform the CCOT about patients who are at risk. Similar models exist throughout the world, and although there are differences in the way such teams are run, they share the common aim of reducing the impact of critical illness on a variety of patient groups.

Interventions delivered by CCOT include haemodynamic support through fluid management, physiotherapy, respiratory support and liaison between parent

Haematology in Critical Care: A Practical Handbook, First Edition. Edited by Jecko Thachil and Quentin A. Hill.
© 2014 John Wiley & Sons, Ltd. Published 2014 by John Wiley & Sons, Ltd.

medical teams and the critical care unit. The clinical evidence to support such interventions is currently lacking, despite attempts to assess the impact of CCOT on morbidity and mortality. The difficulty of conducting an RCT in this area is clear: outcome measures, such as ICU admission rates and mortality, are difficult to link to the activity of a team that provides many different interventions and other supportive actions. As such, there is little evidence in the literature that demonstrates an impact on patient mortality [1]. At the same time, the principles of early recognition and treatment of critical illness underpin CCOT, and these are principles that few would oppose.

Diagnostic strategy in the patient with organ dysfunction: Achieving early diagnosis

In all areas of medicine, early diagnosis is more likely to lead to more effective treatment. This is particularly true when a disease process has progressed to causing organ failure.

Diagnostic strategy in acute respiratory failure

The most common causes of acute respiratory failure in cancer patients are pneumonia, acute lung injury (ALI) and acute respiratory distress syndrome (ARDS), antineoplastic agent-induced lung injury and venous thromboembolism [2]. Admission to intensive care for respiratory failure in these patients carries an overall 50% mortality risk, and this is higher for patients requiring mechanical ventilation [3].

Pneumonia

In the patient with impaired immunity, a wider variety of potential pathogens (bacterial, viral and fungal) can be expected, and accurate early diagnosis is more difficult. If sputum cannot be obtained, it is possible to obtain samples using fibre-optic bronchoscopy and bronchoalveolar lavage. Although this technique is considered safe, even in hypoxaemic patients, the use of non-invasive diagnostic tests is not inferior in yielding accurate diagnostic information [4]. Non-invasive tests are likely to be the safer option when conducted outside the critical care unit.

ALI/ARDS

There are no specific therapeutic interventions that are effective in ALI/ARDS. In particular, there are no ward-based interventions that can slow the progress of this pathology, and the main benefit of early diagnosis of this is to enable prompt referral for management in a critical care area. The syndrome is characterized by acute onset severe hypoxia (ALI, PaO_2/FiO_2 ratio <40 kPa; ARDS, PaO_2/FiO_2 ratio <27 kPa), bilateral infiltrates on chest X-ray and the absence of a cardiogenic cause. In addition, it is necessary to identify a precipitating factor, which can be an intrathoracic or extrathoracic inflammatory process.

Lung injury associated with anticancer agents

Because of the multitude of pulmonary-toxic effects of anticancer therapies, it is never straightforward diagnosing this aetiology of respiratory failure. A diagnosis can be made only by integrating the findings from the clinical history, imaging and biopsy or sampling. Cessation of the suspected trigger, and the judicious use of supplemental oxygen if bleomycin-induced lung injury is suspected, may slow the process and avert ICU admission.

Diagnostic strategy in cardiovascular failure

Early intervention in cardiovascular failure is key to preventing other organ dysfunction. A simple diagnostic approach towards shock states enables prompt treatment, which can be instituted before critical care admission becomes necessary. In all shocked patients, the broad diagnostic categories are as follows:
- Vasodilatory
- Hypovolaemic (including distributive)
- Cardiogenic

Commonly, these conditions will coexist, and a careful clinical approach is necessary to guide early management. Of these, only hypovolaemia can be treated effectively outside of the critical care environment and should be diagnosed as quickly as possible. The accurate diagnosis of hypovolaemia is important, as excessive fluid administration can be harmful, and is frequently encountered when overzealous fluid resuscitation has been carried out in the face of a euvolaemic state. Following a review of fluid balance, a straightforward test of hypovolaemia is the passive leg-raise test: after recording of a patient's pulse and blood pressure, the patient's legs are elevated to an angle of 45°. After 30 s, the observations are repeated. If the blood pressure has improved, hypovolaemia is likely to be a significant component of the shock state [5].

The diagnosis of vasodilatory shock, most commonly seen in sepsis, can be difficult to make. Simple clinical signs of warm peripheries and rapid capillary refill are frequently absent: central vasodilatation of capacitance vessels results in relative hypovolaemia, and microvascular injury may coexist, leading to capillary leakage and thrombosis. Vasodilatory shock must always be suspected in patients with a suspected focus of infection who are euvolaemic.

A useful adjunct to the assessment of shocked patients is the use of bedside echocardiography. The proliferation of handheld cardiac ultrasound systems has enabled clinicians to make rapid assessments of cardiac function by the bedside. Immediate diagnosis of severe left ventricular failure, right ventricular pressure overload, pericardial effusion or gross hypovolaemia can be made, and interventions can be guided accordingly.

Diagnostic strategy in acute kidney injury

Deteriorating renal function is classified according to the risk of renal dysfunction, injury to the kidney, failure of kidney function, loss of kidney function and end-stage kidney disease (RIFLE) classification [6]. The identification of the patient at risk, or with injury to the kidney, may help to prevent subsequent deterioration and requirement for renal replacement therapy (RRT). The definitions of each of these categories are as follows:
• Risk of renal dysfunction: increase in serum creatinine greater than 150% of baseline
• Injury to the kidney: increase in serum creatinine greater than 200% of baseline
• Failure of kidney function: increase in serum creatinine of greater than 300% of baseline

The most common general causes of acute kidney injury in the patients with malignancy are shock states, nephrotoxic drugs and tumour lysis syndrome. Others include sinusoidal obstruction syndrome, haemolytic uraemic syndrome and multiple myeloma [7]. A diagnostic strategy that rapidly targets those causes that may be reversible may avert the need for RRT. Patients with sepsis who do not require RRT have a better outcome than those who do require RRT.

The diagnosis and management of shock states are covered earlier in this chapter and rely on first excluding hypovolaemia where possible. This is of particular importance in acute kidney injury, as it is often the only immediately reversible aetiology in the patient at risk of kidney dysfunction. Cessation or limitation of nephrotoxic drugs, along with strategies to avoid tumour lysis syndrome, has the potential to prevent deterioration into the injury or failure categories of the RIFLE classification, but these interventions do not have an immediate effect. As with the management of hypovolaemia, early and judicious fluid resuscitation is the single most efficacious intervention available to the patient at risk of renal dysfunction.

Unlike in cardiovascular or respiratory failure, the support of the failed kidney with RRT is not likely to halt the progression of other organ dysfunction. Aside from the management of fluid overload in an oliguric patient, RRT cannot, therefore, be considered a strategy to prevent ICU admission and is not discussed in this chapter.

Interventions aimed at preventing ICU admission

These can be divided into diagnostic and treatment interventions. Diagnostic strategies in acute respiratory failure may enable prompt treatment and therefore prevent ICU admission. The two organ systems most amenable to supportive therapy that can prevent the development of further organ dysfunction are the respiratory and cardiovascular systems.

Ward-based respiratory support modalities

The initial support of the patient with hypoxaemic respiratory failure begins on the general ward, at the time when hypoxia is first detected. The action taken can be entirely supportive or may have some therapeutic effect, reducing the need for escalation of care to a critical care area. Any respiratory support that can be administered without endotracheal intubation can be considered noninvasive and can frequently be delivered safely outside of a critical care area.

Supplemental oxygen therapy should always be humidified. Failure to do this may exacerbate sputum retention causing atelectasis and cause dry and potentially inflamed mucous membranes, increasing patient discomfort and potentially the need for invasive respiratory support. Humidification devices can operate at room temperature, using an unheated bubble humidifier (*cold humidification*) or through a water bath heated to 37°C (*warm humidification*). Although warm humidification is the superior standard, it may be unavailable initially, and cold humidification should be commenced as an interim measure. Patients requiring low concentrations of supplemental oxygen can safely receive this through nasal cannulae, enabling humidification of inspired air in the upper respiratory tract. Flows of oxygen over 4 L/min cause excessive drying of nasal mucosa and insufficient humidification. All other scenarios demand warm humidification.

The administration of high-flow oxygen is required for those in need of higher fractional inspired oxygen concentrations (FiO_2). This can deliver humidified oxygen up to a FiO_2 of 1.0 and is practicable as a ward-based respiratory support modality. Such high oxygen concentrations have the potential to cause lung injury, and a rising FiO_2 requirement (e.g. FiO_2 >0.6) should trigger an escalation of respiratory support to a more effective modality.

Non-invasive ventilation: CPAP and BIPAP

Non-invasive ventilation (NIV) can provide an alternative to endotracheal intubation and may obviate the need for it. NIV can be delivered as continuous positive airway pressure (CPAP) and bilevel positive airway pressure (BIPAP). Both of these modalities alleviate respiratory failure by reducing the work of breathing and by restoration and maintenance of functional residual capacity (*recruitment*). The advantages of NIV over invasive ventilation include:

1 Can be delivered outside of critical care with appropriate training
2 Improved patient comfort
3 Earlier respiratory support
4 Continued patient co-operation with physiotherapy, mobilization, eating and drinking
5 Maintenance of upper airway humidification
6 Avoidance of sedation

When a patient first becomes hypoxic, CPAP is an appropriate support, helping to preserve the functional residual capacity and aiding pulmonary mechanics by placing the patient on a favourable part of the pressure–volume curve. If, despite this, the patient develops CO_2 retention, BIPAP may be more appropriate. This mode of NIV provides pressure support to the patient, reducing the work of breathing yet further and reducing CO_2 production.

Early intervention with NIV has been shown to reduce ICU admission. In patients with haematological malignancy with respiratory failure, early application of CPAP, for at least 12 h/day, continued for 4 days, prevents the evolution to ALI and mechanical ventilation [8].

Cardiogenic pulmonary oedema is not uncommon in patients with haematological malignancy, and NIV has been shown to be useful in the early treatment of cardiogenic pulmonary oedema. This is likely to be due not just to a positive effect on respiratory mechanics but also to the improvement in cardiovascular physiology it affords: decreased venous return, reduction in afterload and reduced transmural pressure across the myocardial wall all contribute to a more favourable myocardial oxygen supply/demand ratio. Although it has not been reliably shown to reduce mortality, it does induce more rapid improvement in respiratory failure and metabolic disturbance [9].

The early use of NIV, as an adjunct to the aggressive treatment of pulmonary infection with antibiotics and physiotherapy, has undoubted value in the prevention of admission to critical care. Both CPAP and BIPAP have a role to play, and although these interventions do require some additional resources for a general ward, NIV can be delivered safely outside the critical care environment, especially with the support of the CCOT.

Cardiovascular failure: The initial treatment of shock

As discussed earlier in this chapter, the diagnosis and treatment of hypovolaemia can be carried out on a general ward, but no additional form of cardiovascular support is available outside of the critical care environment. A careful approach to the use of intravenous fluid therapy must be used, and the potential harmful effects of excessive fluid administration cannot be overstated: the evolution of ARDS can be greatly accelerated in the setting of fluid overload, and the requirement for invasive mechanical ventilation is strongly associated with a higher mortality. The following fluid administration (Figure 25.1) algorithm is proposed, as a guide to fluid resuscitation

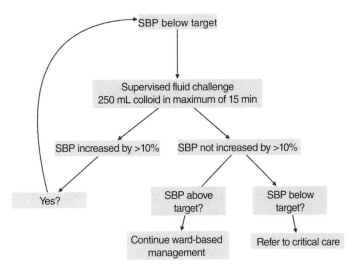

Figure 25.1 Suggested ward protocol for initial fluid resuscitation in the hypotensive patient. Repeated fluid boluses when the patient is volume responsive and cessation of fluid boluses when the patient is not volume responsive ensure maximal oxygen delivery while avoiding fluid overload. SBP, systolic blood pressure.

on the haematology ward. This practical approach is transferable to all areas of clinical medicine and aims to maximize cardiac output and oxygen delivery while avoiding the harmful effects of over-transfusion of fluids. This schema requires an individualized assessment of the patient's target systolic blood pressure (SBP). Precise targets based on urine output, acidosis and cerebration are often difficult to judge accurately, but a mean arterial pressure of at least 65 mmHg is recommended. As the mean arterial pressure may not always be possible to ascertain outside of the critical care environment, a target systolic pressure of 90–100 mmHg is a reasonable initial goal.

Early interventions in the ICU: Preventing deterioration to multiple organ failure

The ward-based interventions described thus far have been aimed at preventing ICU admission. It should be noted, however, that many of these approaches might be carried out more effectively in the critical care environment. Early transfer of patients to ICU may provide several advantages:
- Continuous vital sign monitoring
- Invasive haemodynamic monitoring
- Access to point-of-care testing, e.g. arterial blood gas analysis, haemoglobin, electrolytes and lactate
- Favourable nurse/patient and doctor/patient ratios
- Safer environment for sedation, e.g. to facilitate NIV

In this respect, ICU admission may be considered advantageous, as early management of the deteriorating patient has the potential to be carried out more effectively in the ICU environment. This approach does, of course, place a significant burden on critical care services, and it is rarely possible to admit all patients at risk of deterioration for this purpose.

Summary

Preventing admission to ICU has the potential to improve the outcome in many vulnerable groups of patients. Early recognition of the at-risk patient, prompt assessment and rapid liaison with CCOT give the best chance of reversal of deteriorating organ dysfunction. Ward-based organ support strategies may be sufficient to achieve this, but earlier admission to the ICU allows for closer monitoring, more aggressive treatment and improved patient safety. ICU admission should not be seen as a failure of ward-based therapy in such cases, but as an enhanced quality of care.

References

1 Cuthbertson BH. The impact of critical care outreach: is there one? Crit Care 2007;11(6):179. Epub December 19, 2007.

2 Pastores SM, Voigt LP. Acute respiratory failure in the patient with cancer: diagnostic and management strategies. Crit Care Clin 2010;26(1):21–40. Epub December 1, 2009.

3 Azoulay E, Thiery G, Chevret S et al. The prognosis of acute respiratory failure in critically ill cancer patients. Medicine 2004;83(6):360–70. Epub November 5, 2004.

4 Azoulay E, Mokart D, Lambert J et al. Diagnostic strategy for hematology and oncology patients with acute respiratory failure: randomized controlled trial. Am J Respir Crit Care Med 2010; 182(8):1038–46. Epub June 29, 2010.

5 Monnet X, Rienzo M, Osman D et al. Passive leg raising predicts fluid responsiveness in the critically ill. Crit Care Med 2006;34(5):1402–7. Epub March 17, 2006.

6 Bellomo R, Ronco C, Kellum JA, Mehta RL, Palevsky P. Acute renal failure – definition, outcome measures, animal models, fluid therapy and information technology needs: the Second International Consensus Conference of the Acute Dialysis Quality Initiative (ADQI) Group. Crit Care 2004;8(4): R204–12. Epub August 18, 2004.

7 Benoit DD, Hoste EA. Acute kidney injury in critically ill patients with cancer. Crit Care Clin 2010;26(1):151–79. Epub December 1, 2009.

8 Squadrone V, Massaia M, Bruno B et al. Early CPAP prevents evolution of acute lung injury in patients with hematologic malignancy. Intensive Care Med 2010;36(10):1666–74. Epub June 10, 2010.

9 Gray A, Goodacre S, Newby DE, Masson M, Sampson F, Nicholl J. Noninvasive ventilation in acute cardiogenic pulmonary edema. N Engl J Med 2008;359(2):142–51. Epub July 11, 2008.

CHAPTER 26

Decisions to Intensify Treatment: Who Will Benefit from Intensive Care?

Quentin A. Hill[1] and Peter A. Hampshire[2]

[1] Department of Haematology, Leeds Teaching Hospitals NHS Trust, Leeds, UK
[2] Department of Critical Care, Royal Liverpool and Broadgreen University Hospitals NHS Trust, Liverpool, UK

Patients with haematological malignancy (HM) currently account for 1–2% of admissions to the intensive care unit (ICU) in England and Wales, but the incidence of common HM is increasing. In developed countries, survival of HM patients is also rising. For example, in England and Wales, the 10-year relative survival for patients with non-Hodgkin's lymphoma has more than doubled over the last 40 years from 22% to 51% [1]. Because of this, expectations have also increased, with the potential for cure even after initial relapse and the prospect of remission or effective palliation with third- or fourth-line therapies (usually chemotherapy).

Up to the early 1990s, hospital mortality above 90% was observed in some series of mechanically ventilated cancer patients leading to a perceived reluctance to admit cancer patients. Subsequently, hospital mortality has been falling (Figure 26.1.), and expert opinion now favours a much broader admission policy [2]. Hospital mortality of around 60% has been reported for unselected HM admissions [3] but remains higher in patients requiring invasive mechanical ventilation or multiple organ support.

Decision to admit

Early studies with high mortality led to interest in identifying factors that would help predict poor outcome and avoid inappropriate ICU admission. No variable in isolation is sufficiently reliable to solely exclude an individual patient from admission.

Indicators of a lower mortality risk:
- Bacterial infection as the reason for admission
  Uninformative at admission:
- Disease-related factors (e.g. type of HM, remission status, presence or length of neutropenia) do not predict short-term survival.
- Severity-of-illness scores, e.g. Acute Physiology and Chronic Health Evaluation (APACHE) II score. Although the strongest predictors of outcome, they can only be applied after admission.
- Autologous stem cell transplantation (Auto-SCT). In a systematic review, survival to hospital discharge in SCT patients and mechanically ventilated SCT patients improved from 12–23% and 4–6% pre-1998 to 30–61% and 18–26% post-1998 [4]. When analysed as a risk factor, Auto-SCT does not appear to provide further prognostic information.

Indicators of a higher mortality risk:
- Increasing age (some but not all studies)
- Poor performance status prior to hospital admission (from studies of unselected cancer patients)
- Number and severity of organ failures at point of admission

Haematology in Critical Care: A Practical Handbook, First Edition. Edited by Jecko Thachil and Quentin A. Hill.
© 2014 John Wiley & Sons, Ltd. Published 2014 by John Wiley & Sons, Ltd.

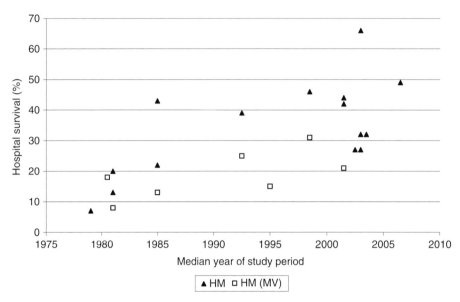

Figure 26.1 Comparison of survival to hospital discharge in studies of patients with haematological malignancy (HM) admitted to intensive care unit (ICU), by the median year of the study period. HM, patients with haematological malignancy; HM (MV), mechanically ventilated patients with haematological malignancy.

• Allogeneic SCT with respiratory failure and hepatic impairment (bilirubin ≥68 μmol/L) or uncontrolled graft-versus-host disease

A number of additional factors should be taken into consideration:

• Understand local guidance on withdrawal or withholding of life-sustaining therapy. This includes the local institution's policy (if available) and the professional and legal principles applicable to that state or country. The following discussion reflects recent guidance from the UK's General Medical Council [5]. While differences exist to (and within) the USA, a recent review suggests that a shared decision-making model is increasingly being adopted [6].

• Understand local, up-to-date audit data on outcomes of HM patients when deciding on the likely benefit of intervention. A limitation of published survival data is its applicability an individual unit, because of differences in patient selection criteria, type of patient and level of ICU support provided.

• Is the patient sick enough?
  ○ Better survival has been noted in myeloma patients with ICU admission early in the course of a hospital admission. Worse survival is associated with late admission [7] and more advanced multi-organ failure, while

in a prospective study of cancer patients referred for ICU admission, 21% of patients considered *too well* for ICU admission died before hospital discharge [8].
  ○ Patients with HM have higher severity-of-illness scores (indicating greater physiological derangement) at admission to ICU than general ICU patients, and this predicts higher mortality. This *risk factor* for poor outcome may potentially be modified by admitting HM patients to critical care units at an earlier stage. The use of physiological early warning scores and outreach services to trigger critical care assessment may reduce APACHE II scores and mortality, suggesting that this approach is beneficial [9].
  ○ Prompt admission allows non-invasive ventilation and intensive monitoring of physiological parameters before the development of irreversible organ failure.
• Is the patient too sick?
  ○ In the same study of referred cancer patients, 30-day survival was 26% among the patients considered *too sick* for ICU admission [8] although similar survival has been reported in unselected patients refused ICU admission because *too sick*.
  ○ Liaise with the treating haematology team to determine the patient's disease-specific prognosis and options for further life-prolonging treatments. Patients

unresponsive to treatment with a terminal and irreversible illness are unlikely to benefit from ICU care.

• What are the patient's wishes? This should have already been explored by the haematology team, but further discussion and ICU expert opinion may still be needed in the context of acute events. There must be a presumption of capacity, and if capacity may be impaired, the patient should be supported to maximize their ability to take part in decision-making.

  ○ *Patients with capacity*: The option of ICU care should be explored with the patient explaining the likely benefits, burdens and risks as well as being open about any underlying uncertainties. The option felt to be best for the patient may be recommended. The patient must weigh up the information provided as well as any non-clinical issues relevant to them and accept or refuse the options provided.

  ○ *Patients without capacity*: The laws surrounding advanced refusals of treatment differ depending on the legal framework of the country. The General Medical Council provides more detailed guidance on how advance directives should be assessed in the UK [5]. Even if not legally binding, advance directives can be taken as an indication of the patient's wishes. The patient may have appointed a legal proxy to make decisions on their behalf while they are incapacitated. Treatment options would then be explained to the legal proxy who can make decisions for a patient who lacks capacity. If there is no appointed legal proxy, consult with those close to the patient and members of the healthcare team (about the patient's known or likely wishes, preferences, feelings, beliefs and values) to help reach a view on what treatment would be of overall benefit to the patient. If there is a reasonable degree of uncertainty about whether a particular treatment will provide overall benefit for a patient who lacks capacity to make the decision, the treatment *should be started* in order to allow a clearer assessment to be made, although treatment may be withdrawn at a later stage if it is ineffective.

Resolving disagreement

Despite good communication about the benefits and burdens of treatment, there may remain disagreement between members of the healthcare team, or between

the healthcare team and the patient or those close to the patient. Doctors are not obliged to provide treatment they consider clinically inappropriate but must explain other options including a second opinion. Disagreement can often be resolved by seeking the advice of a more experienced colleague, obtaining a second opinion or involving an independent advocate. If intensive care support is still being requested, even if the overall benefit is doubtful, a limited trial of ICU support may be helpful in clarifying the clinical picture and achieving consensus.

Continuing care

Shared care involving the patient and their family, with regular input from the haematology team, is the best way to avoid conflict between clinical teams and the patient's family.

Role of scoring systems

The APACHE II and III, the Simplified Acute Physiology Score (SAPS) II and III and the Intensive Care National Audit and Research Centre (ICNARC) model all have reasonable ability to discriminate between surviving and non-surviving HM patients. All scores generally underestimate mortality in HM patients, predominantly in those with low predicted mortality (where APACHE II performs the best [7]). A cancer mortality model, which included certain cancer-specific characteristics (e.g. previous SCT) in addition to weighting physiological derangements, was developed. However, it failed to outperform general scoring systems when tested outside the original study population, again reflecting the failure of cancer-specific variables to predict short-term survival. Organ failure scores can predict mortality, but there are issues of accuracy, calibration and validation such that no scoring system can be used for an individual patient to decide treatment limitation.

How long to treat?

Severity-of-illness scores may also be used to identify patients who are not responding to treatment. Changes over the first days of ICU admission in the Sequential Organ Failure Assessment (SOFA) and SAPS II scores have been shown to predict hospital mortality in ICU patients with HM. However, changes in the scores do not predict individual outcome. Azoulay has advocated that a *trial of intensive care* be provided to most patients, i.e. unlimited organ support for three days with reappraisal of the extent of organ failure after this time [2]. Withdrawal of care should then be considered in those patients who are deteriorating at this point. This approach has the advantages of being objective, has some evidence to support it, maintains the principle of equity of access to intensive care and may limit resource use by restricting treatment to a defined time period. However, this approach assumes that patients destined to survive will unequivocally demonstrate stable or improving organ dysfunction after three days of intensive care treatment, which is not always the case. The length of mechanical ventilation or ICU stay are not in themselves predictors of survival. Decisions to withdraw active treatment must also take into account the emotional, religious and social dimensions that surround the end-of-life decisions as outlined earlier.

Areas of uncertainty

Quality of life and long-term prognosis in survivors

There are scarce data regarding the quality of life of survivors of critical illness with HM. In the study by Yau et al., survivors' quality of life was assessed. Six of seven survivors considered their quality of life to be good, and five had returned to work [10]. However, further larger studies on both long-term outcomes and quality of life are needed.

Why is survival improving and is there an advantage to dedicated haemato-oncology units?

Better survival could simply reflect greater selectivity of HM patients admitted to intensive care or to variations in case mix (e.g. medical vs. surgical). However, prospective data from Azoulay's group with defined admission criteria for mechanically ventilated cancer patients suggested that this is not the only factor. An improved overall standard of care delivered by ICUs may be one reason. There has been a steady reduction in mortality from approximately 30% to 25% over the last 15–20 years across all patients admitted to intensive care, despite the

severity of illness at admission remaining more or less constant. Cancer-specific supportive care may have improved, for example, antimicrobial prophylaxis and recombinant growth factors. More targeted therapies and higher response rates in patients with HM may have resulted in a treated population with better performance status and less treatment-related organ damage. Earlier admission and the increasing use of non-invasive ventilation in immunocompromised patients may have also had a role. Finally, most recent reported outcomes are from *high-volume* specialist cancer centres that treat a greater number of HM patients. Survival appears better in these centres than in general units.

In other areas of cancer and intensive care, a *volume–outcome relationship* has been described, whereby patients have a lower mortality when managed in centres that treat greater numbers of patients with certain conditions. Such relationships have been described for patients receiving invasive mechanical ventilation and cancer surgery. There is evidence for a beneficial volume–outcome relationship in patients with HM who develop respiratory failure and patients with cancer and septic shock [11, 12]. The reasons for this relationship are less clear but are thought to be due to organizational factors or greater clinical experience in high-volume centres.

Conclusion

Survival is improving for patients with HM both outside and following ICU admission, and although mortality remains high in patients requiring invasive mechanical ventilation and in multi-organ failure, a broad admission policy can be justified. Early admission for suitable candidates should be considered to prevent multi-organ dysfunction, preferably to a unit experienced in the care of cancer patients. Those patients with a terminal illness and unresponsive to treatment are unlikely to benefit from ICU care. When considering limitation of life-sustaining therapy either at time of admission or during the ICU stay, the patient (or, when lacking capacity, those close to the patient and the wider healthcare team) should be consulted and their preferences and values considered along with the reversibility of the acute illness when deciding on the overall benefit of treatment.

References

1 Cancer Research UK Cancer Stats. Cancer Research UK 2011 December 16 [cited 2012 Apr 3]. http://info.cancerresearchuk. org/cancerstats (accessed on November 22, 2013).

2 Azoulay E, Soares M, Darmon M, Benoit D, Pastores S Afessa B. Intensive care of the cancer patient: recent achievements and remaining challenges. Ann Intensive Care 2011;1(1):5.

3 Hill QA. Intensify, resuscitate or palliate: decision making in the critically ill patient with haematological malignancy. Blood Rev 2010;24(1):17–25.

4 Naeem N, Reed MD, Creger RJ, Youngner SJ, Lazarus HM. Transfer of the hematopoietic stem cell transplant patient to the intensive care unit: does it really matter? Bone Marrow Transplant 2006;37(2):119–33.

5 The General Medical Council. Treatment and care towards the end of life: good practice in decision making; 2010. http://www.gmc-uk.org/guidance/ethical_guidance/end_ of_life_about_this_guidance.asp (accessed on November 22, 2013).

6 Luce JM. A history of resolving conflicts over end-of-life care in intensive care units in the United States. Crit Care Med 2010;38(8):1623–9.

7 Hampshire PA, Welch CA, McCrossan LA, Francis K, Harrison DA. Admission factors associated with hospital mortality in patients with haematological malignancy admitted to UK adult, general critical care units: a secondary analysis of the ICNARC Case Mix Programme Database. Crit Care 2009;13(4):R137.

8 Thiery G, Azoulay E, Darmon M et al. Outcome of cancer patients considered for intensive care unit admission: a hospital-wide prospective study. J Clin Oncol 2005;23(19):4406–13.

9 Bokhari SW, Munir T, Memon S, Russell NH, Beed M. Impact of critical care reconfiguration and track-and-trigger outreach team intervention on outcomes of haematology patients requiring intensive care admission. Ann Hematol 2010;89(5):505–12.

10 Yau E, Rohatiner AZ, Lister TA, Hinds CJ. Long term prognosis and quality of life following intensive care for life-threatening complications of haematological malignancy. Br J Cancer 1991;64(5):938–42.

11 Lecuyer L, Chevret S, Guidet B et al. Case volume and mortality in haematological patients with acute respiratory failure. Eur Respir J 2008;32(3):748–54.

12 Zuber B, Tran TC, Aegerter P et al. Impact of case volume on survival of septic shock in patients with malignancies. Crit Care Med 2012;40(1):55–62.

SECTION 7

Point-of-Care Testing

CHAPTER 27

The Relevance of Thromboelastography in Intensive Care Patients

Jon Bailey[1] and Nicola S. Curry[2,3]

[1] Oxford University Hospitals, John Radcliffe Hospital, Oxford, UK
[2] Department of Haematology, Oxford University Hospitals, Oxford University, Oxford, UK
[3] Oxford Haemophilia and Thrombosis Centre, Oxford University Hospitals, Oxford, UK

Coagulopathy (hypo- and hypercoagulability) is common in the intensive care setting. Traditionally, coagulation potential has been assessed using plasma-based tests, such as the prothrombin time (PT) or the activated partial thromboplastin time (APTT); but these tests have repeatedly been shown to be poor predictors of bleeding and thrombosis [1]. Reliable prediction and/or diagnosis of clinically relevant clotting dysfunction and subsequent monitoring of effective treatment are important management issues in critically ill patients. Viscoelastic tests, such as TEG® or ROTEM®, are increasingly being used to predict coagulopathy and guide transfusion therapy. This chapter will briefly describe the mechanics of these tests, discuss their potential for use in the critical care setting and touch on the evidence that supports their use.

Viscoelastic tests

Both TEG® (Haemonetics Corp., Braintree, MA, USA) and ROTEM® (Tem International GmbH, Munich, Germany) are viscoelastic haemostatic assay (VHA) devices which assess the global elastic properties of clot formation under low shear stress. Whole blood (native or citrated) is used, and the interaction of coagulation

factors, and their inhibitors, with red blood cells and platelets during clotting and fibrinolysis is evaluated, usually over 60 min. Both devices measure the speed of clot formation, the strength and stability of the clot when formed and the kinetics of clot breakdown (fibrinolysis) (see Figure 27.1 and Table 27.1). VHAs are argued to be better measures of overall *haemostatic potential* than plasma-based tests, providing a more physiologically relevant interpretation of coagulation. However, the results from the two devices, although similar, should not be regarded as directly comparable since different coagulation activators are used (see Table 27.2).

TEG® was originally developed by Hartert in 1948, but it is only recently that the instrument has seen widespread uptake across intensive care units (ICUs), theatres and emergency departments. The TEG® instrument has two measurement channels, each containing an oscillating cup (heated to 37°C) into which a pin, freely suspended by a wire, is inserted. Whole blood for analysis is placed in the cup, and as the clot starts to form, the movement of the pin is coupled to that of the cup. The elasticity and strength of the developing clot is transmitted through the pin and converted into the characteristic TEG® trace (see Figure 27.1). Originally, the TEG® instrument used fresh whole blood, *native TEG®* (see Table 27.2), but the long

Haematology in Critical Care: A Practical Handbook, First Edition. Edited by Jecko Thachil and Quentin A. Hill.
© 2014 John Wiley & Sons, Ltd. Published 2014 by John Wiley & Sons, Ltd.

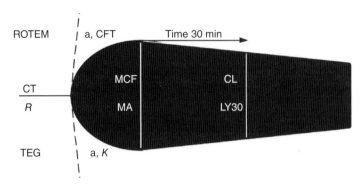

Figure 27.1 Diagram of a typical TEG®/ROTEM® trace.

Table 27.1 TEG and ROTEM variables.

Process studied	Causes of variation	TEG value	ROTEM value
Time until first evidence of clot formation (amplitude of 2 mm reached)	Prolonged by clotting factor deficiencies and heparin	R value (reaction time)	Clotting time (CT)
Rate of clot formation (time for amplitude to increase from 2 to 20 mm)	Decreased by clotting factor deficiencies such as hypofibrinogenaemia and platelet dysfunction or insufficiency	K value and α angle	α angle and clot formation time (CFT
Maximum clot strength	Reduced by platelet dysfunction and hypofibrinogenaemia	Maximum amplitude (MA)	Maximum clot firmness (MCF)
Clot lysis (CL)	Measures degree of fibrinolysis	LY30 – CL at 30 min	CL

A mathematical formula determined by the manufacturer can be used to determine a coagulation index (CI) that takes into account the relative contribution of each of r, K, α and MA into a single complex equation.

Table 27.2 Viscoelastic Haemostatic Assays.

TEG		ROTEM		
Test	Activator	Test	Activator	Diagnostic use
NATEM (native TEG)				Coagulation without added activator
Kaolin-activated TEG	Kaolin	INTEM	Ellagic acid	Defects in the intrinsic pathway of coagulation activation, heparin anticoagulation
		EXTEM	Recombinant TF	Defects in the extrinsic pathway, prothrombin complex deficiency, platelet deficiency
RapidTEG	Kaolin and TF			Defects in the intrinsic and extrinsic pathways
FF reagent	TF and abciximab	FIBTEM	Cytochalasin D	Fibrin-based clot defects, fibrin/fibrinogen deficiency Can help differentiate low fibrinogen values and platelet dysfunction which both cause low EXTEM MCF or low MA
		APTEM	Aprotinin	Evaluates fibrinolysis, when compared to EXTEM values
Kaolin-activated TEG + heparinase	Kaolin and heparinase	HEPTEM	Heparinase	Heparin/protamine imbalance

R time limited its practicability in situations of major haemorrhage, where rapid results are required, and both kaolin and more recently kaolin + tissue factor (TF) (RapidTEG®) are used as activators. Other available tests include functional fibrinogen, a measure of fibrin-based clot function, and Multiplate which evaluates platelet function.

ROTEM® uses similar principles to TEG® – the main difference being that ROTEM® has a rotating pin, not cup. The instrument has four independent measurement channels and uses a variety of activators (see Table 27.2), which like TEG® includes a specific measure of fibrinogen-based coagulation (FIBTEM). One potential advantage of the ROTEM® instrument is that it affords a degree of resilience to mechanical shock, making it more suitable to the clinical setting.

Specific TEG® and TEM® parameters reflect the three phases of the cell-based model of haemostasis: initiation, amplification and propagation. Initiation is represented by *R/clotting time (CT)* (TEG® and ROTEM®, respectively), amplification by *K/clot formation time (CFT)* and the thrombin burst by *α* angle, and the overall stability of the clot is represented by *maximum amplitude (MA)/ maximum clot firmness (MCF)* (see Figure 27.1). VHAs have several advantages over plasma clotting tests: the assessment of global haemostatic potential provides more information than time to fibrin formation, and now with multiple activators, these tests can readily differentiate a coagulopathy due to low fibrinogen from one due to thrombocytopenia. Furthermore, as point-of-care (POC) devices, there is ease of access to the machine, and turna-round times are short, with many results being available within 5–10 min of starting the test. On the flip side, VHA devices are reported to show marked inter-operator variability and poor precision. A UK National External Quality Assurance Scheme (NEQAS) reported coefficients of variance ranging from 7.1% to 39.9% for TEG® and 7.0% to 83.6% for ROTEM® [2].

VHA for evaluation of bleeding risk

Thirty per cent of adult ICU patients have a prolonged PT/INR measurement during their critical care stay, but many do not have associated bleeding. These patients are often viewed as hypocoagulable or at risk of bleeding and may receive blood components, in particular fresh frozen plasma (FFP) to *treat* prolonged clotting tests either prophylactically or prior to routine inter-ventions, such as central venous catheter placement [3]. Conventional clotting tests are poor predictors of bleeding risk, particularly in patients without active bleeding [1], and better predictive methods would be valuable, particularly if a test could differentiate patients at higher risk of bleeding, enabling targeted FFP transfusion. Few data exist about whether VHA devices can be used in this way, and an ongoing UK prospective observational study (ISOC-2, ISRCTN50516147) is set to address some of these questions. This study is evaluating the role of global haemostatic tests (TEG®, ROTEM® and thrombin generation) in ICU patients with prolonga-tion of PT, without clinical bleeding. It will provide information about the haemostatic potential of these patients and the ability for each of these tests to predict bleeding risk.

Certainly, promising results for predicting bleeding risk using thromboelastography have been reported in other patient groups, i.e. those with cirrhosis and acute liver failure. This group has historically been classified as *hypocoagulable*, again due to prolonged PT or INR measurements. The concept of hypocoagulability was recently challenged [4], and it has been demonstrated that haemostasis is in fact *rebalanced*, with an equal loss of pro-and anticoagulant proteins. In accordance with these findings, TEG® traces are normal in stable cirrhotic and acute liver failure patients. Furthermore, TEG® (*r* time, *k* time and *α* angle) has also been shown to be superior to INR and platelet count for estimating the risk of re-bleeding from oesophageal varices in cirrhotics.

VHA evaluation of thrombotic risk

Critical care patients are at significant risk of developing venous thromboembolism (VTE). A hypercoagulable state predisposes to thromboembolic disease, and con-ventional clotting tests have not been shown to reliably predict VTE risk. Viscoelastic tests can detect hyperco-agulable states, and the ability to risk stratify patients using a reliable global coagulation tool is tantalizing. Many observational studies have reported favourable results – showing superiority of VHA over conventional tests, but there is a general lack of agreement about which VHA parameter best defines hypercoagulability; one study evaluating 152 surgical ICU patients reported that *r*-TEG® clot strength (G) predicted VTE, whereas another study found an association between pulmonary embolism (PE) risk and *r*-TEG® MA values, in 2070 trauma patients. A recent systematic review concluded that the best parameter to identify hypercoagulability and predict VTE was MA (TEG®) or MCF (ROTEM®) [5]. This review also concluded that the predictive accuracy of TEG® for post-operative thromboembolic events was highly variable (diagnostic odds ratio ranged between 1.5 and 27.7) and that more prospective studies were needed to establish whether VHAs were a reliable measure of VTE risk.

Uses of VHA devices for treatment guidance

Viscoelastic haemostatic assay devices are widely used during the management of patients with major bleeding. Their use falls into two categories – prediction of transfusion need and guidance of transfusion therapy.

Prediction of transfusion need

The field of trauma and major traumatic haemorrhage has led the way when evaluating the utility of VHA devices in predicting transfusion need. Many observational studies have reported that both TEG® and ROTEM® can detect differences between patients who go on to need significant transfusion support, and it seems that clot strength parameters (i.e. MA or MCF) are the most commonly reported predictors, where low clot strength correlates with higher transfusion need. A recent report evaluating ROTEM® in trauma haemorrhage demonstrated that a single EXTEM clot amplitude measurement at 5 min (EXTEM CA5) of ≤35 mm had a negative predictive value (NPV) of 83% for any red cell transfusion and 99% for massive transfusion (10+ U) (AUC 0.803; 95% CI, 0.635–0.972) [6]. The future use of ROTEM may therefore be better as an early method of *deactivating* massive transfusion protocols in patients, but definitive studies are required.

Transfusion algorithms

TEG® and ROTEM® are increasingly being used as part of standard management for those patients requiring massive transfusion support, to guide the delivery of blood and blood components. TEG® and ROTEM® have been used for many years in cardiac and liver transplant surgery [7] and have been reported in randomized studies to reduce peri-operative transfusion requirements [8] and be a cost-effective tool [9]. In other settings, such as traumatic haemorrhage, TEG® has successfully been used to fine-tune major haemorrhage protocol (MHP), and cohort studies have reported both reduction in transfusion use and mortality [10]. However, thromboelastography is particularly sensitive to changes in fibrin polymerization and platelet count and may therefore be most useful for the early detection of dilutional coagulopathy and for guiding cryoprecipitate or fibrinogen concentrate therapy. Several ongoing randomized studies are evaluating ROTEM®-guided fibrinogen replacement in both obstetric haemorrhage and trauma, and the results are awaited with interest. A small cardiac surgery RCT has reported a significant reduction in allogeneic blood component use (2 U vs. 13 U) using such an algorithm [11].

Viscoelastic haemostatic assay-guided transfusion algorithms may enable clinicians to optimize targeted transfusion therapies, rather than delivering blood and blood components within an empirical MHP. This may reduce unnecessary transfusion administration, reducing transfusion-related adverse outcomes such as acute respiratory distress syndrome, infection and organ failure. A recent Cochrane review however evaluated the use of ROTEM® and TEG® as a method for monitoring transfusion therapy during massive transfusion. Nine trials were found but only covered cardiac and liver transplantation surgery. The authors reported that neither device led to a significant reduction in mortality when compared to standard care, but the use of VHA-guided transfusion algorithms reduced the volume of bleeding. And although many of the included studies reported fewer FFP and platelet transfusions, overall transfusions were not significantly reduced [12]. Large controlled trials comparing strategies of coagulation management and establishing algorithms and VHA cut-off values for transfusion of blood components are needed.

Conclusions

TEG and ROTEM have the potential to offer detailed information about haemostatic potential in critically ill patients, and their use compares favourably to conventional coagulation tests. However, there are few high-quality data as yet that unequivocally support their use.

References

1 Dzik WH. Predicting hemorrhage using preoperative coagulation screening assays. Curr Hematol Rep 2004;3:324–30.

2 Kitchen DP, Kitchen S, Jennings I, Woods T, Walker I. Quality assurance and quality control of thromboelastography and rotational thrombelastometry: the UK NEQAS for blood coagulation experience. Semin Thromb Hemost 2010;36:757–63.

3 Walsh TS, Stanworth SJ, Prescott RJ et al. Prevalence, management, and outcomes of critically ill patients with prothrombin time prolongation in United Kingdom intensive care units. Crit Care Med 2010;38:1939–46.

4 Tripodi A, Mannucci PM. The coagulopathy of chronic liver disease. N Engl J Med 2011;365:147–56.

5 Dai Y, Lee A, Critchley LA et al. Does thromboelastography predict postoperative thromboembolic events? A systematic review of the literature. Anesth Analg 2009;108:734–42.

6 Davenport R, Manson J, De'Ath H et al. Functional definition and characterization of acute traumatic coagulopathy. Crit Care Med 2011;39:2652–8.

7 Coakley M, Reddy K, Mackie I, Mallett S. Transfusion triggers in orthotopic liver transplantation: a comparison of the thromboelastometry analyzer, the thromboelastogram, and conventional coagulation tests. J Cardiothorac Vasc Anesth 2006;20:548–53.

8 Ak K, Isbir CS, Tetik S et al. Thromboelastography-based algorithm reduces blood product use after elective CABG: a prospective randomized study. J Card Surg 2009;24:404–10.

9 Health Technology Assessment Advice 11. The clinical and cost effectiveness of thromboelastography/thromboelastometry. NHS Quality Improvement Scotland, 2008. ISBN 1-84404-896-9. www.healthcareimprovementscotland.org (accessed on December 9, 2013).

10 Johansson PI, Stensballe J. Hemostatic resuscitation for massive bleeding: the paradigm of plasma and platelets – a review of the current literature. Transfusion 2010;50:701–10.

11 Rahe-Meyer N, Hanke A, Schmidt DS, Hagl C, Pichmaier M. Fibrinogen concentrate reduces intraoperative bleeding when used as first-line hemostatic therapy during major aortic replacement surgery: results from a randomized, placebo-controlled trial. J Thorac Cardiovasc Surg 2013;145:S178–85.

12 Afshari A, Wikkelsø A, Brok J, Møller AM, Wetterslev J. Thrombelastography (TEG) or thrombelastometry (ROTEM) to monitor haemotherapy versus usual care in patients with massive transfusion. Cochrane Database Syst Rev 2011;16(3):CD007871.

SECTION 8

Haematology Drugs in Critical Care

CHAPTER 28

Recombinant Activated Coagulation Factor VII (rFVIIa) in Critical Care

Leon Cloherty and Richard Wenstone

Department of Critical Care, Royal Liverpool University Hospital, Liverpool, UK

Background

Factor VII (FVII) is a vitamin K-dependent coagulation factor synthesized in the liver. In 1986, Novo Nordisk began the development of recombinant activated coagulation factor VII, rFVIIa (eptacog alpha [activated], NovoSeven®). Initially developed to treat haemophilia patients with inhibitors against FVIII and FIX, it was granted an EU license in 1996 and gained FDA approval in the USA in 1999. Its potential to treat other haemorrhagic conditions was recognized soon after its clinical introduction, and it has been used *off-label* for a wide variety of conditions, predominantly in the emergency setting.

Between 2000 and 2008, off-label (including prophylactic) use of rFVIIa increased more than 140-fold and, in 2008, accounted for more than 97% of in-hospital use of the drug [1]. During this same period, in-hospital use for haemophilia patients increased only fourfold. However, evidence to support its off-label use is lacking with concerns about an increased incidence of thromboembolic events. A recent Cochrane review [2] of 25 randomized controlled trials (RCTs) (of which 11 examined the therapeutic use of rFVIIa) suggested that its off-label use should be restricted to clinical trials only.

Large trials or smaller series have examined the efficacy and safety of rFVIIa in, for example:
- Trauma (blunt and penetrating)
- Cerebral haemorrhage
- Post-cardiac surgery
- Prostatectomy
- Cirrhosis with gastrointestinal bleeding
- Hepatic surgery
- Major vascular surgery
- Major spinal surgery
- Postpartum haemorrhage
- Post-stem cell transplantation
- Reversal of anticoagulation

Mechanism of action

Following tissue injury, tissue factor (TF, a lipoprotein expressed in the sub-endothelium) is exposed to the circulation and activates FVII. FVIIa induces haemostasis at the injury site by forming a complex with TF derived from injured vessel wall endothelium. This reaction occurs on the surface of the sub-endothelial cells. FVIIa has little proteolytic activity until this complex forms. This *initiation phase* activates factor X (FX) independently of FVIII and FIX. FXa then binds to FVa on the cell surface.

In the *amplification phase*, FXa/FVa complex converts small amounts of prothrombin to thrombin, activating FV, FVIII, FIX and platelets locally. The *propagation phase* occurs on the surface of activated platelets, which bind these factors, with the FVIIIa/FIXa complex activating further FX. The FXa/FVa (prothrombinase) complex

Haematology in Critical Care: A Practical Handbook, First Edition. Edited by Jecko Thachil and Quentin A. Hill.
© 2014 John Wiley & Sons, Ltd. Published 2014 by John Wiley & Sons, Ltd.

now converts large amounts of prothrombin to thrombin during a *thrombin burst*, leading to the formation of a stable fibrin clot.

At pharmacological dose, rFVIIa directly activates FX on the surface of locally activated platelets independent of TF. The quality of the resultant clot is dependent upon adequate concentrations of platelets and clotting factors. rFVIIa also mediates the inhibition of fibrinolysis, stabilizing clot formation.

Theoretically, this reaction should therefore be limited to activated platelets at the site of tissue injury. However, systemic activation has been described, and meta-analyses suggest an increased incidence of thromboembolic events when used off-label.

Presentation and dosing

For licensed (on-label) use, it is given as an intravenous bolus as early as possible in the bleeding episode at a dose of 90 mcg/kg. This dose is then repeated every 2–3 h until haemostasis is achieved (rFVIIa half-life is 2.4–3.2 h).

Off-label use of rFVIIa is somewhat more complicated. Although surgical procedures have used a similar dosing regimen, it is unclear to what extent these dosing guidelines can be applied to a heterogeneous, non-haemophiliac patient population. Reports describe doses of between 5 and 300 mcg/kg being administered for a wide variety of clinical indications [2]. It has been administered prophylactically before major surgery (predominantly cardiac and liver but also in prostate, pelvic and spinal surgery) and as a rescue therapy in uncontrolled haemorrhage [2].

Typical regimens have used an initial dose of 100–200 mcg/kg with up to two further doses depending upon response. However, some reports have suggested an absence of dose–response effect, and the optimum dosing regimen is still unclear. Our own guideline (available from the authors) is an initial dose of 100 mcg/kg followed by, if response is inadequate, one further dose of 120 mcg/kg after 2 h. Failure to respond to an initial dose is likely to indicate futility, and no more doses should be administered without careful consideration. A coagulation screen should be checked immediately before and 15 min after administration (due to the expected consumption of clotting factors), and this will direct further coagulation therapy.

Suggested parameters before rFVIIa use include:
- Correction of acidaemia (to a pH >7.2)
- Correction of hypothermia (>34 °C)
- An adequate number of viable platelets (>50 × 10⁹/L)
- Adequate circulating coagulation factors (especially FX, prothrombin, fibrinogen)
- Haemoglobin level above 7 g/dL

Following the administration of rFVIIa, rapid consumption of coagulation factors, platelets and fibrinogen typically necessitates replacement.

There is no direct way to monitor rFVIIa efficacy. Surrogate markers include a reduction in transfusion requirements and cessation of bleeding. A significant reduction in PT (often to less than the normal range) has been demonstrated within 15 min of the administration of rFVIIa with a concomitant reduction in activated partial thromboplastin time (APTT). However, reduction in PT does not completely reflect the *in vivo* effect of rFVIIa on coagulation and is not a reliable monitor of rFVIIa efficacy, although in rFVIIa-treated patients, prolonged PT values greater than or equal to 18 s were associated with significantly higher 24 h mortality.

Frequently reported off-label use and evidence

Much interest has focused on cardiac surgery, trauma (body and head) and intracerebral haemorrhage. In one study [1], these indications accounted for 69% of off-label use of rFVIIa. It has also been used in liver transplantation, spinal surgery, prostatectomy, obstetric haemorrhage and major vascular surgery.

Trauma
Trauma remains a cause of 1 in 10 deaths worldwide with up to a third of these secondary to refractory haemorrhage. The first use of rFVIIa in trauma was reported in the *Lancet* in 1999 [3]: a soldier with an inferior vena cava bullet wound received a massive transfusion before bleeding finally halted after two doses of rFVIIa. Unfortunately, despite multiple case reports, there has been a failure to replicate these outcomes in larger controlled trials.

The CONTROL trial [4] compared the safety and efficacy of rFVIIa in trauma. Patients with blunt and penetrating trauma were randomized to either three single doses of rFVIIa (200 mcg/kg + 100 mcg/kg + 100 mcg/kg) or placebo after 4–8 U of RBCs had been administered. It failed to establish an improved outcome with rFVIIa and was stopped following an interim analysis (573 patients). Thirty-day mortality and 90-day mortality were similar in both groups. Transfusion requirements were less in both treatment groups although this only reached statistical significance in the blunt trauma group. Thromboembolic events were similar across study cohorts. No trials have demonstrated a mortality benefit although a reduced incidence of ARDS and MOF has been reported [4].

Cardiac surgery

Excessive bleeding post-cardiac surgery is a serious complication. Up to 15% of patients will require allogeneic transfusion in uncomplicated CABG or valve replacement. This figure rises to 80% of patients after complicated surgery. Up to 5% of all patients will require reoperation because of excessive blood loss, and this is associated with an increase in morbidity and mortality. Cardiac surgery in the UK currently uses 5% of all UK donated blood, 17% of platelets and 12% of FFP.

Gill et al. [5] showed that the rates of reoperation and transfusion were reduced when rFVIIa was used but with a trend towards increased thromboembolic events in the treated group. A meta-analysis in 2011 failed to establish a mortality benefit but also found an increased thromboembolic risk. Cardiac surgery, both adult and paediatric, accounts for a large proportion of off-label use of rFVIIa, without a solid evidence base. The risk/benefit ratio should therefore be carefully considered, and, although peri-operative bleeding remains a problem, further high-quality trials are required to establish its efficacy. A useful guide in this setting is the assessment of the APTT, which, if not normalized, should preclude the use of rFVIIa and direct towards the use of blood products or other components (e.g. non-activated prothrombin complex concentrates, which contain multiple coagulation factors).

It has been suggested that the effectiveness of rFVIIa in cardiopulmonary bypass setting may be increased by a concomitant administration of fibrinogen. *In vitro* studies have shown that although the administration of rFVIIa shortened the onset of clot formation, the clot strength was improved using the combination of rFVIIa and fibrinogen [6].

Intracerebral haemorrhage

An RCT published by Mayer et al. in 2008 [7] failed to replicate that group's earlier study which had suggested that rFVIIa may have a place in the treatment of ICH, with a reduction in haematoma growth, reduced mortality and improved functional outcomes. Again, an increase in thromboembolic events was evident in both trials.

Hazards of rFVIIa

Some, but not all, studies have shown an incidence in thromboembolic events, when using rFVIIa outside approved indications, of 1–10%. Levi et al. [8] analysed data from 35 placebo-controlled trials and found an increase in arterial but not venous thrombotic events. They were particularly prevalent in patients over 65 years old, rising further in the over 75 s. Coronary arterial thrombotic events were seen in 2.9% of patients given rFVIIa versus 1.1% of patients given placebo ($p = 0.002$).

Mayer et al. [7] saw similar rates of arterial thrombotic events (absolute increase of 5% vs. placebo), with cerebral infarction and myocardial ischaemia occurring most commonly. A meta-analysis of thromboembolic events from pooled data published by the manufacturer states an arterial risk of 5.6% versus 3% for placebo. The side effect profile is certainly different to that seen in haemophiliac patients with inhibitors (its licensed indication) and must be balanced against potential benefit.

Administration

It is unclear at what point in the transfusion process rFVIIa should be considered. rFVIIa is dependent upon other parts of the clotting cascade, i.e. adequate platelet count and fibrinogen to form stable clot. For this reason, it is imperative that abnormalities in these parameters are corrected first, before considering rFVIIa. The currently available routine tests of coagulation are limited in their ability to find the cause of bleeding and may even be normal despite continued bleeding. The decision to use rFVIIa is therefore based upon clinical judgement. Indeed, as most case reports attest, rFVIIa is usually considered a *rescue therapy* once standard transfusion protocols have been followed and failed.

Although we don't know what the ideal time point is at which to use rFVIIa, there is evidence suggesting when its administration would be futile. Studies have shown a raised PT, high Revised Trauma Score and acidosis to be independent risk factors for failure to respond to rFVIIa. Other adverse factors include massive transfusion, hypothermia and significant co-morbidities.

Despite rFVIIa use, a large proportion of patients will still die, if not from haemorrhage then from subsequent multi-organ failure. Clearly, because of the expense and side effect profile, it is desirable to avoid futile administration of rFVIIa. Numerous authors have tried to identify the factors that predict whether rFVIIa will work or not and to incorporate them into a scoring system. Measures of organ dysfunction, illness severity and clinical and laboratory variables have all been used to give simple predictive scores of mortality. Unfortunately, none of these scoring systems has been validated. Indeed, Bowles et al. [9] suggest that an urgent prospective study of these factors is required to move away from the 'present indiscriminate uncontrolled use of rFVIIa in critically ill patients'.

The simplest prognostic scoring system with corresponding mortality can be seen in the following (Table 28.1 and Figure 28.1), although this retrospective analysis incorporated just 36 patients [10]. Patients were stratified into risk groups according to score: low risk (score ≤1), intermediate risk (>1 but <3) and high risk (≥3).

Economics

rFVIIa is expensive (£3500–£5000 per patient episode), and, even if adequate evidence of mortality and morbidity benefit be shown in the future, this may limit widespread use. Attempts have been made to quantify the overall cost with respect to potential savings, i.e. shorter intensive care stay and reduced transfusion requirements. Ridley

Table 28.1 Prognostic scoring system [10].

Characteristic	Score
Coagulopathy, defined as any of: Platelet count ≤50 × 109/L Fibrinogen ≤1·0g/L PT/APTT ≥1·5 × ULN	1
Renal impairment, defined as: Creatinine ≥120 μmol/L	1
Hypothermia, defined as: Core temperature ≤35°C	1
≥10 U of red cell transfusion	1
Age ≥60 years	1
Obstetric indication	−1

Source: Biss and Hanley [10]. Reproduced with permission of John Wiley & Sons, Ltd.
APTT, activated partial thromboplastin time; ULN, upper limit of reference range; PT, prothrombin time.

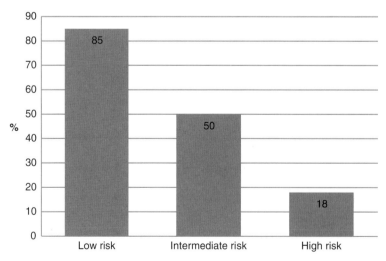

Figure 28.1 Prognostic score. Survival according to prognostic score. Survival expressed as percentage surviving to discharge from hospital (low risk, *n* = 13; intermediate risk, *n* = 6; high risk, *n* = 17). Source: Biss and Hanley [10]. Reproduced with permission of John Wiley & Sons, Ltd.

et al. [11] found that the incremental costs per quality-adjusted life year (QALY) gained for rFVIIa relative to placebo were £18,825, i.e. below the maximum recommended by the National Institute for Clinical Excellence of £20,000–30,000. Although this suggests that the treatment may be cost-effective (for the NHS), the economic model was based upon the initial work by Boffard et al. [4], which was subsequently superseded by more negative clinical data. The authors point out that as mortality risk reduction is reduced with respect to placebo, rFVIIa becomes less cost-effective. The work by Loudon et al. suggested that rFVIIa only became cost-effective after 14 U of RBCs had been transfused and at best may be cost neutral [12].

Summary

In summary, there is no strong published evidence to support the use of rFVIIa in the critically ill. However, rFVIIa has the potential to be a useful drug when used *off-label*, and it is likely to be effective in certain subgroups of patients rather than something that should be used indiscriminately. Identifying these groups remains a challenge as study design has obvious limitations in acute uncontrolled haemorrhage.

A common theme in the literature is a reduction in bleeding and transfusion requirements. Although desirable, this must be tempered by a lack of evidence to suggest a reduction in mortality and a trend towards increasing thromboembolic events. Dosing and monitoring remain problematic and, to a large extent, are based upon initial trial data for haemophilia patients. The significant economic cost and higher than expected incidence of thromboembolic events must also be acknowledged. Despite the evidence, rFVIIa was used off-label in an estimated 70,000 in-hospital cases in the USA between 2000 and 2008. Strong psychological, moral and ethical factors continue to dominate physicians' decision-making [13]. When faced with the exsanguinating patient and a failure of traditional resuscitation, the 'rules of evidence-based medicine' may be overridden by urgency and the demands of context'.

Unfortunately, it is unlikely that further large-scale trials will be performed in the near future. rFVIIa will remain a drug of last resort, in consultation with haematology and other colleagues.

References

1 Logan A, Yank, V, Stafford S. Off-label use of recombinant factor VIIa in U.S. hospitals: analysis of hospital records. Ann Intern Med 2011;154:516–22.

2 Stanworth SJ, Birchall J, Doree CJ, Hyde C. Recombinant factor VIIa for the prevention and treatment of bleeding in patients without haemophilia. Cochrane Database Syst Rev 2009:CD005011.

3 Kenet G, Walden R, Eldad A, Martinowitz U. Treatment of traumatic bleeding with recombinant factor VIIa. Lancet 1999;354:1879.

4 Hauser CJ, Boffard K, Dutton R et al. Results of the CONTROL trial: efficacy and safety of recombinant activated factor 7 in the management of refractory haemorrhage. J Trauma 2010;69:489–500.

5 Gill R, Herbertson M, Vuylsteke A et al. Safety and efficacy of recombinant activated factor VII. A randomized placebo-controlled trial in the setting of bleeding after cardiac surgery. Circulation 2009;120:21–27.

6 Tanaka KA, Taketomi T, Szlam F, Calatzis A, Levy JH. Improved clot formation by combined administration of activated factor VII (NovoSeven) and fibrinogen (Haemocomplettan P). Anesth Analg 2008;106:732–38.

7 Mayer SA, Brun NC, Begtrup K et al. Efficacy and safety of recombinant activated factor VII for acute intracerebral haemorrhage. N Eng J Med 2008;358:2127–37.

8 Levi M, Levy J, Anderson H, Truloff D. Safety of recombinant activated factor VII in randomized clinical trials. N Eng J Med 2010;363:1791–800.

9 Bowles KM, Park GR. Predicting response to recombinant factor VIIa in non haemophiliac patients with severe haemorrhage. Br J Anaesth 2007;98(5):690–91.

10 Biss T, Hanley J. Recombinant activated factor VII (rFVIIa/NovoSeven®) in intractable haemorrhage: use of a clinical scoring system to predict outcome. Vox Sang 2006;90(1):45–52.

11 Morris S, Ridley S, Munro V. Cost effectiveness of recombinant activated factor VII for the control of bleeding in patients with severe blunt trauma injuries in the United Kingdom. Anaesthesia 2007;62:43–52.

12 Loudon B, Smith MP. Recombinant factor VII as an adjunctive therapy for patients requiring large volume transfusion: a pharmacoeconomic evaluation. Intern Med J 2005;35:463–7.

13 Lipworth W, Kerridge I, Little M, Day R. Evidence and desperation in off label prescribing: recombinant factor VIIa. BMJ 2012;343:d7926.

CHAPTER 29

The Use of Haemostatic Drugs in Post-operative Bleeding

Catharina Hartman[1] and Nigel Webster[2]

[1] Intensive Care Unit, Aberdeen Royal Infirmary, Aberdeen, UK
[2] Anaesthesia and Intensive Care, Institute of Medical Sciences, University of Aberdeen, Aberdeen, UK

Introduction

Post-operative bleeding can occur because the primary insult was not adequately addressed, as a complication of surgery or because of a multifactorial systematic coagulopathy. The first consideration after diagnosing post-operative bleeding is whether further surgical or trans-vascular intervention is indicated to arrest the haemorrhage. Deciding on the most appropriate course of action should be done in consultation with an experienced surgeon and/or interventional radiologist. If a systemic coagulopathy is suspected, an attempt should be made to understand the cause of the coagulopathy so that it can be addressed appropriately.

Most of the therapies discussed here have been studied in the context of pre- and intra-operative interventions to reduce the need for peri-operative blood transfusion or as treatment for patients with inherent disorders of coagulation. Recently, a lot of work has been reported on the coagulopathy of trauma, its influence on mortality and how to treat it. It is acknowledged that patients admitted to the ICU with post-operative bleeding may not exactly resemble these scenarios, but a pragmatic approach is advocated. It is necessary to pause briefly and describe the clotting process as we currently understand it.

In its unprovoked *in vivo* state, blood does not clot due to the prevailing anticoagulant effects of antithrombin on activated factors IX, X and XI; thrombomodulin–protein

S–protein C complex on activated factors V and VIII; and tissue factor pathway inhibitor (TFPI) on the crucial haemostasis initiating activation of factor X (FXa) through activated factor VII (FVIIa) and tissue factor (TF).

When an injury occurs, robust haemostasis is dependent on an adequate number of functional platelets and the generation of a sufficient burst of thrombin. Injuring endothelial cells exposes collagen and von Willebrand factor (vWF), which facilitates platelet adhesion. The platelet membrane provides a crucial support structure and many essential molecules for the coagulation process. TF is presented and combines with FVIIa that activates both factor IX and factor X. This TF pathway provides the initial thrombin burst. The addition of activated factor VIII (FVIIIa) and activated factor IX (FIXa) subsequently activates factor X (FXa).

The FXa complexes formed thus are also called *tenases* and combine with activated factor V (FVa) and activate factor II (prothrombin) to form thrombin. Thrombin further stimulates its own production by activating factor XI, but the ultimate goal is for thrombin to convert fibrinogen to fibrin. Fibrin strands provide a meshwork for platelets to aggregate in and plug the hole in the injured blood vessel. The fibrin mesh is stabilized by factor XIII cross links.

Thrombin also switches off the clotting process by altering the configuration of thrombomodulin, which then interacts with protein S and protein C, while

Haematology in Critical Care: A Practical Handbook, First Edition. Edited by Jecko Thachil and Quentin A. Hill.
© 2014 John Wiley & Sons, Ltd. Published 2014 by John Wiley & Sons, Ltd.

antithrombin and TFPI are stoichiometric inhibitors. Fibrin converts plasminogen to plasmin, which dissolves the clot and hence re-establishes blood flow.

General measures

Hypothermia and acidosis along with coagulopathy have been described as the *lethal triad* or *bloody vicious cycle* of haemorrhagic shock. Simple measures such as avoiding excessive exposure and an appropriate ambient temperature are usually enough to maintain normothermia but are easily overlooked. Heated air blankets are also useful in the ICU. Always ensure that the patient has been rewarmed and that the temperature is maintained at 37 °C. Acidosis should be corrected through adequate resuscitation. Hypocalcaemia due to chelation of calcium ions with citrate in packed red cell units is common after blood transfusion and inhibits clotting. Give calcium if the ionized calcium level is less than 0.9 mmol/L [1].

These measures will ensure the optimum haemostatic milieu. The term *damage control resuscitation* has been coined in the trauma literature, but the approach is equally important in the non-traumatic bleeding patient.

Monitoring

Conventional clotting tests

The traditional measures of clotting through the prothrombin time (PT) and activated partial thromboplastin time (APTT) are used to monitor anticoagulant therapy with warfarin and heparin, respectively. Although abnormal results may be seen when a coagulopathy is present, these tests do not aid understanding of the cause of the problem. In general terms, a prolonged PT indicates a deficiency of the TF pathway and a prolonged APTT an abnormality of the contact pathway or final common pathway.

Fibrinogen levels can be measured and will identify insufficient fibrinogen levels or hyperfibrinolysis as the cause of a coagulation deficit. Platelet counts although useful do not indicate normal platelet function.

Thromboelastography/ thromboelastometry (see Chapter 27)

In our view, these tests provide a clearer picture of any coagulation deficit. The problem can be identified as related to platelet dysfunction (too few or non-functional), low clotting factors or hyperfibrinolysis. The near-patient nature of the test also allows ongoing monitoring once the deficit has been corrected.

Antifibrinolytics

Antifibrinolytic drugs interfere with the binding of plasminogen to fibrin, thereby preventing fibrinolysis. Tranexamic acid and ε-aminocaproic acid (EACA) are lysine analogues and block the fibrin binding site of plasminogen. Aprotinin is a serine protease inhibitor and, unlike tranexamic acid and EACA, interferes only with plasminogen unbound to fibrin and hence does not prevent the dissolution of clots in the small vessels.

Tranexamic acid

Tranexamic acid forms a reversible complex that displaces plasminogen from fibrin, resulting in the inhibition of fibrinolysis; it also inhibits the proteolytic activity of plasmin. The early use of tranexamic acid has consistently shown a reduction in transfusion requirements in urological, orthopaedic and cardiac elective surgery. Different dosing regimens have been described depending on the clinical scenario, but the common message is to give it sooner rather than later. In severely injured patients, give 1 g infused over 10 min as soon as possible, followed by 1 g infused over the next 8 h [2]. A single dose of 1 g appears to decrease the incidence of postpartum haemorrhage after vaginal delivery or caesarean section [3]. Topical administration of this agent may be beneficial in areas where excessive fibrinolysis contributes to bleeding like the oral cavity. A solution of tranexamic acid (1 g in 100 mL saline) was also effective being poured into the peritoneal cavity and mediastinal tissues before closure in the cardiac surgery setting. Most trials report no evidence of a statistically significant increase in adverse thrombotic events, but tranexamic acid is associated with non-ischaemic seizures (especially with higher doses) thought to be due to an inhibitory effect on GABA receptors. The use of this drug is absolutely contraindicated in cases where secondary fibrinolysis predominates (e.g. DIC), where fatal thromboembolism can result. In patients with haematuria, antifibrinolytics can precipitate clot colic since it inhibits urokinase.

ε-Aminocaproic acid (EACA)

The less potent of the lysine analogues, EACA binds competitively to plasminogen, thereby preventing its conversion to plasmin and resulting in the inhibition of fibrinolysis. EACA did not have the same blood-sparing effect as tranexamic acid in one randomized controlled trial in patients undergoing cardiac surgery [4]. Different dosing regimens exist, but commonly, a bolus dose of approximately 150 mg/kg is given initially followed by an infusion at 15 mg/kg/h. Rapid administration can lead to hypotension, and prolonged high-dose oral administration (>28 days) of the drug has been associated with myonecrosis and rhabdomyolysis (due to the inhibition of carnitine synthesis).

Aprotinin

Aprotinin is a broad-spectrum serine protease inhibitor that attenuates the coagulation, fibrinolytic and inflammatory pathways by interfering with the chemical mediators thrombin, plasmin and kallikrein. Additionally, it protects platelet-expressed glycoproteins from mechanical shear forces. This preserves normal haemostatic activity through protease receptor-independent mechanisms (e.g. via ADP and glycoprotein IIb/IIIa) while blocking thrombin-mediated aggregation. Aprotinin was associated with increased mortality compared with tranexamic acid in a large randomized trial in high-risk cardiac surgery, which led to its withdrawal from the market. Lysine analogues have been recently identified to be a cost-effective and safer alternative to aprotinin.

Desmopressin (DDAVP)

Desmopressin is a synthetic vasopressin analogue with an agonist effect at the V2 (antidiuretic) but not V1 (vasopressor) receptor. It induces the release of vWF and factor VIII from endothelial cells. A dose of 0.3 μg/kg of the intravenous preparation will take effect after approximately 30 min peaking at 90–120 min, and the effect usually lasts for 6–12 h. It is mostly used in the setting of known type I von Willebrand disease or mild haemophilia but has also been used in patients with platelet dysfunction due to uraemia or treatment with aspirin.

Desmopressin can cause mild facial flushing, headache, palpitations and hypotension. It has potent antidiuretic effects and can cause water retention, hyponatraemia and seizures. It should be used with caution in pregnancy as it can induce premature labour and has also been linked with an increased risk of myocardial infarction. Arterial thrombosis can be precipitated by its use in individuals at risk of cardiovascular disease. Fluid restriction in the first 24 h after the administration of DDAVP may decrease the risk of hyponatraemia. Repeated use may cause tachyphylaxis, and electrolyte monitoring is advisable in such cases to prevent significant hyponatraemia.

Recombinant activated factor VII (rFVIIa)

It is a vitamin K-dependent glycoprotein and promotes haemostasis by replacing deficient FVIIa, which then complexes with TF and activates factor X and factor IX. Factor Xa converts prothrombin to thrombin, which is a key step in the formation of a haemostatic platelet plug as described earlier. rFVIIa was developed and is licensed for use in patients with haemophilia and antibody inhibitors to factor VIII or factor IX. It is given at supraphysiological doses in order to induce a sufficient thrombin burst to initiate platelet plug formation.

Interest in its use in the exsanguinating patient continues, fuelled by dramatic case reports of successful use. No evidence of a survival benefit has yet been documented in controlled trials. Safety evaluation of thromboembolic events in all published randomized, placebo-controlled trials of rFVIIa used on an off-label basis noted higher rates of arterial thromboembolic events, particularly among those who were 65 years of age or older (9.0% vs. 3.8%), although the venous thromboembolic rates were similar [5].

It is worth noting the CONTROL trial investigating the use of rFVIIa in massive haemorrhage [6]. This phase 3 randomized controlled trial was terminated prematurely because of a much lower than expected mortality rate in the treatment and control arms. There was no statistically significant difference in mortality for patients with blunt or penetrating trauma. It has been postulated that the overall good haemostatic resuscitation advocated by the investigators led to the decrease in mortality and strengthens the argument for such practices and against the use of rFVIIa.

Factor VIII inhibitor bypassing activity (FEIBA)

Factor VIII inhibitor bypassing activity (FEIBA) is also used in haemophiliacs with inhibitors and like rFVIIa has much lower activity than the relatively absent clotting factors. Recent reports suggest its use in patients with life-threatening haemorrhage while receiving new oral anticoagulants especially dabigatran.

Recommended course of action

The importance of providing a favourable environment to enhance platelet activity is emphasized. Do not allow the patient to become hypothermic and pay close attention to ionized calcium levels especially when blood products have been administered. If a coagulopathy is suspected, take initial blood samples for full blood count and thromboelastography/thromboelastometry (or APTT, PT and fibrinogen if no alternative) and give an antifibrinolytic. It is difficult to give advice on what constitutes and adequate number of platelets as effective function is more important. In hyperfibrinolysis, cryoprecipitate or fresh frozen plasma (FFP) can be used, and antifibrinolytic therapy should be continued. Give FFP if there is a clotting factor deficiency. We do not advocate the use of rFVIIa until all of the aforementioned have been corrected.

References

1 Lier H, Krep H, Schroeder S, Stuber F. Preconditions of hemostasis in trauma: a review. The influence of acidosis, hypocalcemia, anemia, and hypothermia on functional hemostasis in trauma. J Trauma Inj Infect Crit Care 2008;65(4):951–60.

2 CRASH-2 trial collaborators, Shakur H, Roberts I et al. Effects of tranexamic acid on death, vascular occlusive events, and blood transfusion in trauma patients with significant haemorrhage (CRASH-2): a randomised, placebo-controlled trial. Lancet 2010;376(9734):23–32.

3 Novikova N, Hofmeyr GJ. Tranexamic acid for preventing postpartum haemorrhage. Cochrane Database Syst Rev 2010;7:007872.

4 Rahman Z, Hoque R, Ali A, Rahman M, Rahman MS. Blood conservation strategies for reducing peri-operative blood loss in open heart surgery. Mymensingh Med J 2011; 20(1):45–53.

5 Levi M, Levy JH, Andersen HF, Truloff D. Safety of recombinant activated factor VII in randomized clinical trials. N Engl J Med. 2010;363(19):1791–800.

6 Hauser CJ, Boffard K, Dutton R et al. Results of the CONTROL trial: efficacy and safety of recombinant activated Factor VII in the management of refractory traumatic hemorrhage. J Trauma 2010;69(3):489–500.

CHAPTER 30

Delivering Chemotherapy on Intensive Care

Arvind Arumainathan[1] and Daniel Collins[2]

[1] Department of Haematology, Royal Liverpool University Hospital, Liverpool, UK
[2] Department of Pharmacy, Royal Liverpool University Hospital, Liverpool, UK

Introduction

The majority of patients with haematological malignancy who need intensive care unit (ICU) admission do so because of treatment-related complications. However, on occasion, newly diagnosed patients require organ support. Causes of ICU admission at initial presentation and their usual sequelae may include:

• Acute tumour lysis: renal failure and gross electrolyte disturbance
• Leukostasis: central nervous system complications, ventilatory failure and thromboses
• Hyperviscosity: central nervous system complications, ventilatory failure and thromboses
• Myeloma and renal failure
• Highly proliferative lymphoma: organ infiltration and acute tumour lysis
• Acute leukaemia: organ infiltration and sepsis

In these situations, intensive supportive care alone is generally insufficient, and definitive treatment in the form of chemotherapy may need to be initiated on the ICU.

Patients with haematological malignancies (acute leukaemia or lymphoma) comprise the majority of cancer patients requiring chemotherapy on the intensive care at their initial presentation [1]. Chemotherapy may be given with curative intent or for disease control. In the latter case, many patients will achieve remission for several years or more with treatment. Expert consensus opinion

recommends that newly diagnosed patients should have full access to ICU and that for patients suitable for ICU requiring chemotherapy, this should be delivered, along with life-sustaining therapies, until that chemotherapy becomes effective [1]. In a retrospective study of 37 patients with haematological malignancy requiring intravenous chemotherapy in ICU, in-hospital mortality was 43% and 6-month mortality 67%. Hospital mortality was not predicted by whether chemotherapy was given at diagnosis or relapse [2]. In a prospective study of 100 cancer patients requiring chemotherapy in ICU at diagnosis, hospital mortality was 41% and 6-month mortality was 51% [3].

Broadly, traditional cytotoxic chemotherapy interferes with cell division and replication. These effects are usually not specific to the malignant cells and are thus responsible for some of the generic side effects of chemotherapy, such as bone marrow suppression and gut irritation. Newer approaches include the use of monoclonal antibodies and targeted molecular therapies, which tend to lack these generic complications, but can still cause significant problems in the acutely ill patient, for example, infusion-related reactions.

Understandably, few data to guide best practice in this area exist. The decision to initiate chemotherapy on the ICU must thus be made after a careful assessment of the risks and benefits to the patient and close discussion between the haematology and intensive care teams [4].

Haematology in Critical Care: A Practical Handbook, First Edition. Edited by Jecko Thachil and Quentin A. Hill.
© 2014 John Wiley & Sons, Ltd. Published 2014 by John Wiley & Sons, Ltd.

Families – and patients where possible – must also be closely involved and made aware of the associated risks. Chemotherapy can be teratogenic and may also reduce fertility in the longer term. The possibility of pregnancy must be considered and issues of fertility sensitively explored. Issues of consent are discussed in Chapter 26. Staff familiar with cytotoxics must perform chemotherapy administration, and close pharmacy support is mandatory [5].

Steroids alone can have a significant effect on treatment naïve, highly proliferative haematological malignancies. Some critically ill patients will not be diagnosed until after their ICU admission. Consider the need to obtain diagnostic samples and tumour lysis prophylaxis in patients with a suspected haematological malignancy before prescribing steroids. For example, the 200–300 mg hydrocortisone per day (equivalent to approximately 50–60 mg prednisolone) for 5–7 days suggested by the surviving sepsis campaign for vasopressor and fluid refractory hypotension would be a therapeutic dose for some high-grade lymphomas, although without consolidation with combination chemotherapy, any response would not be sustained.

Approach to the patient

Multidisciplinary discussion

After the patient is stabilized, consideration must be given to the specific interventions that may be possible for the underlying disorder. For example, in ventilatory failure caused by leukostasis, therapeutic leukapheresis may also be required.

Discussions about initiating chemotherapy must also take place between the intensive care and haematology teams. If initiating chemotherapy, this should take place as soon as is feasible and safe. The haematology team should ensure that the intensive care team is aware of the regimen and drugs used, common and significant complications of these drugs and procedures for safe handling. Specialist cytotoxic and intensive care pharmacists play a valuable role and must be closely involved in discussion at all stages.

These situations are dynamic, and clear communication, ideally at consultant level, must take place regularly, particularly in respect to patients' prognosis in light of their clinical progress.

Venous access

An important practical aspect of chemotherapy administration is good venous access. Patients in the ICU are likely to have central venous access, which is also useful for concomitant administration of supportive measures such as hydration and antimicrobials. In patients likely to need medium- to longer-term access (such as patients with acute leukaemia), consideration should be given to early insertion of a tunnelled catheter. Central venous access is not always necessary as some chemotherapy agents can be given peripherally.

Psychosocial support

Admission to the ICU, coupled with a new diagnosis of cancer, is an incredibly difficult time for patients and families. Communication, respect and compassion have been demonstrated to be as important as good medical care in improving family satisfaction on the ICU [6]. The support of trained counsellors and psychologists may be useful.

Chemotherapy administration

Chemotherapy selection and dose attenuation

The initial chemotherapy regimen may be tailored to minimize toxicity, depending on the degree of physiological disturbance and organ dysfunction. Care must be taken to avoid drug interactions, especially in patients receiving antimicrobial therapy. For example, plasma methotrexate levels are increased in patients receiving co-trimoxazole or trimethoprim and itraconazole potentiates the neuromuscular side effects of vincristine. Prescribing of chemotherapy should follow an agreed treatment protocol [7, 8]. Most agreed protocols contain information for prescribers on dose modification of chemotherapy for impaired organ function, such as in renal or hepatic impairment.

It is crucial that prescribers refer to these protocols when initiating chemotherapy for patients on ICU. Specialist haemato-oncology pharmacists can play a crucial role in the verification of dose attenuations and may sometimes refer to alternative resources for further clarification [9]. Examples of chemotherapy that may require attenuation include:
- Renal impairment – high-dose methotrexate
- Hepatic impairment – vinca alkaloids
Table 30.1 later presents the agents used most commonly in haemato-oncology practice and some of their major

Table 30.1 Cytotoxic agents commonly used in haemato-oncology and associated common or major side effects (abbreviations in the succeeding text).

Class	Drugs	Nausea/vomiting	Mucositis	Dose in renal impairment	Dose in hepatic impairment	Class-specific effects	Drug-specific side effects
Alkylating agents	Bendamustine	Mild	Uncommon	Clinical decision in severe impairment	Dose reduce if Bil>20 μmol/L		
	Bleomycin	Mild	High doses	Dose reduce if CrCl<50 mL/min	Clinical decision in severe impairment		Pneumonitis
	Carmustine	Moderate	High doses	Dose reduce if CrCl<60 mL/min	Clinical decision in severe impairment		
	Cyclophosphamide	Moderate	High doses	Dose reduce if CrCl<20 mL/min	Clinical decision in severe impairment		Haemorrhagic cystitis
	Ifosfamide	Severe	Uncommon	Dose reduce if CrCl<60 mL/min	Clinical decision in severe impairment		Haemorrhagic cystitis, encephalopathy
	Melphalan	Moderate	High doses	Dose reduce if CrCl<50 mL/min	No dose reduction necessary		
Purine analogues	Cladribine	Mild	Uncommon	Clinical decision in severe impairment	Clinical decision in severe impairment		T-cell dysfunction
	Fludarabine	Mild	Uncommon	Dose reduce if CrCl<70 mL/min	No dose reduction necessary		T-cell dysfunction
	Nelarabine	Moderate	Stomatitis	Clinical decision in severe impairment	Clinical decision in severe impairment		Neurotoxicity
	Gemcitabine	Mild	Uncommon	Dose reduce if CrCl<30 mL/min	Dose reduce if Bil>27 μmol/L		Pneumonitis
	Pentostatin	Moderate	Uncommon	Dose reduce if CrCl<60 mL/min	Clinical decision in severe impairment		T-cell dysfunction
Antimetabolites	Cytarabine	Moderate	High doses	High doses only: dose reduce if CrCl<60 mL/min	Dose reduce if Bil>34 μmol/L		Cerebellar syndrome (at high doses), rash, conjunctivitis
	High-dose methotrexate	Moderate	Severe	Dose reduce if CrCl<80 mL/min	Dose reduce if Bil>50 μmol/L or AST>180 U/L		Renal impairment
Anthracyclines	Daunorubicin	Moderate	Mild	Dose reduce if CrCl >105 μmol/L	Dose reduce if Bil>20 μmol/L	Cardiotoxicity	
	Doxorubicin	Moderate	Mild	Clinical decision in severe impairment	Dose reduce if Bil>20 μmol/L		
	Liposomal doxorubicin	Moderate	Stomatitis	No dose reduction necessary	Dose reduce if Bil>20 μmol/L		
	Epirubicin	Moderate	Moderate	Clinical decision in severe impairment	Dose reduce if Bil>24 μmol/L		
	Idarubicin	Moderate	Moderate	Dose reduce if CrCl >100 μmol/L	Dose reduce if Bil>40 μmol/L		

Platinum	Carboplatin	Moderate	Moderate	Use Calvert equation for dosing	No dose reduction necessary	Renal failure
	Cisplatin	Severe	Moderate	Dose reduce if CrCl<60mL/min	No dose reduction necessary	Ototoxicity
Vinca alkaloids	Vinblastine	Mild	Mild	No dose reduction necessary	Dose reduce if Bil>26μmol/L or AST>60 U/L	Peripheral neuropathy
	Vinorelbine	Mild	Mild	No dose reduction necessary	Dose reduce if Bil>26μmol/L or AST>60 U/L	Constipation
	Vincristine	Mild	Mild	No dose reduction necessary	Dose reduce if Bil>2×UNL or AST>5×UNL	
Monoclonal antibodies	Alemtuzumab	Uncommon	N/A	No dose reduction necessary	No dose reduction necessary	Anaphylaxis
	Rituximab	Uncommon	N/A	No dose reduction necessary	No dose reduction necessary	
Immunomodulatory agents	Thalidomide	Mild	N/A	No dose reduction necessary	No dose reduction necessary	Thrombogenicity
	Lenalidomide	Uncommon	N/A	Dose reduce if CrCl<50mL/min	Clinical decision in severe impairment	
	Pomalidomide	Uncommon	N/A	Clinical decision in severe impairment	Clinical decision in severe impairment	
Others	Amsacrine	Moderate	Moderate	Dose reduce if CrCl<60mL/min	Dose reduce if Bil>34μmol/L	
	Asparaginase	Uncommon	N/A	No dose reduction necessary	Clinical decision in severe impairment	Thrombosis
	All-trans-retinoic acid (ATRA)	Uncommon	N/A	No dose reduction necessary	No dose reduction necessary	ATRA syndrome (see table footnotes), pseudotumour cerebri, hepatotoxicity
	Bortezomib	Mild	N/A	Clinical decision in severe impairment	Clinical decision in severe impairment	Peripheral neuropathy, constipation
	Dacarbazine	Severe	Mild	Dose reduce if CrCl<60mL/min	Clinical decision in severe impairment	Flu-like symptoms
	Etoposide	Moderate	Mild	Dose reduce if CrCl<50mL/min	Dose reduce if Bil>26μmol/L or AST>60 U/L	
	Mitoxantrone	Moderate	Moderate	No dose reduction necessary	Clinical decision in severe impairment	

ATRA syndrome is characterized by fever, dyspnoea, acute respiratory distress, weight gain, pulmonary infiltrates and pleural and pericardial effusions. If not treated early, it can progress to hepatic, renal and multi-organ failure.

CrCl, creatinine clearance; Bil, bilirubin; N/A, not applicable; UNL, upper limit of normal range; AST, aspartate transaminase.

side effects. Immunosuppression would also be expected with the majority of cytotoxic drugs but will vary with class and dose.

Nursing staff

Appropriately trained nursing staff must be involved in the administration of all cytotoxic chemotherapy [7, 8]. However, the practicalities of this can be frustrating for all staff involved. Nursing staff on the ICU can feel vulnerable and undertrained, while nurses from haemato-oncology feel a duty of care to patients on their own wards. The key principle to overcoming these practicalities is the establishment of good working relationships. Regular communication must also be undertaken to ensure any issues that develop are resolved quickly.

In our experience, it is the nurses from haemato-oncology areas that administer the chemotherapy, while the nurses from the ICU monitor these procedures. Future developments for ICU departments may include the appropriate training of a core number of staff to deal with these situations.

Renal replacement therapy

The timing of chemotherapy is crucial for patients on any form of renal replacement therapy. As with other medicines, dialysis has the ability to modify drug bioavailability and metabolism, and it is crucial therefore that thorough checks are carried out using appropriate resources [10]. This may include the involvement of nephrologists and renal pharmacists and, on occasion, direct contact with drug manufacturers. As with dose attenuation of chemotherapy, specialist haemato-oncology pharmacists should be involved in decisions.

Supportive care

The toxicity and side effects of chemotherapy merit generic and drug-specific supportive measures. Most patients will need intervention to cover these side effects, such as hydration and anti-emetics. However, patients on ICU may require more aggressive intervention. Local policy should include measures for the following areas:
• Antimicrobial prophylaxis: bacterial, fungal and viral infections
• Tumour lysis prophylaxis: role of rasburicase, allopurinol and aggressive hydration

• Granulocyte colony-stimulating factor (G-CSF), e.g. filgrastim, lenograstim and pegfilgrastim: primary prophylaxis is recommended for *high-risk* patients [11]:
  ○ Patient age greater than 65 years
  ○ Poor performance status
  ○ Previous episodes of febrile neutropenia
  ○ Bone marrow involvement by tumour, producing cytopenias
  ○ Poor nutritional status
  ○ The presence of open wounds or active infections
  ○ Other serious co-morbidities

Adverse events (including chemotherapy extravasation)

Staff on the ICU must also be made aware of potential side effects of chemotherapy by haemato-oncology staff. The scope of this chapter is inadequate to provide a comprehensive list of toxicities related to chemotherapy, but staff must be conscious that side effects can occur in the short term (within 24 h of administration) or longer term (days and weeks). Grading of side effects should be documented in patients care notes using an appropriate tool [12] as they may affect future treatment.

Chemotherapy extravasation is the leakage of a vesicant drug or fluid from a vein into the surrounding tissue during intravenous administration. A vesicant drug (e.g. anthracyclines, vinca alkaloids) is one which can result in tissue necrosis, which can lead to functional impairment or disfigurement [13]. Irritants (e.g. platinum compounds, taxanes) will cause inflammation but not necrosis although the degree of tissue injury also depends on the volume and concentration of extravasated drug.

Staff administering chemotherapy must be aware of the potential risk of extravasation and should report a suspected event immediately to an appropriately experienced clinician. Initial signs and symptoms include leakage of fluid around the infusion site, pain, discomfort, inflammation and erythema, but onset may occur days or weeks later. Vesicant-induced ulceration and tissue necrosis of surrounding tissue may take several days to develop and worsen for weeks or months.

Local haemato-oncology units will have robust and detailed polices on the prevention and management of extravasation, and it is recommended that any clinical area that administers chemotherapy has access to these policies as well as an *extravasation kit*. Immediate actions include cessation of the infusion, an attempt to aspirate

Table 30.2 Indications for irradiated blood components with respect to malignancy and chemotherapy in adult patients [14, 15].

Situation	Indication
Allogeneic haematopoietic stem cell transplant (HSCT)	All allogeneic HSCT recipients from time of conditioning therapy, continued while patient is receiving graft-versus-host disease (GvHD) prophylaxis
	If chronic GvHD present or taking immunosuppressants irradiated components required indefinitely
Autologous stem cell transplant	Patients undergoing autologous stem cell transplantation from start of conditioning therapy until 3 months post transplant (6 months if total body irradiation was used)
Hodgkin's lymphoma	All individuals with Hodgkin's lymphoma at any stage
Aplastic anaemia	Patients with aplastic anaemia receiving anti-thymocyte globulin (ATG) and/or alemtuzumab
Purine analogue therapy	After purine analogues (fludarabine, cladribine and pentostatin)*
After alemtuzumab (anti-CD52)	All patients, including those with autoimmune disease and solid organ transplant recipients who have received alemtuzumab. Duration unclear at present
Stem cell harvests	Patients undergoing bone marrow or peripheral blood stem cell *harvesting* for future autologous reinfusion during and for 7 days before harvesting

Source: National Cancer Institute [12] and Lewis et al. [13]. Reproduced with permission of John Wiley & Sons, Ltd.
*Situation with other purine analogues and related agents, such as bendamustine and clofarabine, is currently unclear, but use of irradiated components is recommended as mode of action similar.

fluid from the extravasation site through the access device and elevation of the affected limb [13]. Subsequent management will depend on the drug and local policy but may involve the use of topical cooling, topical warming, topical DMSO, subcutaneous hyaluronidase injections or the use of steroids. Significant peripheral extravasation events and those involving a central line may also require involvement of a plastic surgeon.

Patients with Hodgkin's lymphoma, allogeneic stem cell transplant recipients and patients treated with purine analogues are at risk of transfusion-associated graft-versus-host disease (GvHD) and should receive irradiated blood products. The hospital transfusion laboratory should be alerted to this.

Table 30.2 above summarizes the indications for irradiated blood products.

Illustrative case study 1

A 40-year-old man presents to the emergency department with a three week history of progressive breathlessness and rash. On examination, he is hypoxic, has a widespread petechial rash and has marked gum hypertrophy. The full blood count shows Hb 63 g/L, WCC 350×10^9/L and platelets 12×10^9/L. A plain chest radiograph shows bilateral pulmonary infiltrates. Blood film examination shows numerous blasts with monocytic differentiation. He deteriorates rapidly and requires intubation and mechanical ventilation. Immunophenotyping on the peripheral blood confirms acute monocytic leukaemia, and a diagnosis of pulmonary failure secondary to leukostasis and leukaemic infiltration is made.

The patient is commenced on urgent therapeutic leukapheresis. After two sessions, the peripheral WCC is 230×10^9/L, but he is no better. A decision is therefore made to commence him on induction therapy for acute myeloid leukaemia in the form of daunorubicin 50 mg/m^2 (once daily, days 1, 3 and 5) and cytarabine 100 mg/m^2 (twice daily, days 1–10).

The patient is married with two young children. They are closely supported by his parents. At all times, the intensive care and haematology teams keep his family informed of the diagnosis and clinical progress. At this point, the need for cytotoxic chemotherapy, and the associated risks, is explained to them. They are made aware that the treatment is potentially life-saving and agree that it should be given.

The chemotherapy achieves rapid cytoreduction. On day 8 of his induction therapy, he is extubated and is discharged from the ICU 3 days later.

Illustrative case study 2

A 56-year-old woman presents to her general practitioner with general malaise. She has routine bloods done, which demonstrate advanced kidney injury (eGFR 5). She is duly admitted for investigation. Renal ultrasound demonstrates enlarged kidneys bilaterally, suspicious of an infiltrative process. She undergoes a renal biopsy and is commenced on haemodialysis via a tunnelled central venous catheter.

She subsequently has a computed tomography (CT) scan, which demonstrates large nodal masses in the abdomen, mediastinum, pelvis and lung infiltrates and is felt to be suspicious of lymphoma. Over the course of the next 2 days, she deteriorates and requires invasive ventilation and continuous venovenous haemofiltration on the ICU. At that point, her biopsy is reported to show a diffuse large B-cell lymphoma. There is no obvious cause for her deterioration other than rapidly proliferative lymphoma.

She is commenced initially on high-dose corticosteroids with pre-emptive rasburicase. She develops features of acute tumour lysis syndrome, manifesting primarily as hyperkalaemia, and requires aggressive renal replacement therapy. A decision to commence her on combination treatment with rituximab, cyclophosphamide, doxorubicin, vincristine and prednisolone (R-CHOP) is made. After discussion between the renal, haematology, intensive care and pharmacy teams, her renal replacement therapy is timed to take place 12 h after completion of the intravenous chemotherapy. She is also given primary prophylaxis with recombinant human G-CSF.

Following her chemotherapy, she makes a slow improvement and is extubated after a further week. Her renal function does not improve significantly, though an interval CT scan demonstrates excellent regression of her lymphadenopathy. She goes on to complete a total of six cycles of treatment.

Summary

The aforementioned case studies illustrate that patients with haematological malignancy can present acutely unwell due to their illness. In these instances, treatment of the illness may be merited, in less than ideal circumstances.

With careful discussion of the potential risks, benefits and safety considerations, chemotherapy can be administered safely on the intensive care setting.

References

1 Azoulay E, Soares M, Darmon M, Benoit D, Pastores S, Afessa B. Intensive care of the cancer patient: recent achievements and remaining challenges. Ann Intensive Care 2011;1:1–5.

2 Benoit D, Depuydt P, Vandewoude K et al. Outcomes in severely ill patients with haematological malignancies who received intravenous chemotherapy on the intensive care unit. Intensive Care Med 2006;32:93–9.

3 Darmon M, Thiery G, Ciroldi M et al. Intensive care in patients with newly diagnosed malignancies and a need for cancer chemotherapy. Crit Care Med 2005;33:2488–93.

4 Song J, Suh G, Chung M et al. Risk factors to predict outcome in critically ill cancer patients receiving chemotherapy in the intensive care unit. Support Care Cancer 2011;19:491–5.

5 Pitello N, Treon M, Jones KL, Kiel PJ. Approaches for administering chemotherapy in the intensive care unit. Curr Drug Saf 2010;5:22–32.

6 Henrich N, Dodek P, Heyland D. Qualitative analysis of an intensive care unit family satisfaction survey. Crit Care Med 2011;39:1000–1005.

7 National Chemotherapy Advisory Group. Chemotherapy Services in England: Ensuring Quality and Safety. 2009. http://www.dh.gov.uk/prod_consum_dh/groups/dh_digital-assets/documents/digitalasset/dh_104501.pdf (accessed on November 20, 2013).

8 National Cancer Peer Review Programme. Manual for Cancer Services: Chemotherapy Measures ver 1.0. 2011. http://www.cquins.nhs.uk/?menu=resources (accessed on November 20, 2013).

9 Daniels S, Summerhayes M, Gabriel S, Chambers P, Riches E. UCLH – Dosage Adjustment for Cytotoxics in Hepatic & Renal Impairment Version 3 – Updated January 2009.

10 Ashley C, Currie A. Renal Drug Handbook. 3rd edition. Oxford: Radcliffe Publishing; 2009.

11 Smith T, Khatcheressian J, Lyman G, et al. 2006 Update of ASCO Recommendations for the Use of Haematopoietic Colony-Stimulating Factors. J Clin Oncol 2006;24:3187–3205.

12 National Cancer Institute. Common Terminology Criteria for Adverse Events (CTCAE) and Common Toxicity Criteria (CTC) v4.0. 2009. http://ctep.cancer.gov/protocolDevelopment/electronic_applications/ctc.htm#ctc_40 (accessed on November 20, 2013).

13 Lewis M, Hendrickson A, Moynihan T. Oncologic emergencies: pathophysiology, presentation, diagnosis, and treatment. CA Cancer J Clin 2011;61:287–314.

14 Treleavan J, Gennery A, Marsh J et al. Guidelines on the use of irradiated blood components prepared by the British Committee for Standards in Haematology transfusion task force. Br J Haematol 2011;152:35–51.

15 BCSH transfusion task force. Addendum: Guidelines on the Use of Irradiated Blood Components Prepared by the British Committee for Standards in Haematology Transfusion Task Force. 2010. http://www.bcshguidelines.com/documents/BCSH_TTF_addendum_irradiation_guidelines_final_6_11_12.pdf (accessed on November 20, 2013).

SECTION 9

Haematology in Paediatric and Neonatal Intensive Care

CHAPTER 31

Neonatal Anaemia

Michael Richards

Department of Paediatric Haematology, Leeds Children's Hospital, Leeds, UK

Normal development of red cell production during the foetal and neonatal period

Red cell production in the foetus occurs initially in the liver but shifts to the bone marrow during the third trimester of gestation. It is responsive to the effect of the glycoprotein hormone erythropoietin, production of which moves from the liver to the kidney near term. Erythropoietin concentrations fall following delivery, remaining depressed until 6–8 weeks of age; the resulting decreased rate of erythropoiesis results in a reduction in haemoglobin concentrations with a nadir around 10–12 weeks that rarely falls below 100 g/L [1]. The normal range of haemoglobin concentrations during the neonatal period varies according to the gestational age of the infant at birth and the postnatal age of the infant. Increasing erythropoietin levels lead to a rise in the haemoglobin concentration until 6 months of age. This dynamic process makes it essential to refer to the appropriate age-adjusted normal range for haemoglobin concentration in the interpretation of test results during the first 6 months of life [2].

Normal blood values and impact of technical issues

The peak haemoglobin concentration occurs during the first day following delivery, this level being higher than that seen in cord blood samples. The haemoglobin concentration subsequently declines as does the mean red corpuscular volume (MCV). The percentage reticulocyte count decreases from 3–7% on day 1 to 0–1% on day 7 [2]. Examination of the blood film is notable by the presence of nucleated red cells on day 1, which have largely disappeared by the third day of life and are absent in normal older infants.

Blood samples obtained by a skin prick represent capillary blood and have a higher haemoglobin concentration than blood obtained by venous sampling. In the first hours following delivery, this difference averages approximately 35 g/L, but in some patients, this difference may exceed 100 g/L [3]. This difference is most notable in premature infants and those who are clinically unstable displaying acidosis or hypertension. The impact of the sampling technique becomes less significant as infants approach full-term gestation and by the end of the first week of life.

The blood volume and red cell mass of the infant are influenced by the treatment of the umbilical cord blood vessels. Shortly after birth, the mean blood volume of term infants has been determined at 85 mL/kg, ranging from 50 to 100 mL/kg. Placental blood vessels contain 75–125 mL of blood at birth, which represent 25–75% of the foetal blood volume. The umbilical arteries generally constrict after delivery; however, the umbilical veins remain dilated; newly delivered infants held below the level of the placenta therefore gain blood from the umbilical vein; however, those who are held above the placenta may bleed into it. Early clamping of the umbilical cord will result in a reduction in the volume of

Haematology in Critical Care: A Practical Handbook, First Edition. Edited by Jecko Thachil and Quentin A. Hill.
© 2014 John Wiley & Sons, Ltd. Published 2014 by John Wiley & Sons, Ltd.

blood transfused from the placenta to the neonatal circulation. Usher et al. reported that infants for whom the clamping of the cord was delayed had an average blood volume of 93 mL/kg at an age of 72 h compared to 82 mL/kg in those following immediate cord clamping [4]. There is some evidence suggesting that reduced blood volume is associated with increased mortality in premature infants; conversely, delayed clamping may lead to circulatory overload and congestive cardiac failure.

Anaemia of prematurity

Premature infants (<37 weeks of gestation) experience an earlier (4–6 weeks) and lower nadir concentration of haemoglobin (70 g/L if birth weight <1000 g) than full-term babies, resulting in a normochromic, normocytic anaemia with a low reticulocyte count that is mostly due to impaired erythropoietin production and phlebotomy blood loss [1]. Some premature infants tolerate this anaemia well, but others especially the very low-birth-weight and sick infants demonstrate adverse signs such as tachycardia, tachypnoea, apnoea, poor weight gain, increased oxygen requirement, diminished activity and pallor.

Management options for these infants have included red cell transfusion and the use of exogenous recombinant erythropoietin. There are no data to suggest that recombinant erythropoietin dramatically decreases or eliminates the need for red cell transfusions in preterm infants although there is a suggestion that its use may prevent red cell transfusion in extremely low-birth-weight infants (birth weight <1000 g) after 1 month of age [5]. There are limited, non-corroborated data that suggest that retinopathy of prematurity (a disorder of vascular proliferation) may be exacerbated by recombinant erythropoietin. Red cell transfusion remains the mainstay of treatment for anaemia of prematurity; recent developments have concentrated on the need to restrict the use of transfusions to cases which satisfy strict criteria. Specific haemoglobin targets vary according to postnatal age and cardiorespiratory status. Ensure the infant is iron replete, especially if breastfed. Strategies to reduce red cell loss include delayed clamping of the umbilical cord and reducing the frequency and volume of blood sampling.

Anaemia in the neonate

As in older patients, anaemia in the neonate may be categorized into pathology leading to bleeding or haemolysis, and disorders that compromise production of red cells from the bone marrow. The causes of anaemia are summarized in Table 31.1, and an approach to the investigation of anaemia in neonatal intensive care is outlined in Figure 31.1. The role of transfusion in neonatal intensive care is discussed in Chapter 34.

Neonatal blood loss

Neonatal blood loss may occur during, before or soon after delivery. Bleeding occurring *in utero* may be caused by internal blood loss or bleeding into the maternal or accompanying twin circulations.

Foetal to maternal haemorrhage. Foetal to maternal haemorrhage is minimal in the majority of cases. Foetal to maternal transplacental haemorrhages of at least 80 mL of foetal blood have been reported with an incidence of one in 1146 pregnancies and of 150 mL or more with an incidence of one in 2813 pregnancies [6]. Contributors to this event include abdominal trauma to the mother, third trimester amniocentesis, external cephalic version, placental tumours, abruptio placentae and manual removal of the placenta.

The impact on the neonate depends on the volume and rate of blood loss. Rapid blood loss will lead to physiological decompensation in the infant, whereas chronic bleeding will lead to less evidence of acute compromise, but there may be evidence of congestive heart failure including hepatomegaly. Pallor will be evident following both events. Anaemia is invariably present following a chronic bleed; however, the initial haemoglobin may be maintained in cases of acute blood loss before declining during the first 24 h of life as haemodilution occurs. A hypochromic microcytic red cell picture reflecting low serum iron levels is common in infants born following chronic blood loss, whereas acute blood loss more typically presents with normochromia and macrocytosis. Infants born following acute blood loss require emergency resuscitation and red cell transfusions, whereas chronic blood loss may require red cell transfusions and possibly oral iron treatment.

The diagnosis of a foetal to maternal bleed requires the identification of foetal blood in the maternal circulation. The most common methodology used is the acid elution

Table 31.1 Causes of neonatal anaemia.

Inadequate production	Foetal/neonatal blood loss	Increased red cell consumption
Exaggeration of physiological anaemia as seen in premature infants	Twin-to-twin transfusion, foetal to maternal haemorrhage, placenta praevia	Immune-mediated haemolysis secondary to Rhesus disease of the newborn and other red cell antigen incompatibilities, maternal autoimmune haemolytic anaemia
Bone marrow failure syndromes, e.g. Diamond–Blackfan anaemia, Fanconi anaemia, Down's syndrome	Early clamping of the umbilical cord	Microangiopathic haemolytic anaemia secondary to arteriovenous malformation
Haematinic deficiency iron deficiency, rarely B12 and folate deficiency	Significant internal haemorrhage including intracranial haemorrhage and cephalohaematoma	Red cell membrane disorders
Disorders of haemoglobin synthesis including severe alpha thalassaemia	Venous sampling for investigations	Red cell enzyme deficiency
Infiltration of the bone marrow by leukaemia, lymphoma, neuroblastoma, osteopetrosis		Vitamin E deficiency
Bone marrow suppression by viruses, notably parvovirus		Parasitaemia

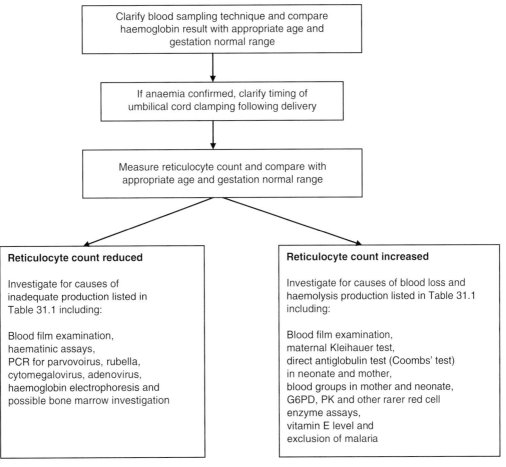

Figure 31.1 Approach to investigating anaemia on neonatal intensive care.

method for staining cells that contain foetal haemoglobin in a maternal blood sample. This technique, described as the Kleihauer–Betke technique, may be confounded by conditions where there is an increased level of baseline maternal foetal haemoglobin such as hereditary persistence of foetal haemoglobin or sickle cell disease. In these circumstances, alternative techniques can be used to detect foetal red cells including flow cytometry.

Twin-to-twin transfusions. Twin-to-twin transfusions are observed in monozygotic twins who share a single placenta. The frequency of twin-to-twin transfusion syndrome in pregnancies where there is a monochorial placenta has been estimated between 5% and 15% [7]. Transfusion of blood from one twin to the other leads to anaemia in the donating foetus and polycythaemia in the recipient; the difference in haemoglobin concentrations may exceed 70 g/L. The anaemic infant may suffer consequences of chronic anaemia including congestive cardiac failure. The anaemia is managed by transfusion as required when the condition is recognized following birth. The recipient twin may present with plethora, hyperviscosity, disseminated vascular coagulation and hyperbilirubinaemia (see Chapter 4 for management of neonatal polycythaemia).

Obstetric accidents. Obstetric accidents that can lead to blood loss include abnormalities of the umbilical cord or placenta and obstetric interventions. Umbilical cord pathology may include rupture of either a normal or an abnormal cord, a haematoma of the umbilical cord and rupture of anomalous blood vessels. Placenta praevia and rupture of the placenta are both associated with neonatal blood loss. Intrauterine manipulation of the foetus, caesarean section and placental damage during caesarean section may also lead to significant blood loss and anaemia.

Internal haemorrhage. Bleeds involving the head of the infant may lead to a volume of blood loss sufficient to lead to shock. Bleeds may occur in the intracranial, subdural or subarachnoid spaces. A cephalohaematoma describes blood loss in the sub-periosteal space of one of the cranial bones; a greater volume of blood loss may enter the sub-aponeurotic area of the scalp because the bleeding is not limited to an area overlying a single skull bone. Bleeds involving the head tend to occur more frequently after trauma including instrumental assistance such as the use of forceps or a ventouse suction device. Significant neonatal bleeding may also occur in the adrenal glands, spleen, kidneys, liver and retroperitoneal area. Bleeding in these sites is more likely to occur following traumatic delivery including breech delivery. Other risk factors for neonatal haemorrhage include congenital bleeding disorders, haemorrhagic disease of the newborn, thrombocytopenia, viral infections and haemangiomata of the skin or gastrointestinal tract.

Blood sampling. Anaemia caused by blood sampling for investigation is frequently recognized in neonates. Given the small total blood volume, a blood sample taken for investigations may comprise 1–2% of the blood volume in a significantly premature infant. Blood transfusion is not infrequently required to replace blood losses consequent on these necessary investigations.

Haemolysis

The normal red cell lifespan in a term infant is 60–80 days but is shorter for a premature infant [2]. Haemolysis in the neonatal period causes a reduced red cell survival. It may present with an increased reticulocyte count with or without a drop in haemoglobin in the absence of haemorrhage. The presence of haemolysis may also be inferred if, in the absence of bleeding, there is a rapidly falling haemoglobin concentration in the presence of an increased reticulocyte count. Haemolysis is usually accompanied by hyperbilirubinaemia.

There are a number of causes of a haemolytic process in the neonatal period, some of which are unique to this stage of life:

• *Immune mediated.* Foetal to maternal red cell antigen incompatibility including Rhesus, ABO and other minor blood groups; maternal autoimmune haemolytic anaemia; drug-induced haemolytic anaemia (for further details, see Chapter 32).

• *Infection.* Bacterial, syphilis, malaria, cytomegalovirus, adenovirus, rubella, toxoplasmosis and disseminated herpes. Congenital malaria and parasitaemia at birth are strongly associated with low haemoglobin at delivery.

• *Microangiopathic anaemia.* Disseminated intravascular coagulation, cavernous haemangiomata or haemangioendotheliomata, large vessel thrombi, renal artery stenosis and severe coarctation of the aorta.

• *Metabolic disorders.* Galactosaemia and prolonged or recurrent metabolic or respiratory acidosis.

• *Haemoglobin abnormalities.* Alpha thalassaemia syndromes, alpha chain structural abnormalities, gamma thalassaemia syndromes and gamma chain structural abnormalities.

The haemoglobin molecule consists of a haem group consisting of an iron ion held in a heterocyclic ring known as porphyrin. This is surrounded by a tetrahedral arrangement of two pairs of globin proteins. There are four principal globin proteins that contribute to the three principal forms of haemoglobin present in the neonatal period: alpha (α), beta (β), gamma (γ) and delta (δ) chains. Each form of haemoglobin contains two alpha chains; these are combined with two beta chains to form haemoglobin A ($\alpha_2\beta_2$), two gamma chains to form haemoglobin F ($\alpha_2\gamma_2$) and two delta chains to form haemoglobin A2 ($\alpha_2\delta_2$). The principal haemoglobin molecule at birth is haemoglobin F, the proportion of which reduces during the first 6 months of life to be replaced by haemoglobin A. A small proportion of haemoglobin A2 is synthesized during the first 6 months such that by 6 months of age, the normal relative proportions of haemoglobin are haemoglobin A, 95%; haemoglobin A2, 1.5–3.5%; and haemoglobin F, less than 1%.

- *Structurally abnormal haemoglobin molecules.* Abnormal forms of alpha (α) and gamma (γ) chains may result in mild clinical abnormalities. These include unstable alpha-globin chains such as haemoglobin Hasharon and rare unstable gamma-globin chains. These present with mild disorders of infancy, which spontaneously resolve as the switch from haemoglobin F to haemoglobin A occurs. Clinical expression of beta-globin abnormalities is usually but not exclusively restricted to infants over 6 months of age by which time the gamma to beta chain switch has occurred. However, if there has been a significant loss of neonatal red cells due to haemolysis or blood loss in the early months of life, replacement by new red cells containing newly synthesized haemoglobin A may lead to an increased proportion of haemoglobin A and an earlier clinical expression of a beta-globin disorder. Sickle cell disease is one such disorder and normally presents beyond the age of 6 months for the aforementioned reasons, but rare cases of significant sickling have been described within the first month of life due to sickle cell anaemia.
- *Defects in haemoglobin synthesis.* Defects in the synthesis of alpha and gamma-globin chains may result in clinical problems in the neonatal period. The synthesis of alpha-globin chains is controlled by four genes; alpha thalassaemia syndromes may result from the deletion or mutations affecting one, two, three or four of these genes. One- or two-gene deletions lead to alpha thalas-

saemia trait, which is not clinically significant but may cause a mild microcytic anaemia. Deletion of three genes leads to haemoglobin H disease characterized by a significant microcytic anaemia with ongoing haemolysis and large quantities of haemoglobin Barts (γ_4) and some haemoglobin H (β_4) in the newborn period. As the infant matures, the haemoglobin Barts disappears but the haemoglobin H remains. Deletion of all four alpha gene leads to death of the untreated affected foetus, a condition known as hydrops foetalis. The sole form of haemoglobin in these cases is haemoglobin Barts (γ_4) with occasional remnants of earlier haemoglobin forms such as haemoglobin Portland. The infant has severe anaemia, and oxygen delivery is poor because of the left-shifted oxygen dissociation curve characteristic of haemoglobin Barts. If the disorder is detected *in utero*, it is possible to treat by *in utero* red cell transfusions, which are then continued after delivery.

- Gamma thalassaemia is rarely recognized, which may reflect the multiple genes for gamma gene synthesis and the spontaneous resolution of any symptoms during the haemoglobin switching period. Beta thalassaemia does not present in the neonatal period but later during the switch from haemoglobin F to haemoglobin A, and there are no red cell abnormalities at birth. Early presentations with beta thalassaemia minor or major may follow shortened red cell survival in the foetal or neonatal period.

• *Congenital methaemoglobinaemia and drug-induced methaemoglobinaemia* may present in the neonatal period. Acquired methaemoglobinaemia may present during this period as a consequence of nitrate oxide inhalation for reduction of pulmonary vascular resistance; it has also been described in association with diarrhoea.

• *Congenital disorders of the red cell membrane.* Congenital disorders of the red cell membrane may result in haemolysis and anaemia in the neonate. Structural disorders of the red cell membrane may lead to abnormal-shaped red cells, which may have clinical presentations during the neonatal period. These disorders include hereditary spherocytosis, hereditary elliptocytosis, hereditary stomatocytosis and hereditary xerocytosis. Patients with hereditary spherocytosis have a baseline haemoglobin lower than age-matched controls. These patients may develop a significant anaemia during the neonatal period and given the blunted reticulocyte response may require red cell transfusion. They may also present with neonatal jaundice.

• *Red cell enzyme deficiencies.* Glucose-6-phosphate dehydrogenase deficiency and pyruvate kinase deficiencies are the most common enzyme disorders that lead to haemolysis and may both present in the neonatal period. Other examples include 5′ nucleotidase deficiency and glucose phosphate isomerase deficiency.

Impaired red cell production

Congenital disorders leading to reduced red cell production can all present during the neonatal period. These syndromes include Diamond–Blackfan anaemia, which leads to pure red cell aplasia and variable other cellular deficiencies. Neonates with this disorder may have low birth weight and associated morphological abnormalities including macrocephaly, cleft palate, abnormalities of the eye, a webbed neck and deformity of the thumb. Pearson's syndrome is a disorder characterized by exocrine pancreatic dysfunction, sideroblastic anaemia and vacuolization of bone marrow precursors; it is thought to be secondary to an abnormality in mitochondrial DNA. A macrocytic neonatal anaemia has also been described in some cases of cartilage hair hypoplasia, and congenital dyserythropoietic anaemia may present in infancy. Exogenous causes of impaired red cell production that may present with neonatal anaemia include congenital infections such as rubella, cytomegalovirus, adenovirus and parvovirus. Bone marrow infiltration such as congenital leukaemia and osteopetrosis may also lead to anaemia due to inadequate red cell production as in many cases of Down's syndrome may

be associated with anaemia. Impaired red cell production will manifest as a reduced reticulocyte number compared to the age-adjusted normal range. Many cases of neonatal anaemia resolve with observation during supportive care; however, a bone marrow examination would be indicated if the abnormality persists. Morphological appearances associated with the possible diagnoses will be evident.

References

1 Strauss RG. Anaemia of prematurity: pathophysiology and treatment. Blood Rev 2010;24:221–225.

2 Nathan DG, Oski FA. The neonatal erythrocyte and its disorders. In Nathan DG, Orkin SH, Ginsburg D, Look AT (eds), Hematology of Infancy and Childhood. 6th edition. Philadelphia: Saunders, 2003.

3 Oetinger L, Mills WB. Simultaneous capillary and venous haemoglobin determinations in newborn infants. J Pediatr 1949;35:362–365.

4 Usher R, Shephard M, Lind J. The blood volume of the newborn infant and placental transfusion. Acta Paediatr 1963;52:497–512.

5 Von Kohorn I, Ehrenkranz R. Anemia in the preterm infant: erythropoietin versus erythrocyte transfusion—it's not that simple. Clin Perinatol 2009;36:111–123.

6 de Almeida V, Bowman JM. Massive fetomaternal hemorrhage: Manitoba experience. Obstet Gynecol 1994;83:323–328.

7 Seng YC, Rajadurai V. Twin-twin transfusion syndrome: a five year review. Arch Dis Child Fetal Neonatal Ed 2000;83:F168–70.

CHAPTER 32

Haemolysis

Michael Richards

Department of Paediatric Haematology, Leeds Children's Hospital, Leeds, UK

Haemolysis describes the pathological process whereby red cells are destroyed resulting in a shortened lifespan. Most haemolytic processes result in extravascular red cell removal in the reticuloendothelial tissues (mainly liver and spleen). Clinical features include variable anaemia and jaundice, splenomegaly, occasional hepatomegaly and the formation of bile pigment gall stones. Haemolysis may also occur within the bone marrow tissue when unstable red cell precursors are destroyed prior to release into the circulation (e.g. thalassaemia major). Intravascular haemolysis is generally more severe and may require critical care support. Patients may develop back or loin pain, acute renal injury and, in severe cases, cardiovascular collapse. Important causes of intravascular haemolysis are:

• Mismatched blood transfusion usually involving the ABO group
• Glucose-6-phosphate dehydrogenase (G6PD) deficiency
• Paroxysmal nocturnal haemoglobinuria (PNH)
• Paroxysmal cold haemoglobinuria (PCH)
• Severe autoimmune haemolytic anaemia (AIHA)
• Septicaemia due to *Clostridium perfringens*
• Blackwater fever due to malaria
• Microangiopathic processes

Both haemolysis within the intravascular compartment and in the reticuloendothelial tissues will result in a rise in the levels of unconjugated bilirubin and urobilinogen in the faeces and urine. Intravascular haemolysis results in the release of free haemoglobin into the plasma, which may occasionally be detected but is usually conjugated to haptoglobin, which then reduces the concentration of free haptoglobin. Haptoglobin concentrations may be increased during an acute-phase response, and production is reduced in infancy; therefore, reduced haptoglobin levels are not always a reliable marker of haemolysis. Rarely, haemoglobin is excreted through the kidney and can be detected in the urine as free haemoglobin and later as haemosiderin within the urine. The serum lactate dehydrogenase (LDH) is typically raised. Examination of the blood film may show abnormal red cell morphology, the nature of which depends on the particular process leading to haemolysis.

The pathogenesis of haemolysis in the infant and child encompasses similar generic considerations as are encountered in adults (see Chapter 1). Inherited disorders and maternal/foetal interactions, however, play an increased role compared to pathology that is more relevant to adults. Assessment of the cause of haemolysis requires focus on the family history especially adverse outcomes in previous siblings and a focus on dysmorphic somatic physical features that may indicate a specific syndrome.

Categorization of haemolytic processes

The causes of haemolysis may be differentiated into pathology that is intrinsic or extrinsic to the red cell and whether it is a congenital or acquired disorder (Table 32.1).

Haematology in Critical Care: A Practical Handbook, First Edition. Edited by Jecko Thachil and Quentin A. Hill.
© 2014 John Wiley & Sons, Ltd. Published 2014 by John Wiley & Sons, Ltd.

Table 32.1 Causes of haemolysis.

	Congenital	Acquired
Intrinsic to red cell	Membrane abnormalities Enzyme deficiencies Haemoglobin abnormalities Thalassaemia Haemoglobinopathies	Paroxysmal nocturnal haemoglobinuria (PNH)
Extrinsic to red cell		Immune Autoimmune Alloimmune Microangiopathic haemolysis Infections Malaria Babesiosis

Immune-mediated haemolytic anaemia

Immune haemolysis occurs as a consequence of binding of immunoglobulin molecules to the red cell surface followed by interaction with monocytes and complement and removal of these erythrocytes. Alloimmune haemolysis may occur as a consequence of incompatibility of the red cell of the neonate with maternal red cells in haemolytic disease of the newborn (HDN), or haemolysis of incompatible red cells following transfusion. Autoimmune haemolysis occurs when the host immune system becomes sensitized to its own red cell antigens.

Haemolytic disease of the newborn

Maternal sensitization to an incompatible foetal blood group antigen results in transfer of immunoglobulin IgG from the maternal to the foetal circulation, leading to haemolysis. Severely affected foetuses may have foetal hydrops. This is characterized by severe anaemia leading to foetal heart failure, progressively greater extramedullary erythropoiesis, hepatomegaly and splenomegaly. Hypoalbuminaemia, pericardial and pleural effusions and associated polyhydramnios may also occur. In mild disease, there may be no anaemia or anaemia well compensated for *in utero*. The resulting neonatal unconjugated hyperbilirubinaemia may lead to neurotoxicity, a condition known as kernicterus. The principle treatments for unconjugated hyperbilirubinaemia

are phototherapy or exchange transfusions. Anaemia may be treated by top-up or exchange transfusions.

The specific red cell antigens that may lead to severe haemorrhagic disease in the newborn include Rhesus D and c, Kell and Fya. Other antigen systems cause milder disorders; these include Rhesus E, C, Kpa, k and S. Anti-Kell antibodies may lead to the suppression of erythropoiesis. ABO group haemolysis is mild and has a negative or only weakly positive direct antiglobulin test (DAT) but prominent spherocytosis [1].

Treatment for HDN during the perinatal period depends on the severity of the condition. Significant hyperbilirubinaemia may develop within the first 24 h after birth, which may require phototherapy to avoid kernicterus. Severe anaemia and resistant hyperbilirubinaemia will require transfusion including possible exchange transfusion.

Autoimmune haemolytic anaemia (AIHA)

AIHA can be divided into a primary state or secondary to a discrete underlying pathology. Primary AIHA is commonly due to warm reactive IgG autoantibodies, frequently with Rhesus antigen specificity that cause extravascular haemolysis predominantly in the spleen. The DAT is positive with anti-IgG. PCH follows the binding of the Donath–Landsteiner antibody, an IgG antibody that has specificity to the P red cell antigen. It binds in the peripheral circulation where temperatures are cooler (<30°C), but complement activation and intravascular haemolysis occur when the red cells pass to the warmer central circulation. The DAT results at room temperature are positive with anti-C3 (complement) but negative with anti-IgG. Cold agglutinin disease is characterized by the binding of IgM to the I or i red cell antigen at temperatures below 37°C and leads to avid complement fixation. Haemolysis may be either intravascular or extravascular.

Spherocytes are most prominent in cases of warm autoantibodies. Red cell agglutination may be seen in cold AIHA. Reticulocytosis is common, but reticulocytopaenia may occur in approximately 10% of paediatric patients with AIHA. Very rarely a negative DAT can occur in a disorder that otherwise fits with an AIHA.

Evan's syndrome is characterized by AIHA, thrombocytopenia and rarely neutropenia, a severe disorder in which aggressive treatment is required.

Warm AIHA and PCH frequently follow a viral-type illness. Cold AIHA is seen more commonly in adults and may follow mycoplasma infection. Most cases of AIHA have a good prognosis, and a proportion will remit spontaneously. In those cases with cold-reacting antibodies, maintenance of adequate body temperature including the peripheries is important. Treatment modalities for persistent AIHA include the use of red cell transfusions for significant anaemia. This is frequently technically challenging because the autoantibody may potentially mask a significant alloantibody during the crossmatching process. Treatment to alter the disease process includes immunosuppressives including corticosteroids and intravenous immunoglobulin and in IgM disorders exchange transfusion or plasmapheresis. Splenectomy has been used in chronic cases. There has been increasing evidence of the efficacy of rituximab, a therapeutic anti-CD20 antibody that leads to the lysis of B lymphocytes [2].

Secondary AIHA is associated with another underlying disease state. It may occur as part of a broader immune dysregulation state as seen in disorders such as systemic lupus erythematosis, Sjögren's syndrome, scleroderma, dermatomyositis, ulcerative colitis, rheumatoid arthritis, autoimmune thyroiditis and autoimmune lymphoproliferative syndrome. Malignancy such as Hodgkin's disease and non-Hodgkin's lymphoma may be associated with AIHA. Congenital immune deficiency may be associated with AIHA as is acquired immune deficiency following immunodeficiency virus infection. Infections that may lead to autoimmune haemolysis include large number of viruses, *Mycoplasma pneumoniae*, Epstein–Barr virus, measles, varicella, mumps, rubella and parvovirus. Acute bacterial infections may lead to exposure of the cryptic T antigen on red cells which may lead to haemolysis, especially in neonates affected by necrotizing enterocolitis. Previous transfusion practice was to provide T antibody-negative transfusions for these infants, but this is now not recommended. Drugs that may cause secondary AIHA include the following: methyldopa, penicillin, cephalosporin, erythromycin, probenecid, acetaminophen and ibuprofen.

The treatment of cases of secondary autoimmune haemolysis focuses on removal of the precipitant or treatment of the underlying condition. Additional therapy will follow that described for idiopathic cases.

Paroxysmal nocturnal haemoglobinuria (PNH)

PNH is an acquired clonal stem cell disorder caused by a somatic mutation in the gene encoding phosphatidylinositol glycan A (*PIG-A*), an enzyme required for the synthesis of glycosyl-phosphatidylinositol (GPI), a molecule that anchors the surface proteins CD55 and CD59 on blood cells. Without these proteins, cells are vulnerable to attack by the terminal complement pathway giving rise to chronic intravascular haemolysis. There may be other cytopenias as PNH can arise on a background of bone marrow failure. Other symptoms include dysphagia, lethargy, erectile failure, abdominal pain and haematuria worst in the morning and clearing through the day. Thrombosis, which is the leading cause of mortality, is usually venous with a predilection for intra-abdominal and cerebral veins. PNH can be readily diagnosed by peripheral blood flow cytometric analysis. Its treatment has been revolutionized by the use of eculizumab, a humanized monoclonal antibody which prevents cleavage of C5, preventing intravascular haemolysis.

Pitfalls in PNH management

• Not thinking of it. Consider testing patients with unexplained haemolysis, thrombosis at atypical sites or underlying bone marrow failure.
• Plasma products such as fresh frozen plasma contain complement. Patients receiving C5 blockade may develop breakthrough haemolysis if given plasma products. Discuss care with an expert treatment centre.
• Patients receiving C5 blockade are at increased risk of meningococcal infection. This should be considered in such patients if presenting unwell with a fever.

Microangiopathic haemolytic anaemia

This group of anaemias are characterized by the presence of schistocytes in the peripheral blood film. In childhood, the most common cause is haemolytic uraemic syndrome characterized by anaemia, variable thrombocytopenia and renal dysfunction. Generally, this requires renal support and the haematological manifestations of the disorder are self-limiting. Thrombotic thrombocytopenic purpura (TTP) is characterized by anaemia, thrombocytopenia, microangiopathy, fever and neurological deterioration. It is predominantly seen in adults as an acquired disorder. It is associated with deficiency of the enzyme ADAMTS13 (a disintegrin and metalloproteinase with a thrombospondin type 1 motif, member 13). This proteinase cleaves high-molecular-weight multimers of von Willebrand factor, thus controlling the platelet endothelial interaction. The absence of a control on this process leads to arteriolar fibrinoid deposition, platelet trapping and schistocyte formation. In adults, an antibody has been found to the ADAMTS13 proteinase, which explains the acquired nature of the disorder. Mutations have been detected in children, leading to congenital deficiency of this protein, but other paediatric cases have occurred secondary to an antibody [3]. Treatment in the acquired disorder includes plasma exchange and immunosuppression. In the congenital disorder, it is necessary to replace the deficient proteinase with plasma coagulation factor concentrates. Microangiopathic haemolytic anaemia may also occur in association with immune vasculitis, disseminated malignancy, pregnancy and malignant hypertension. Microangiopathy may also be associated with large blood vessel disorders including haemangiomas, which may be associated with haemolytic anaemia, intravascular coagulation and severe thrombocytopenia (Kasabach–Merritt syndrome). Red cell lysis may occur in association with valvular heart disease, most notably after the insertion or failure of a prosthetic heart valve. A variety of drugs have also been associated including cocaine, quinine, ciclosporin and tacrolimus. Treatment of microangiopathic disorders associated with other conditions is focussed on management of the primary disorder or removal of the precipitant.

Red cell membrane disorders

The red cell membrane is composed of a phospholipid bilayer with interspersed glycolipids, cholesterol and proteins. The protein red cell membrane skeleton is positioned internal to the lipid bilayer.

Disturbance of the bilayer may lead to increased interaction with the vascular endothelium as is seen in sickle cell disease and patients with diabetes, membrane projections (echinocytosis) or invagination of the membrane forming cup-shaped red cells (stomatocytosis). Abnormalities in the band 3 membrane protein have been

associated with disorders such as hereditary spherocytosis (HS) and Southeast Asian ovalocytosis.

Pathological states consequent on disorders of the erythrocyte membrane.

HS is an inherited disorder characterized by haemolysis and sphere-shaped red cells (spherocytosis). It affects approximately 1 person in 5000 in northern Europe. There is a typical autosomal dominance in two-thirds of patients; the remainder have a nondominant inheritance. The disorder is consequent on defects in the proteins that bind the lipid bilayer to the membrane skeleton including spectrin, ankyrin, protein 4.2 and band 3. Since spherocytes have less cellular deformability, they have a shortened half-life resulting in haemolysis.

The typical features of HS include the clinical and biochemical evidence of haemolysis with spherocytosis observed on a peripheral blood film and confirmed by *in vitro* tests including increased osmotic fragility. There is frequently an informative family history. There is a spectrum of severity, which appears to correlate with the degree of spectrin deficiency of the red blood cells. The DAT is negative.

Recommended screening tests include the cryohaemolysis test and eosin-5-maleimide (EMA) binding. Clinical features of HS include neonatal jaundice and anaemia and rare cases of hydrops foetalis. Complications of the disorder include bile pigment gallstones, exacerbation of haemolysis usually following viral infections and aplastic crises usually caused by the parvovirus B19 infection. Red cell production may be limited by a megaloblastic erythropoiesis due to folate deficiency especially in patients recovering from an aplastic crisis.

Splenectomy reduces the rate of haemolysis, anaemia and symptoms in the vast majority of patients with clinically significant HS. Splenectomy should be performed in children with severe HS, considered in those who have moderate disease, and should probably not be performed in those with mild disease [4] but ideally should be performed after the age of 6 years. Red cell transfusions may be required for patients undergoing an aplastic crisis and rarely during the exaggeration of the physiological fall in haemoglobin seen in the first 6 months of life.

Hereditary elliptocytosis (HE) is characterized by the appearance of elliptical or oval red cell on a peripheral blood smear. It is inherited predominantly in an autosomal dominant manner; it is most common in people of African and Mediterranean ancestry. The majority of HE

Table 32.2 Miscellaneous red cell haemolytic disorders characterized by predominant morphological abnormality.

Morphological abnormality	Red cell disorders
Spherocytes	Hereditary spherocytosis (HS), ABO incompatibility in neonates, autoimmune haemolytic anaemia (AIHA), acute oxidant injury, haemolytic transfusion reactions. *Clostridium perfringens* sepsis, severe burns, spider and snake venoms, severe hypophosphataemia, hypersplenism
Bizarre-shaped red cells	Red cell fragmentation syndromes, acute oxidant injury, hereditary pyropoikilocytosis (HPP), homozygous hereditary elliptocytosis (HE), hereditary stomatocytosis, Rhesus null blood group, thalassaemia, irreversibly sickle cells, sickle cell anaemia
Intra-erythrocyte parasites	Malaria, bartonellosis, babesiosis
Prominent basophilic stippling	Thalassaemia and unstable haemoglobinopathies, lead poisoning, pyrimidine-5'-nucleotidase deficiency
Target cells	Haemoglobins S, C, D and E; HS; thalassaemia
Spiculated or crenated red cells	Acute hepatic necrosis, uraemia, red cell fragmentation syndromes, infantile pyknocytosis, Embden–Meyerhof pathway defect, vitamin E deficiency, abetalipoproteinaemia, McLeod blood group, post-splenectomy, anorexia nervosa
Non-specific* or normal morphology	Enzyme defects and unstable haemoglobinopathies, PNH, dyserythropoietic anaemia, copper toxicity (Wilson's disease), cation permeability defects, erythropoietic porphyria, vitamin E deficiencies, haemolysis with infections, Rhesus haemolysis in newborns, PCH, cold haemolytic disease, hypersplenism, AIHA

*These conditions may present without abnormal morphology but may also present with typical morphological features.

disorders are as a consequence of alpha or beta spectrin abnormalities.

Hereditary pyropoikilocytosis (HPP) is an uncommon disorder mostly seen in patients of African origin, which may lead to severe anaemia. A peripheral film reveals markedly abnormal shapes and sizes of red cells including budding red cells, fragmented cells, spherocytes and increased red cell thermal sensitivity. The underlying molecular defect leads to a severe deficiency in spectrin.

Management of HE and HPP is similar to the treatment of HS.

Southeast Asian ovalocytosis is a disorder that is inherited in an autosomal dominant fashion common in Malaysia, Indonesia and the Philippines that results in a mild haemolytic anaemia. The underlying molecular abnormality is a band 3 mutation, which also leads to a protection against malaria.

Hereditary stomatocytosis is characterized by red cells with a mouth-shaped area of central pallor, which occurs as a consequence of red cell swelling due to the increased permeability of the membrane to potassium and sodium ions. Haemolysis can be severe, and the dehydrated form may present with pseudohyperkalaemia and potentially lethal perinatal oedema. Splenectomy is usually avoided due to the increased risk of thrombosis.

Hereditary xerocytosis results in mild anaemia characterized by dehydrated red cells that appear contracted and speculated. Stomatocytosis and spherocytosis may occur as a consequence of the absence of Rhesus antigen on the red cell membrane (Rhesus null) (Table 32.2).

Enzyme deficiencies leading to haemolysis

The critical enzymes in maintaining erythrocyte viability are those that are involved in the glycolytic production of adenosine triphosphate (ATP) and the enzymes that protect the cell from oxidative damage. Enzyme deficiency results in haemolysis, which is rarely associated with spherocytosis. Although splenectomy is recommended for some enzymopathies, not all disorders may benefit from this intervention. Disorders of glycolysis generally have a recessive inheritance; G6PD deficiency is sex linked. Investigation of glycolytic pathway defects requires specific assays of the intermediate compounds of the metabolic pathways. Confounding factors in the assay of these metabolites include recent red cell transfusions and reticulocytosis.

Pyruvate kinase deficiency is the most common glycolytic enzyme disorder. It has an incidence of up to 50 cases per 100,000 in the white population and causes variable anaemia. Blood film examination reveals macrocytes, occasional shrunken spiculated erythrocytes and acanthocytes. Inheritance is usually autosomal recessive. Splenectomy may be partially effective in cases with a severe phenotype.

Pyrimidine-5'-nucleotidase deficiency is associated with a moderate lifelong chronic haemolytic anaemia, which may be associated with splenomegaly. Blood films may reveal prominent basophilic stippling in as much as 5% of all red cells. Inheritance is autosomal recessive. Lead poisoning may give similar red cell morphological appearances.

Other rare glycolytic enzyme deficiencies may be associated with systemic manifestations including neurodevelopmental disorders and specific facial features.

Glucose-6-phosphate dehydrogenase deficiency is a key enzyme in the pentose phosphate pathway, which leads to the production of glutathione, which protects the cell from oxidative damage. G6PD deficiency may lead to acute haemolytic anaemia following an oxidative challenge, which may lead to intense intravascular haemolysis and very dark urine. The haemoglobin may be moderately or severely reduced with levels of 25 g/L recorded. Peripheral film red cell morphology is characterized by irregularly contracted cells, cells with an uneven distribution of haemoglobin and *bite* cells. The reticulocyte count is increased, and a supravital stain will reveal Heinz bodies within the red cell consisting of denatured haemoglobin. Precipitants of this oxidative stress include fava beans; drugs especially the antimalarials, chloroquine and primaquine; sulphonamide antibacterial agents including dapsone and septrin; other antibacterial compounds such as nitrofurantoin; analgesia such as aspirin and phenacetin; anthelmintic such as beta naphthol, stibophen and niridazole; and miscellaneous drugs such as vitamin K analogues, naphthalene, probenecid, dimercaprol and methylene blue. G6PD deficiency may also lead to neonatal jaundice and a chronic low-grade non-spherocytic haemolytic anaemia. Measurement of red cell G6PD may be confounded by a reticulocytosis and leukocyte contamination. The G6PD gene is situated on the X chromosome, and female carriers may have deficient levels of the enzyme. Patients from Africa have milder disorders than patients from the Mediterranean and Southeast Asia. Patients must be advised to avoid the precipitants of haemolysis. Supportive measures and red cell transfusion may be needed in the case of acute haemolytic anaemia. Neonatal jaundice may require phototherapy or rarely exchange transfusion. Folic acid supplementation is indicated for patients with chronic non-spherocytic haemolytic anaemia as well as advice regarding avoidance of precipitants of haemolysis. Splenectomy has on occasions been beneficial.

Haemoglobinopathies and thalassaemia

Patients who have inherited a quantitative deficiency of a globin chain – alpha or beta thalassaemia – or a structural abnormality, the haemoglobinopathies, have red cells that are more vulnerable to lysis. These result in chronic haemolytic states with acute exacerbations. Beta-globin abnormalities will cause clinical sequelae in children over 3 months of age and most notably after 6 months. The other clinical manifestations of these disorders overshadow the chronic haemolytic states that result.

References

1 Nathan DG, Oski FA. Immune hemolytic disease. In Nathan DG, Orkin SH, Ginsburg D, Look AT (eds), Hematology of Infancy and Childhood. 6th edition. Saunders, 2003.

2 Zecca M, Nobili B, Ramenghi U et al. Rituximab for the treatment of refractory autoimmune hemolytic anemia in children. Blood 2003;101:3857–61.

3 McDonald V, Liesner R, Grainger J, Gattens M, Machin SJ, Scully M. Acquired, noncongenital thrombotic thrombocytopenic purpura in children and adolescents: clinical management and the use of ADAMTS 13 assays. Blood Coagul Fibrinolysis 2010;21:245–50.

4 Bolton-Maggs PHB, Stevens RF, Dodd NJ, Lamont G, Tittensor P, King MJ on behalf of the General Haematology Task Force of the British Committee for Standards in Haematology. Guidelines for the diagnosis and management of hereditary spherocytosis. Br J Haematol 2004;126:455–74.

CHAPTER 33

Approach to Thrombocytopenia

Amrana Qureshi

Paediatric Haematology and Oncology Children's Hospital, John Radcliffe Hospital, Oxford, UK

General approach to thrombocytopenia

Causes of thrombocytopenia are varied in paediatric and neonatal intensive care [1]. Causes of thrombocytopenia may be primary (e.g. immune thrombocytopenic purpura) or part of an existing condition and the reason for admission to ITU (e.g. leukaemia) or secondary to sepsis/disseminated intravascular coagulation (DIC). Broadly, all causes may be divided into those with a predominant immune or non-immune aetiology. Although there is overlap of causes of thrombocytopenia in adults and children, many conditions are either specific to neonates and children, such as prematurity, neonatal allo- and autoimmune thrombocytopenia and congenital causes, or have a different natural history, such as immune thrombocytopenia, which is usually self-limiting.

In this chapter, the approach to thrombocytopenia for patients developing thrombocytopenia in neonatal and paediatric intensive care is reviewed with particular focus on practical approaches to diagnosis and management. The mainstay of management remains transfusions of platelets. A specific section at the end describes an approach to use of platelets in neonatal and paediatric critical care. This will provide practical guidelines on transfusion practice for both prophylaxis prior to procedures in patients with thrombocytopenia and for (less commonly) bleeding in association with thrombocytopenia. For certain clinical conditions, platelet transfusions are not indicated, for example, thrombotic thrombocytopenic purpura (TTP) in childhood. In the face of major bleeding and if the predominant mechanism for thrombocytopenia is immune (ITP), platelet transfusions are likely to be less effective, and immunomodulatory therapy with steroids and immunoglobulins will be warranted.

More common causes of childhood thrombocytopenia in ITU

Non-immune mediated
Microangiopathic haemolytic anaemias
Disseminated intravascular coagulation (DIC)

In the ITU setting, sepsis is the most common cause of thrombocytopenia, which may also result in DIC and platelet consumption. Bacterial, viral and fungal infections can cause DIC. Meningococcal meningitis/septicaemia remains the most frequent cause of severe DIC in children. Other causes of DIC include malignancy, trauma, burns and liver disease. Pathogenesis and laboratory diagnosis of DIC are explained in Chapter 9.

Management of DIC

As DIC is a secondary event, the underlying cause should be treated. Replacement therapy with blood products is reserved for bleeding patients or prior to an invasive procedure. Fresh frozen plasma (FFP) can be given (15 mL/kg) with cryoprecipitate (5 mL/kg) and platelets to maintain a fibrinogen greater than 1 g/L and platelet count of 50×10^9/L in bleeding patients. The use of heparin and thrombolytic therapy in DIC is controversial. Protein C concentrate has been used in severe DIC secondary to meningococcal sepsis although there are no randomized control trial to prove its efficacy.

Haematology in Critical Care: A Practical Handbook, First Edition. Edited by Jecko Thachil and Quentin A. Hill.
© 2014 John Wiley & Sons, Ltd. Published 2014 by John Wiley & Sons, Ltd.

Haemolytic uraemic syndrome/TTP

Haemolytic uraemic syndrome (HUS) is a combination of microangiopathic haemolytic anaemia (MAHA), thrombocytopenia and acute renal failure. In children, HUS is most often caused by *E. coli* toxin (0157), which predominantly damages glomerular endothelial cells. Most cases recover without sequelae. Management is supportive but may require plasma exchange. Thrombocytopenia in HUS is caused by platelet aggregation, and platelet transfusion is relatively contraindicated as this may further increase microvascular thrombosis.

Acquired TTP is rare in children and most likely secondary to ciclosporin post-transplant (see also Chapter 11 on TTP). Emergency treatment with plasma exchange is required. More recently, rituximab (an anti-CD 20 antibody), which inhibits antibody formation, has been tried with success. Platelet transfusions, again, are relatively contraindicated. Congenital TTP results from deficiency of the ADAMST 13 enzyme, and treatment involves regular plasma infusions.

Haemophagocytic lymphohistiocytosis

This is a primary or secondary disorder which results from pathological and uncontrolled macrophage and T-cell activation from cytokine production. It is defined by bilineage (two blood cell lines), cytopenia (at least), fever, hepatosplenomegaly, deranged clotting, low fibrinogen, high ferritin and fasting triglycerides and histopathological evidence of haemophagocytosis in the skin, liver and bone marrow. In congenital type, presentation is often in infancy or early childhood, and the child can present with haemodynamic shock and acidosis. Urgent treatment with chemotherapy and steroids is required. Secondary cases mostly occur in older children, due to sepsis, and EBV is often causal in the older age group, sometimes in association with immunodeficiency. Treatment of the underlying cause is the mainstay of treatment. Chemotherapy may be required in severe cases. Platelet transfusion may be indicated in the case of bleeding.

More common causes of neonatal thrombocytopenia in ITU

Thrombocytopenia is common in the intensive care setting, and up to 35% of all neonates will develop platelet counts less than 50×10^9/L [2]. In premature and low-birth-weight

neonates, the incidence of thrombocytopenia is as high as 80%. The strongest predictors of thrombocytopenia are prematurity and antenatal factors, resulting in physiological stress to the neonate due to either placental insufficiency or infection [3].

The likely cause of thrombocytopenia can be postulated from the timing from birth.

Non-immune causes

In the premature neonate, or small-for-gestation age, in the first 72 h after birth, thrombocytopenia is likely to be due to antenatal and maternal factors (placental insufficiency and antenatal/perinatal infection), which results in suppressed production of platelets.

After 72 h, thrombocytopenia is most likely due to postnatally acquired infection, often bacterial, or necrotising enterocolitis and involves both suppression of platelet production due to cytokine release and increased consumption, often as part of DIC. Profound thrombocytopenia can develop quickly in this setting.

In the term, neonate thrombocytopenia usually results from sepsis and DIC. Further rare causes are mentioned in the Table 33.1 later.

Rarer causes of thrombocytopenia in ITU
Immune-mediated causes
Childhood
Immune thrombocytopenia (ITP)
Childhood ITP is a self-limiting autoimmune disorder and has an incidence of between 4.0 and 5.3 per 100,000. But the clinical condition may occasionally be associated with major bleeding and intracranial haemorrhage, which requires therapy in intensive care.

Acute, abrupt-onset ITP is seen mainly in childhood and often follows a viral illness or immunization. The majority of children require no treatment, and in 80–85% of cases, the disorder resolves within 6 months. Some 15–20% of children develop a chronic form of ITP, which, in some cases, resembles the more typical adult disease. Chronic ITP in childhood has an estimated incidence of 0.46 per 100,000 children per year. It can occur at any age, but after age of 10 years, the condition can be associated with other autoimmune conditions and is more likely to follow a chronic course.

0.5–1% of children may develop an intracranial haemorrhage, and bleeding from another site is a predictor in

Table 33.1 Causes and investigation of thrombocytopenia in the neonate in intensive care.

Cause	Investigation
Placental insufficiency	History (of pre-eclampsia, IUGR, abruption)
Perinatal asphyxia	History (evidence of hypoxic–ischaemic encephalopathy)
Sepsis	
Perinatal infection:	
Bacterial (group B Strep)	Blood cultures
Congenital infection	TORCH screen
Late-onset sepsis	Blood cultures
Necrotising enterocolitis	Clinical diagnosis
Disseminated intravascular coagulation (DIC)	Blood film – left shift, toxic granulation, fragments
	Prolonged APTT, PT, reduced fibrinogen (although different normal values in neonates)
Other causes of hypercoagulability	
Cyanotic congenital heart disease	Clinical, echocardiogram
Rhesus incompatibility	Anaemia, jaundice, positive Coombs' test
Anticoagulant deficiency (antithrombin) Proteins C and S Thrombosis	Thrombosis, serum levels of inhibitor
Immune causes (see next section)	
Neonatal alloimmune thrombocytopenia	History of severe thrombocytopenia in a well neonate within 48 h of birth. Check for HPA antibodies
Rare causes	
Familial thrombocytopenia (see succeeding text)	Family history, blood film platelet function studies
Metabolic disease	Organic aciduria, metabolic acidosis, bone marrow replacement/evidence of storage disease
Propionic and methylmalonic acidaemia, Gaucher's disease, Niemann–Pick disease, osteopetrosis	
Kasabach–Merritt syndrome	Evidence of haemangioma consumptive picture: increased PT, APTT, low fibrinogen, high D-dimers
Transient abnormal megakaryopoiesis	History of Down's syndrome, blood film, GATA 1 mutation
Congenital leukaemia	Blood film/bone marrow
Inherited bone marrow failure, e.g. congenital megakaryocytic leukaemia (CAMT)	Bone marrow, genetic studies

30% of patients and is a major reason for managing bleeding symptoms aggressively [4]. If the child does not respond to treatment or has an atypical presentation, bone marrow examination should be carried out to confirm the diagnosis.

The diagnosis of ITP is suspected from the clinical presentation and is a diagnosis of exclusion. There is usually an acute presentation of bruising, and sometimes bleeding in an otherwise well child, and clinically there are no positive findings except bruising or bleeding. The blood count will reveal an isolated low platelet count, usually in the single digits. The blood film examination will confirm thrombocytopenia, with often large platelets. In the UK, children are not treated unless there are bleeding symptoms, which can occur in 3–4% of cases.

In this instance, treatment is with steroids (prednisolone 4 mg/kg for 4 days or 1–2 mg/kg for 14 days) or immunoglobulin (0.8 g/kg once) [5]. In the event of life-threatening haemorrhage, platelet transfusion is also required.

Term neonate

In the term neonate, early and profound thrombocytopenia is most likely due to immune destruction of platelets by maternally derived antibodies.

Neonatal alloimmune thrombocytopenia

Neonatal alloimmune thrombocytopenia (NAIT), in the majority of proven cases, results from maternally derived anti-human platelet antigen (HPA)-1a or HPA-5b platelet antibodies. When an otherwise well neonate presents with severe thrombocytopenia within 48 h of birth, NAIT should be strongly suspected. Neonates can present with petechiae/bruising or bleeding. Serology testing of mother and baby through monoclonal antibody-specific immobilization of platelet antigen (MAIPA) can detect maternal HPA antibodies, and parents and infants can be genotyped for common HPA antigens. Specific antibodies can be detected in 20% of cases. Once identified, or if there is a strong clinical suspicion, the parents should be informed that future pregnancies are at risk of severe foetal thrombocytopenia and these should be closely monitored in a foetomaternal unit. In 80% of cases, an antibody may not be detected. If there is a strong clinical suspicion, there may be an indication to test further for low-frequency HPA antigens and antibodies, but this needs discussion with a paediatric haematologist.

In terms of clinical management, the baby should be transfused immediately if the platelet count is less than 30×10^9/L with HPA-1a- and HPA-5b-negative platelets if available, otherwise with random platelets as these have a role in absorbing circulating antibody, although they may be consumed quickly. Cranial ultrasound to exclude intracranial haemorrhage should be performed. If there is evidence of bleeding, a higher platelet threshold of greater than 50×10^9/L should be maintained. The platelet count should be maintained above this threshold until there is a sustained increase in platelet count. Most cases improve within 7–10 days, although rarely thrombocytopenia can persist up to 8–12 weeks. Intravenous immunoglobulin can have a role in the management of NAIT.

Neonatal autoimmune thrombocytopenia

Neonatal autoimmune thrombocytopenia is the second most common cause of profound thrombocytopenia in an otherwise well neonate. In the majority of cases, there is a known history of maternal ITP. This non-specific platelet antibody transfers across the placenta to the foetal circulation and cause a profound and sometimes prolonged thrombocytopenia. The neonates' blood count should be checked at birth and, if normal, 2–3 days later. If the thrombocytopenia is unexpected, the maternal platelet count should be checked. Normally, the platelet count in the neonate will rise within a week as the antibody levels fall. However, as in NAIT, the thrombocytopenia can persist up to 12 weeks. If the platelet count is less than 30×10^9/L in the first week of life and then less

than 20×10^9/L thereafter, treatment with IVIG, or steroids and occasional platelet transfusion to absorb the autoantibody, may be helpful.

Other causes of isolated thrombocytopenia in children include

1 Familial thrombocytopenia

Although present from birth, this condition is usually diagnosed in early childhood, due to bruising or bleeding or associated factors. It should be thought as a differential diagnosis, if thrombocytopenia is persistent in a young child. There are many types and extensive details are beyond the scope of this chapter [6, 7]. In the majority of cases, the platelet count is either mildly or moderately affected, and bleeding manifestations are uncommon. However, bleeding can be severe in Wiskott–Aldrich, and thrombocytopenia with absent radii (TAR syndrome), due to low platelet count, and Chediak–Higashi and Bernard–Soulier, due to marked platelet dysfunction. Diagnosis can be made by noting associated systemic features, blood film examination, platelet function assay, flow cytometry and genetic studies

2 Bone marrow infiltration

Infiltration with leukaemia, neuroblastoma or sometime storage diseases like Gaucher's or Niemann–Pick disease can cause thrombocytopenia. In these cases, additional clinical features will be present, including bone pain, hepatosplenomegaly, abdominal mass and other cytopenias.

3 Bone marrow failure syndromes

Fanconi anaemia can present with isolated thrombocytopenia. This is a rare autosomal recessive condition where a mutation in the FANC gene results in a defect in the Fanconi anaemia repair pathway, which is crucial in chromosomal repair. This results in a marked propensity for malignancy. There is phenotypic heterogeneity and skeletal abnormalities in the radial bone; short stature and skin pigmentation are the most common clinical features. A cardinal feature is the gradual onset of bone marrow failure, firstly with thrombocytopenia and eventual bone marrow aplasia. The median age for development of haematological abnormalities is about 5 years. The treatment for bone marrow failure is with androgens or bone marrow transplant.

4 Massive splenomegaly leading to hypersplenism

5 Chemotherapy

6 Vasculitides such as Henoch–Schönlein purpura

Management of thrombocytopenia

Transfusions of platelets form the mainstay of treatment for bleeding associated with thrombocytopenia or to prevent bleeding in thrombocytopenic patients, for example, pre-procedure. There are no clinical trials to establish the safe platelet threshold to avoid bleeding. However, clinical observation and consensus in the British Committee for Standards of Haematology state that the threshold for prophylactic platelet transfusion in a well child is $10 \times 10^9/L$. In an unwell/haemodynamically unstable child (which is the case in the intensive care setting), it is $20 \times 10^9/L$. In a bleeding child, platelets should be administered for non-immune causes if the platelet count is less than $50 \times 10^9/L$. Table 33.2 gives guidance on threshold platelet counts for different settings [8].

All neonates should currently receive apheresed (single donor), CMV-negative platelets. The dose of platelets should be 10–20 mL/kg, administered usually over 30 min. All prescriptions should be in millilitres rather than 'pools'; otherwise, it can result in inappropriate

and dangerously large volume transfusion (transfusion associated circulatory overload). Most platelet bags contain 200–300 mL of platelets, but it can be available as a paediapack (50 mL to 1 U divided into four), which reduces donor exposure. Attempts should be made to avoid wastage when prescribing platelets. At the time of writing, one (adult) platelet transfusion costs £133 (see also Chapter 13 on blood components).

References

1 Slichter SJ. Relationship between platelet count and bleeding risk in thrombocytopenic patients. Transfus Med Rev 2004; 18(3):153–67.

2 Roberts I, Murray NA. Neonatal thrombocytopenia: causes and management. Arch Dis Child Fetal Neonatal Ed 2003;88: 359–64.

3 Chakravorty S, Roberts I. How I manage neonatal thrombocytopenia. Br J Haematol 2011;156:155–62.

4 Psaila B, Petrovic A, Page LK, Menell J, Schonholz M, Bussel JB. Intracranial hemorrhage (ICH) in children with immune thrombocytopenia (ITP): study of 40 cases. Blood 2009;114(23):4777–839.

5 Provan D, Stasi R, Newland AC et al. International consensus report on the investigation and management of primary immune thrombocytopenia. Blood 2010;115:168–86.

6 Arceci RJ, Hann IM, Smith OP. Pediatric Haematology. 3rd edition. New York: Blackwell Publishing, 2006 (Section 6 Chapters 22–25 Pages 507–79).

7 Cines DB, Bussel JB, McMillan RB, Zehnder JL. Congenital and acquired thrombocytopenia. Hematology Am Soc Hematol Educ Program 2004; 1390–406.

8 Gibson BE, Todd A, Roberts I, et al. Transfusion guidelines for neonates and older children. Br J Haematol 2004;124:433–53.

Table 33.2 Platelet thresholds for transfusion in neonates and children.

	Platelet threshold
All neonates (up to 1 month of age)	$20 \times 10^9/L$
<1 kg, <1 week of age	$30 \times 10^9/L$
Sick preterm or term neonate	
Well child	$10 \times 10^9/L$
Unwell/haemodynamically unstable child	$20 \times 10^9/L$
Active bleeding	$50 \times 10^9/L$

CHAPTER 34

Blood Component Therapy in Children and Neonates

Anne Kelly[1], Simon J. Stanworth[2,3] and Helen V. New[4]

[1] Department of Haematology, Division of Transfusion Medicine, University of Cambridge/NHS Blood and Transplant Cambridge, Cambridge, UK
[2] NHS Blood and Transplant/Oxford University Hospitals NHS Trust, John Radcliffe Hospital, Oxford, UK
[3] Department of Haematology, University of Oxford, Oxford, UK
[4] Department of Paediatrics, Imperial College Healthcare NHS Trust/NHS Blood and Transplant, London, UK

Introduction

The paediatric population receiving blood transfusions in critical care comprises two main groups of recipients: neonates and patients admitted to paediatric intensive care. The age and weight ranges of recipients are therefore very broad, from babies less than 400 g and 25 weeks gestation, to adolescents weighing over 100 kg. As for all interventions in paediatric practice, blood transfusion has risks alongside perceived benefits, and the balance between these factors may vary across the wide differences in physiology, co-morbidities and reasons for admission from preterm neonates up to 'small' adults.

Traditionally, the evidence supporting transfusion recommendations in neonatal and paediatric intensive care has been patchy and in some cases derived from adult practice. No one would now doubt the limitations of extrapolating from adult to neonatal medicine and the need for specialist transfusion input into paediatric and neonatal issues. Specific clinical studies in these patient groups are now starting to emerge, which will attempt to provide more rational recommendations for practice. In this chapter, we will discuss key aspects of transfusion in paediatric and neonatal critical care including the risks, special transfusion requirements, specific indications and the volumes to prescribe.

Risks of transfusion

Transfusion has played a core role as part of the supportive therapy for sick neonates and children and enabled the survival of increasingly premature neonates and sick children. But blood for transfusion is not without risk, as well as being a costly and scarce resource. Important information on adverse outcomes of transfusion is available from national haemovigilance schemes such as the UK Serious Hazards of Transfusion (SHOT) reporting scheme, although it is difficult to accurately assess the prevalence of these outcomes. Over the last few years, a specific chapter in the SHOT annual report has been devoted to neonatal and paediatric issues. Key points relevant to paediatric transfusion practice from the SHOT and other data include:
• There have been a disproportionate number of reports from patients less than 18 years by comparison to reports in adults [1] and moreover from transfused neonates when compared to children.

Haematology in Critical Care: A Practical Handbook, First Edition. Edited by Jecko Thachil and Quentin A. Hill.
© 2014 John Wiley & Sons, Ltd. Published 2014 by John Wiley & Sons, Ltd.

• In the most recent SHOT report [2], 35/122 (29%) of paediatric reports were in infants (babies under 1 year of age), of whom 15/35 (43%) were neonates less than 4 weeks old.

• A significant proportion of all reports in children and neonates were related to transfusion errors, including transfusion of an incorrect blood component.

• Common errors are in the correct identification of neonates and children, potentially due to lack of name bands or moving cots in neonatal units, as well as errors in the selection and administration of blood components.

• There are repeated reports of over-transfusion of children as the result of prescribing transfusions as 'units'. It is therefore recommended that paediatric transfusions are prescribed in mL and that the rate or length of time of the transfusion is specified [3].

• In recent years, there has been an increase in the number of reports to SHOT of paediatric acute transfusion reactions, including anaphylactic reactions, probably due to a change in reporting patterns.

• Other risks may be more common in small neonates receiving large volume transfusions, e.g. metabolic effects such as hyperkalaemia.

• There are limited data from neonates on other potentially serious complications of transfusion, such as transfusion-associated lung injury (TRALI) and transfusion-associated circulatory overload (TACO), these being generally better defined and recognized in critically ill adults.

• The incidence of transfusion transmission of infections, in particular viral infections, is (reassuringly) very low, but it is important that clinicians are aware of the possibility of transmission of bacterial infections particularly from platelet components, which are stored at room temperature and therefore are an excellent 'broth' for culture.

• Blood transfusions may cause fluid overload, and routine transfusion volumes as mL/kg body weight are often higher in neonates when compared to average adults. There is some evidence for persistent echocardiographic abnormalities in anaemic infants following a transfusion.

It is important to emphasize that blood for transfusion is a biological agent with potential immunomodulatory effects. There may be additional unrecognized risks from transfusion in critically ill neonates and children, which are not well captured by current definitions of transfusion adverse outcomes. Unrecognized immunomodulatory effects could be manifested by small but nevertheless clinically significant increased rates of infection in critical care or complications such as necrotizing enterocolitis (NEC). However, evidence for causal relationships between transfusion and such outcomes is currently lacking.

The reason for transfusion should be discussed with parents and documented, although formal written consent is not a requirement in many hospitals.

Special requirements

Given the potential for full life expectancy in transfused neonates and sick children who are discharged home, a number of additional safety measures have been introduced in the UK and other countries to further reduce the already low risks of transfusion transmission of pathogens. For example, donations for children and neonates are collected from donors who have been screened and tested for microbiological infections on multiple occasions, to minimize any risks that collection of blood from donors occurs during a 'window period' of an infection. There have been four confirmed cases of transmission of the prion disease variant CJD (vCJD) through blood transfusion in the UK. To minimize risks of transfusion transmission of vCJD, in addition to universal leukcodepletion of blood components for all recipients, plasma and cryoprecipitate for children and neonates are currently sourced from the either Austria or the USA where the population rates of vCJD are essentially zero.

Additional clinical special requirements may be required for specific groups of recipients. When this is the case, the requirements should be notified to the blood transfusion laboratory and included as part of the transfusion prescription and administration checks.

Irradiated cellular components
Several groups of patients are immunologically at risk of transfusion-associated graft-versus-host disease (TA-GVHD) if transfused with cellular components, which contain functionally active T lymphocytes. In order to remove this risk, the components are irradiated, reducing the shelf life of red cells to 14 days (24 h for red cells for neonatal exchange and large volume

transfusions) due to increased leakage of potassium. Patient groups requiring irradiated components who may be admitted to either paediatric or neonatal intensive care units (PICUs or NICUs) include those undergoing stem cell transplantation (until T-cell recovery or discontinuation of GVHD prophylaxis), with Hodgkin's disease or T-cell immunodeficiencies, taking certain drugs (purine analogues, alemtuzumab) and receiving post-intrauterine transfusions (for 6 months post delivery) and neonatal exchange transfusions where possible (see [4] for further details). On PICU, it is important to consider the need for irradiated components for patients undergoing cardiac surgery who could have DiGeorge's syndrome and associated T-cell immunodeficiency.

Cytomegalovirus (CMV) negative components

Patients who are immunodeficient and naïve to cytomegalovirus (CMV) infection are at risk of disseminated CMV. Leukcodepletion has, however, vastly reduced the risk of CMV transmission via component transfusion. Recent recommendations from the Advisory Committee on the Safety of Blood, Tissues and Organs (SaBTO) reduced the number of patient groups who should receive CMV seronegative components to foetuses, neonates up to 28 days post expected delivery date, seronegative pregnant women undergoing elective transfusions and recipients of granulocyte transfusions. Leukcodepletion alone is considered adequate for stem cell transplant patients, organ transplant patients and those with immunodeficiency (inherited or acquired).

HLA-matched platelets

Not infrequently, concerns arise as to the effectiveness of platelet transfusion, triggered by poor or poorly sustained count increments. Causes of platelet refractoriness can be divided into non-immunological and immunological, due to anti-HLA antibodies. Non-immunological causes are more common, including sepsis and medications such as antifungals. However, if these non-immune factors are excluded, then a screen for human leukocyte antigen (HLA) antibodies should be sent and platelets, which are matched for the patient's HLA type, may be requested. It is important to monitor platelet increments post transfusion of HLA-matched

platelets in order to identify the most effective donors for each individual recipient.

Transfusions in paediatric critical care

Red cells
Indications for transfusion and transfusion triggers

Decisions about whether or not to transfuse red cells require consideration of the balance between maintenance of adequate haemoglobin (Hb) to ensure tissue oxygenation and limitation of unnecessary red cell transfusion. There are two main categories of indication for red cell transfusion in children: either in the setting of acute blood loss to restore circulating blood volume or, more usually, to restore Hb levels above a certain threshold. Measures to reduce the need for transfusion include optimization of iron status prior to surgery, cell salvage during major surgery and minimizing iatrogenic blood loss from frequent blood sampling of inpatients.

Research in the adult intensive care field has suggested that a more restrictive transfusion programme results in improved outcomes for patients [5]. Attempt has been made to examine this issue within the paediatric population. A large randomized study (TRIPICU) performed in stable PICU patients comparing a restrictive trigger of 70 g/L with a liberal trigger of 95 g/L showed that the more restrictive transfusion practice (mean Hb level 87 g/L in the restrictive vs. 108 g/L in the liberal group) was associated with less blood use and no increase in adverse outcomes [6]. Although it is not clear whether the results of this trial can be extrapolated to unstable patients, in general, a transfusion threshold of 70 g/L in stable patients on PICU is considered reasonable.

Dose

The dose of red cells required can either be calculated as 10–20 mL/kg bodyweight or by using a formula based on the pre-transfusion and desired Hb levels. A commonly used formula is

Volume to transfuse (mL)
$$= \frac{\text{desired Hb (g/L)} - \text{actual Hb (g/L)} \times \text{weight (kg)} \times \text{factor}}{10}$$

A factor of 3 is frequently used in the equation, but some studies suggest that a factor of 5 may be more appropriate for critically ill children.

Note: the formula has been modified to take into account the recent change the units used in reporting of Hb results – now in g/L rather than g/dL.

Patient groups

In the recent UK National Comparative Audit of paediatric transfusion [7], the main groups of patients transfused with red cells in PICU were cardiac and those with infection/sepsis. There is limited data from studies to guide red cell transfusion on PICU for children following cardiac surgery although subgroup analysis of the TRIPICU data also supported a Hb threshold of 70 g/L for noncyanotic patients [8].

Haemoglobinopathies

Children with haemoglobinopathies are frequently transfused, and patients with sickle cell disease in particular are at risk of development of antibodies to red cell antigens (red cell alloimmunization). They should have extended red cell phenotyping performed prior to their first transfusion and should be provided with red cells matched for Rhesus (Rh) and Kell.

Patients with acute sickle cell complications such as splenic or hepatic sequestration or aplastic crises are generally managed with top-up red cell transfusions. However, the patient most likely to present to the critical care units will have an acute chest crisis or stroke, and exchange transfusion may be necessary. This is generally a 1.5 times blood volume exchange and can be performed either as multiple manual procedures or as a single automated procedure using an apheresis machine. The aim is usually to bring the percentage of sickle Hb down to less than 20%.

Trauma/massive haemorrhage

Trauma or management of massive haemorrhage is one area where there has been a huge increase in evidence for transfusion management, particularly for adults but also impacting on paediatric management. There has been particular interest in early and aggressive correction of coagulopathy and an increase in the ratio of plasma to red cells [9].

Platelets

Indications

The aetiology of thrombocytopenia within the PICU population is heterogeneous, and children present with a variety of different clinical scenarios, e.g. severe sepsis, post cardiac surgery or post chemotherapy. In terms of management, the use of platelet transfusions can be split into two broad categories: firstly, as prophylaxis where transfusion is used to increase the count to above a prespecified level, aiming to prevent bleeding including prior to an invasive procedure, and, secondly, for treatment of thrombocytopenia with active bleeding, including the setting of a massive blood transfusion.

For platelet transfusions in thrombocytopenic children with haemorrhage, there is, in general, an aim to increase the platelet count to between 50 and 75×10^9/L. However, the exact platelet count target that should trigger a prophylactic transfusion and indeed whether prophylaxis is necessary in an otherwise stable child remains uncertain due to lack of evidence. Of note, recent age group analysis of large platelet transfusion trial (looking at dose of platelets) suggested that paediatric patients have an increased risk of bleeding compared to adult patients with the same platelet count [10], and thus, extrapolation from adult studies should be done with caution. For adults, studies in patients with haematological malignancies indicate a safe prophylactic threshold of 10×10^9/L in stable patient and above 20×10^9 if febrile or with other risk factors. Most PICUs will have agreed local thresholds for transfusion, but individual practice varies widely. Suggestions of procedure-specific transfusion thresholds exist (see Table 34.1 for suggested thresholds).

Dose

In general, the dose is 10–20 mL/kg of platelet concentrate up to a maximum of a single apheresis pack (~200 mL).

Fresh frozen plasma (FFP)

Therapeutic use of fresh frozen plasma (FFP) in the setting of major haemorrhage will be discussed in Chapter 15.

With regard to prophylactic use of FFP in a child, it should be noted that screening blood tests such as prothrombin time (PT) or activated partial thromboplastin time (APTT) do not correlate well with bleeding risk.

Table 34.1 Summary table of neonatal and paediatric components.

Component	Component specification	Suggested thresholds for transfusion	Dose of component required	Special considerations
Red cells	**Volume**: 220–340 mL (278 mL mean) **Haematocrit**: 0.5–0.7 (for neonatal exchange transfusion 0.5–0.6; 0.5–0.55 from NHSBT, England) Suspended in SAG-M (saline, adenine, glucose, mannitol) (citrate phosphate dextrose for neonatal exchange) Stored for 35 days at 4°C ± 2°C	**Neonate:** First 24 h – 120 g/L Transfuse for >10% acute loss Neonate needing ITU – 120 g/L Chronic oxygen dependency – 110 g/L Late anaemia – 70 g/L **Paediatric:** 70 g/L in stable patients	**Top-up transfusions:** 10–20 mL/kg or via formula e.g. Volume (mL) = body weight (kg) × desired Hb increment (g/dL) × transfusion factor (3–5) **Neonatal exchange:** 80–100 mL/kg (anaemia) 160–200 mL/kg (hyperbilirubinaemia) **Typical administration rates:** Neonatal top-up 5 mL/kg/h Paediatric 5 mL/kg/h (usual max rate 150 mL/h)	**Red cells for neonatal use:** From regular donors (at least one previous donation negative for the mandatory microbiological markers) **Red cells for neonatal exchange:** Group O (compatible with baby and mother plasma) RhD neg, K Neg, 5 days old or less, HbS screen negative, CMV neg and irradiated
Platelets	Produced via apheresis from a single donor (used in preference over pooled units) **Volume:** Mean volume of adult pack 202 mL 50 mL packs available Screened for bacterial contamination Stored for 7 days at 22°C	**Neonate:** 50 × 10⁹/L preterm/term with bleeding 30 × 10⁹/L sick term or preterm not bleeding; NAIT 20 × 10⁹/L stable preterm or term not bleeding **Paediatric:** <10 × 10⁹/L stable patient <20 × 10⁹/L febrile/unwell patient, severe mucositis, disseminated intravascular coagulation (DIC), anticoagulants, likely to fall to <10, risk of bleeding due to tumour infiltration <20–50 × 10⁹/L – DIC, hyperleukocytosis, LP or central line	10–20 mL/kg, max single apheresis pack (for these, still prescribe precise volume in mL) Typical administration rate 10–20 mL/kg/h	ABO identical where possible (or negative for high titre antibodies) Rh-negative patients should receive Rh-negative units where possible and if a positive unit is given to a female then anti-D should be given HPA-1a and HPA-5b negative platelets available for cases of NAIT

(Continued)

Table 34.1 (*Continued*)

Component	Component specification	Suggested thresholds for transfusion	Dose of component required	Special considerations
Fresh frozen plasma	Methylene blue (MB)-treated single-donor plasma from non-UK donors 50 mL aliquots for neonates/small children 200 mL volume for larger children	Abnormalities of coagulation with bleeding/or significant risk of bleeding	10–20 mL/kg Typical administration rate 10–20 mL/kg/h	Solvent–detergent (SD)-treated FFP is commercially available for use for TTP (plasma exchange. Used by some hospitals rather than MB-treated FFP for neonates and children)
Cryoprecipitate	Small volumes (single units), each unit = 20–50 mL. Frequently supplied as a pre-pooled component with five pools per pack, i.e. 100–250 mL per pack	Low fibrinogen (<0.8–1 g/L) and risk of bleeding	5–10 mL/kg. Transfusion of this volume of MB cryoprecipitate is estimated to raise the plasma fibrinogen by ~0.5–1.4 g/L Typical administration rate 10–20 mL/kg/h (i.e. over ~30 min)	

Source: Information in table largely derived from [3] and [11]. Component volumes taken from NHS Blood and Transplant component specification 2010. Reproduced with permission of John Wiley & Sons, Ltd.

The clinical status of the patient and other factors such as the platelet count and fibrinogen level should be taken into account. Overall, the evidence for use of FFP in children is very limited [12], and there is doubtful benefit for trying to correct mild or moderate abnormalities of PT or APTT. In the absence of better evidence, the use of FFP should be reserved for children with significant risk of bleeding and significant coagulation abnormalities.

The dose of FFP should be 10–20 mL/kg, and coagulation testing should be undertaken post infusion to assess the outcome of treatment.

Cryoprecipitate

Cryoprecipitate is manufactured from FFP by controlled thawing to precipitate high-molecular-weight proteins. It is a source of fibrinogen, factor VIII and von Willebrand factor. Cryoprecipitate can be used to raise the fibrinogen level in a hypofibrinogenaemic patient and is indicated when the serum fibrinogen is less than

1 g/L in a patient at risk of bleeding. As FFP also contains fibrinogen, cryoprecipitate may not be needed in addition to FFP. The dose of cryoprecipitate is 5–10 mL/kg, and the fibrinogen level should be rechecked post transfusion.

Transfusions in neonatal intensive care

Red cells

Extremely preterm neonates are recipients of significant numbers of red cell transfusions. These are often given to maintain a particular Hb threshold as a *top-up* transfusion for anaemia, partly caused by frequent blood sampling or because of the presence of surrogate markers of anaemia in the baby such as poor growth, lethargy or increased apnoeas. Potential benefits of transfusion in this group include improved tissue oxygenation and a need for a lower cardiac output to maintain the same level of oxygenation. Occasionally, large volume exchange transfusions are needed for severe anaemia or hyperbilirubinaemia.

To reduce donor exposure, red cells for neonatal top-up transfusions are generally provided as splits of a full-sized donation divided into 6–8 smaller packs (*paediapacks*). This is of particular use for the preterm neonate who is likely to need multiple transfusions over the course of admission on a neonatal unit.

Red cells for neonatal transfusion and for the first 4 months of life must be compatible with the neonate's ABO and Rh group and the mother's antibody screen. Thus, a sample from both the mother and baby is required. If the antibody screen is negative, there is no need for further compatibility testing for the first 4 months of life.

Transfusion thresholds/indications for transfusion

There has been much interest in the appropriate transfusion threshold for neonatal red cell transfusion. Specific Hb targets vary according to the cardiorespiratory status and postnatal age of the infant, partly following the normal trend to decreased Hb over the first few weeks of life (see Table 34.1). Several studies have attempted to determine whether a restrictive or more liberal transfusion policy is superior. A recent Cochrane review [13] summarized the literature, finding that a more restrictive policy resulted in a modest reduction in red cell usage and Hb levels with no significant impact on morbidity or mortality. This conclusion was based on four studies, which examined data from 614 babies in total. Hb triggers for the sickest babies ranged from 115 g/L at the most restrictive to 156 g/L at the most liberal, reducing down to 75 g/L in the restrictive and 130 g/L in the liberal group for stable babies who were self-ventilating in air. However, the authors stated that there is still some uncertainty and that Hb levels below the minimum thresholds used in the studies should be avoided. In practice, individual units tend to have their own particular agreed thresholds depending upon clinical status of the infant.

Dose

The volume of blood to be transfused is based upon weight, usually 10–20 mL/kg, or using a transfusion formula (see preceding text).

Red cells for exchange transfusion

The availability of intensive phototherapy for hyperbilirubinaemia in the neonate together with the reduction in haemolytic disease of the newborn following routine antenatal anti-D for RhD negative women has reduced the incidence of exchange transfusions in the neonate. If red cells are needed for exchange transfusion, it is important for clinicians to liaise with the hospital transfusion laboratory. The standardized specification for red cells for neonatal exchange transfusion is shown in Table 34.1. A double volume exchange is advised (160–200 mL/kg) for hyperbilirubinaemia, aiming to remove both the bilirubin and the infant's red cells, which have been coated with maternal antibody. A single volume exchange (80–100 mL/kg) may be used for severe neonatal anaemia. It is important that NICUs have local protocols in place for exchange transfusions.

Platelets

Platelets for neonatal use are supplied in small packs with a volume of around 50 mL containing $60–90 \times 10^9$/L of platelets.

Thresholds and indications

Thrombocytopenia is common within the neonatal intensive care population, and incidence increases with prematurity. However, the evidence for use of particular platelet thresholds is very limited and has generally been extrapolated from adult practice, with overall higher thresholds being used in view of the increased risk of intracranial haemorrhage in this patient group. There is wide international variation in the exact choice of threshold in neonates. Current research in this area is exploring whether minor symptoms of bleeding in neonates can predict more severe bleeding and thus whether the role for prophylactic transfusion can be limited to those babies who are at increased risk of bleeding [14].

In general, a platelet count of 50×10^9/L in a bleeding infant, 30×10^9/L in a sick preterm or term non-bleeding infant and 20×10^9/L in a stable preterm or term infant are suggested thresholds [11]. However, thresholds of 50×10^9/L may be used for sick or bleeding preterm infants, and again individual units use a variety of thresholds in practice. For babies with evidence of intraventricular haemorrhage (IVH), the counts are generally maintained at $50-100 \times 10^9$/L. In the setting of uncomplicated neonatal alloimmune thrombocytopenia, the platelet count should be maintained above 30×10^9/L in view of the reduction in platelet function.

Neonatal alloimmune thrombocytopenia (NAITP)

This can occur in utero due to a mismatch between the mother's platelet antigen type and the baby's. The most common type is when a HPA-1a-negative mother is carrying a HPA-1a-positive foetus. As for Rh disease, this condition can become worse in subsequent pregnancies. Affected babies can be severely thrombocytopenic at birth and require provision of a specialized platelet component, HPA-1a-/5b-negative platelets, which are unlikely to be affected by the maternal antibodies. If NAITP is suspected, it is important to liaise with transfusion specialists in order to ensure correct investigations of the baby and parents and provision of the correct platelets.

FFP and cryoprecipitate

The indications for FFP use in the neonate require an understanding of the normal ranges, which are dependent on gestational age. However, as for older children, there is no indication for FFP treatment of mild abnormalities of PT or APTT alone. In addition, there is no evidence for using FFP prophylaxis to try to prevent IVH in preterm neonates.

Definite indications for FFP include vitamin K deficiency with bleeding (prothrombin complex concentrate can also be used), disseminated intravascular coagulation (DIC) with bleeding and congenital coagulation factor deficiency for which there is not an adequate recombinant product [11].

In general, the FFP dose used is 10–20 mL/kg as for paediatric and adult practice. The coagulation should be rechecked post transfusion.

For fibrinogen replacement, a dose of 5–10 mL/kg of cryoprecipitate is recommended.

Key points

• Benefits of transfusion need to balance against risks.
• Education and training of all staff involved should be maintained to ensure that errors do not occur.

• Evidence for transfusion practice in paediatrics and neonates is increasing.
• Specific component requirements exist for children and neonates.
• Transfusion prescriptions should specify component, any special indications, volume and rate.

References

1 Stainsby D, Jones H, Wells AW, Gibson B, Cohen H, SHOT Steering Group Adverse outcomes of blood transfusion in children: analysis of UK reports to the serious hazards of transfusion Scheme 1996–2005. Br J Haematol 2008; 141(1):73–9.

2 Knowles S (ed.), Cohen H, on behalf of the Serious Hazards of Transfusion (SHOT) Steering Group. The 2010 Annual SHOT Report. 2011. http://www.shotuk.org/wp-content/uploads/2011/07/SHOT-2010-Report.pdf (accessed on November 21, 2013).

3 Harris AM, Atterbury CLJ, Chaffe B et al. Guideline on the Administration of Blood Components. 2009. http://www.bcshguidelines.com/4_HAEMATOLOGY_GUIDELINES.html (accessed on November 21, 2013).

4 Treleaven J, Gennery A, Marsh J et al. Guidelines on the use of irradiated blood components prepared by the British Committee for Standards in Haematology blood transfusion task force. Br J Haematol 2011;152(1):35–51.

5 Herbert PC, Wells G, Blajchman MA et al.. A multicenter, randomized, controlled clinical trial of transfusion requirements in critical care. N Engl J Med 1999;340:409–17.

6 Lacroix J, Hébert PC, Hutchison JS et al. Transfusion strategies for patients in pediatric intensive care units. N Eng J Med 2007;356(16):1609–19.

7 National Comparative Audit of the use of Red Cells in Neonates and Children . 2010. http://hospital.blood.co.uk/library/pdf/NCA_red_cells_neonates_children.pdf (accessed on November 21, 2013).

8 Willems A, Harrington K, Lacroix J et al. Comparison of two red-cell transfusion strategies after pediatric cardiac surgery: a subgroup analysis. Crit Care Med 2010; 38(2): 649–56.

9 Hendrickson JE, Shaz BH, Pereira G et al. Implementation of a pediatric trauma massive transfusion protocol: one institution's experience. Transfusion 2012;52:1228–36.

10 Josephson CD, Granger S, Assmann SF et al. Bleeding risks are higher in children versus adults given prophylactic platelet transfusions for treatment-induced hypoproliferative thrombocytopenia. Blood 2012;120:748–60.

11 Gibson BES, Todd A, Roberts I et al. Transfusion guidelines for neonates and older children. Br J Haematol 2004;124(4): 433–53.

12 Yang L, Stanworth S, Hopewell S, Doree C, Murphy M. Is fresh frozen plasma clinically effective? An update of a systematic review of randomised controlled trials. Transfusion 2012;52:1673–86.

13 Whyte R, Kirpalani H. Low versus high haemoglobin concentration threshold for blood transfusion for preventing morbidity and mortality in very low birth weight infants. Cochrane Database Syst Rev 2011;(11):CD000512. Review.

14 Stanworth SJ, Clarke P, Watts T et al. Prospective, Observational Study of Outcomes in Neonates with Severe Thrombocytopenia. Pediatrics 2009;124(5):e826–e834.

10

SECTION 10
Haematological Emergencies

CHAPTER 35

Haematological Emergencies

Quentin A. Hill[1] and Amin Rahemtulla[2]

[1] Department of Haematology, Leeds Teaching Hospitals NHS Trust, Leeds, UK
[2] Department of Haematology, Imperial College Healthcare NHS Trust, Hammersmith Hospital, London, UK

Haematological emergencies will often result in an unstable patient who requires intensive support. A number of these conditions have been dealt with in other chapters, but some additional topics are covered, including tumour lysis syndrome (TLS), superior vena cava (SVC) syndrome, chemotherapy- or radiotherapy-induced lung injury, malignant spinal cord compression (MSCC), renal failure following high-dose methotrexate, inadvertent administration of intrathecal vincristine and lymphoma with pericardial involvement.

Tumour lysis syndrome (TLS)

Tumour lysis syndrome is a life-threatening complication that arises when the rapid lysis of tumour cells leads to the release of intracellular cytokines, nucleic acids (catabolized to uric acid) and metabolites (phosphorus, potassium) into the circulation. This overwhelms the body's normal homeostatic mechanisms resulting in hyperkalaemia, hyperphosphataemia, hyperuricaemia and secondary hypocalcaemia [1]. TLS can occur within a few hours or even before chemotherapy but is most commonly seen 12–72h after initiation of treatment. It can result in renal failure, seizures, cardiac arrhythmia, multi-organ failure and death.

Diagnosis

Cairo and Bishop classified TLS according to clinical and laboratory features. In laboratory TLS [2], there is an abnormality in two or more of the metabolic complications below occurring within 3 days before or up to 7 days after chemotherapy:

Uric acid	$\geq 476\,\mu mol/L$ or 25% increase from baseline
Potassium	$\geq 6.0\,mmol/L$ or 25% increase from baseline
Phosphate	$\geq 1.45\,mmol/L$ or 25% increase from baseline
Corrected calcium	$\leq 1.75\,mmol/L$ or 25% decrease from baseline

Clinical TLS was defined as laboratory TLS plus one or more of the following:
- Creatinine greater than $1.5 \times$ upper level of normal
- Cardiac arrhythmia/sudden death
- Seizure

Pathophysiology and clinical manifestations:
- Hyperkalaemia can cause lethargy, nausea, vomiting, diarrhoea, muscle weakness, paraesthesiae and ECG changes such as tall *tented* T waves, widened QRS complex and ventricular arrhythmias, which may be fatal.
- Hyperphosphataemia and secondary hypocalcaemia can cause anorexia, vomiting, confusion, carpopedal

Haematology in Critical Care: A Practical Handbook, First Edition. Edited by Jecko Thachil and Quentin A. Hill.
© 2014 John Wiley & Sons, Ltd. Published 2014 by John Wiley & Sons, Ltd.

spasm, tetany, seizures and arrhythmias. Calcium pyrophosphate crystals may precipitate in various organs and contribute to acute kidney injury.

• Hyperuricaemia may cause non-specific symptoms such as nausea, vomiting, anorexia and lethargy. It causes renal injury by crystal-dependent mechanisms. Uric acid nephropathy develops when uric acid crystals get deposited in the renal tubules and collecting ducts.

• Renal impairment reduces urinary excretion of potassium and phosphate, leading to fluid retention, pulmonary oedema and a metabolic acidosis. This predisposes to further renal urate deposition, and multi-organ failure may ensue.

Risk factors:

• Tumour type – Burkitt lymphoma (BL), diffuse large B-cell lymphoma (DLBCL), lymphoblastic lymphoma (LL), acute lymphoblastic leukaemia (ALL) and highly proliferative and treatment-sensitive solid organ tumours

• Tumour burden – bulky disease, extensive bone marrow infiltration, high white blood count (WBC) (in acute leukaemia) and raised lactate dehydrogenase (LDH) (>2× ULN)

• Other factors – renal impairment, elevated uric acid, oliguria, hypotension, dehydration and nephrotoxic drugs

Management

The best management of this condition is prevention, and ensuring good hydration and urine output is central to this. The initial assessment of all newly presenting patients should include tumour type, burden and cell lysis potential. Also, review the WBC, LDH, uric acid, phosphate, potassium, calcium, creatinine, urine output and cardiovascular status.

Patients who do not already have clinical TLS can then be categorized into low, intermediate and high risk. Several expert groups recently constructed algorithms defining risk and recommending a risk-stratified management approach to TLS [1, 3] (Table 35.1).

Preventative strategies for high-risk patients:

• Monitor urine output, fluid balance and electrolytes. Biochemistry every 6 h initially, de-escalating dependent on clinical response.

• Adequate hydration by IV fluids (usually 3 L/m²/day, avoid potassium) and aim for a urine output of 100 mL/h. Where urine output remains poor, a loop diuretic may be considered [1].

• Consider deferral of chemotherapy for 24–48 h to ensure adequate hydration and urine output depending on clinical urgency. Alternatively, consider a lower-intensity *prephase* treatment, e.g. initial steroid monotherapy for patients with ALL.

• Rasburicase (0.2 mg/kg in 50 mL normal saline infused over 30 min) for up to 7 days. This recombinant urate oxidase catalyzes the oxidation of uric acid to allantoin, which is soluble and readily excreted by the kidneys. Uric acid levels can be reduced within 4 h, improve renal function and thereby reduce phosphate. In contrast, allopurinol takes 24–72 h before effectively preventing uric acid formation and cannot actively remove uric acid already formed. Usually, 1–3 days of rasburicase is adequate. No dose adjustment is required for renal or hepatic impairment. Side effects include rash and urticaria due to allergy. Rasburicase is contraindicated in patients with methaemoglobinaemia, glucose-6-phosphate dehydrogenase (G6PD) deficiency and conditions, which can cause haemolytic anaemia.

• Allopurinol can be given orally or IV after completing rasburicase therapy. Allopurinol blocks the conversion of xanthines to uric acid. Since this would reduce the effect of rasburicase, they should not be given together.

Prevention for moderate-risk patients should include adequate hydration with IV fluids. Hospital in-patient, monitoring of urine output is recommended with biochemical monitoring, initially every 12 h. Allopurinol should be started 1–2 days before treatment and continue for 3–7 days afterwards. Allopurinol can be given orally or IV at a dose of 300 mg/m²/day (maximum 600 mg/day) in one to three divided doses [4]. Dose reductions for renal or liver impairment are required. Low-risk patients are usually managed on an outpatient basis, and hydration can be achieved orally.

Urinary alkalinization (e.g. with sodium bicarbonate) has been used to increase excretion of uric acid but decreases calcium phosphate solubility and lacks evidence of benefit. It is no longer recommended and should be avoided in established TLS, if rasburicase has been used or phosphate elevated.

Established TLS:

• *Renal management*: the treatment of TLS employs the same modalities as prevention, and rasburicase is recommended. Monitoring of electrolytes should initially be 4–6 hourly with continuous cardiac monitoring. Fluid balance should be optimized, aiming for a urine

Table 35.1 Tumour lysis syndrome (TLS) recommendations based on TLS risk.

Low-risk disease (LRD)	Intermediate-risk disease (IRD)	High-risk disease (HRD)
ST*	N/A	N/A
MM	N/A	N/A
CML	N/A	N/A
Indolent NHL	N/A	N/A
HL	N/A	N/A
CLL†	N/A	N/A
AML and WBC <25 × 10^9/L and LDH <2 × ULN	AML with WBC 25–100 × 10^9/L AML and WBC <25 × 10^9/L and LDH ≥2 × ULN	AML and WBC ≥100 × 10^9/L
Adult intermediate-grade NHL and LDH <2 × ULN	Adult intermediate-grade NHL and LDH ≥2 × ULN	N/A
Adult ALCL	Childhood ALCL stage III/IV	N/A
N/A	Childhood intermediate-grade NHL stage III/IV with LDH <2 × ULN	N/A
N/A	ALL and WBC <100 × 10^9/L and LDH <2 × ULN	ALL and WBC ≥100 × 10^9/L and/or LDH ≥2 × ULN
N/A	BL and LDH <2 × ULN	BL stage III/IV and/or LDH ≥2 × ULN
N/A	LL stage I/II and LDH <2 × ULN	LL stage III/IV and/or LDH ≥2 × ULN
N/A	N/A	IRD with renal dysfunction and/or renal involvement
		IRD with uric acid, potassium and/or phosphate > ULN
Prophylaxis recommendations		
Monitoring	Monitoring	Monitoring
Hydration	Hydration	Hydration
±Allopurinol	Allopurinol	Rasburicase‡

Source: Cairo et al. [3]. Reproduced with permission of John Wiley & Sons, Ltd.
ST, solid tumours; MM, multiple myeloma; CML, chronic myeloid leukaemia; NHL, non-Hodgkin's lymphoma; HL, Hodgkin's lymphoma; CLL, chronic lymphoid leukaemia; AML, acute myeloid leukaemia; WBC, white blood cell count; LDH, lactate dehydrogenase; ULN, upper limit of normal; ALCL, anaplastic large cell lymphoma; N/A, not applicable; ALL, acute lymphoblastic leukaemia; BL, Burkitt lymphoma/leukaemia; LL, lymphoblastic lymphoma.
*Rare ST, such as neuroblastoma, germ cell tumours and small cell lung cancer or others with bulky or advanced stage disease, may be classified as IRD.
†CLL treated with fludarabine and rituximab, and/or those with high WBC (≥50 × 10^9/L) should be classified as IRD.
‡Contraindicated in patients with a history consistent with glucose-6-phosphate dehydrogenase deficiency (G6PD). In these patients, rasburicase should be substituted with allopurinol.

output greater than100 mL/h. If fluid replete, a loop diuretic may be considered. Indications for renal replacement therapy are similar to other causes of acute kidney injury but with a lower threshold given the potential for a rapid rise in potassium [1]. Indications would include early renal failure, recalcitrant electrolyte disturbances, volume overload resistant to diuretics and symptoms due to pericarditis or encephalopathy secondary to uraemia. Continuous venovenous techniques (haemofiltration, haemodiafiltration or haemodialysis) use filters with a larger pore size and may allow more rapid phosphate clearance compared to conventional dialysis [1].

- *Hyperkalaemia*: requires continuous cardiac monitoring. Consider repeating the sample to exclude a fictitious result [4]. A rapid reduction in potassium (e.g. if $K^+ > 6.5$ or associated ECG changes) can be achieved with 50 mL of 50% dextrose containing 20 U of human Actrapid insulin over 1 h. Regular monitoring is necessary. Calcium gluconate (10 mL of 10% over 2–3 min) may also be used in the setting of cardiac arrhythmias, but the effect is transient and dialysis may be required.
- *Hypocalcaemia and hyperphosphataemia*: asymptomatic hypocalcaemia does not require treatment (treatment risks precipitation of calcium phosphate), but cardiac monitoring is required. If symptomatic, short-term control can be achieved with calcium gluconate 10 mL of 10% over 10 min. Cardiac monitoring is needed during the infusion, and dialysis should be considered. Initial management of asymptomatic hyperphosphataemia is optimal renal support. Phosphate binders such as aluminium hydroxide (50–100 mg/kg per day orally for 1–2 days maximum) or sevelamer (2.4–4.8 g/ day) can be considered but may be poorly tolerated. Dialysis is required for severe hyperphosphataemia.

Superior vena cava (SVC) syndrome

Superior vena cava syndrome most often results from compression by lymphoma or solid organ malignancies (e.g. lung, breast or germ cell tumours), especially in the elderly. Less common causes include thymoma, post-radiation fibrosis, sarcoidosis or infection (e.g. tuberculosis, actinomycosis or histoplasmosis resulting in fibrosing mediastinitis) [5]. Thrombosis is an increasingly common cause of SVC syndrome, usually associated with an indwelling venous catheter. SVC syndrome often presents subacutely such that there is time to organize diagnostic procedures to guide therapy and less than 5% of cases present with life-threatening features [5].

Symptoms may be worse lying flat. Symptoms and signs include:
- Facial plethora, arm oedema and distended jugular veins (increased venous pressure).
- Dilated collateral veins may be visible on the chest wall.
- Syncope, *fullness* in the head, headaches and confusion (cerebral oedema).
- Cough and dyspnoea.

- Interstitial oedema or compression may cause stridor, hoarseness or dysphagia.

Investigations:
- Chest XR may show a mediastinal mass. Cavitating lesions suggest infection.
- Contrast CT or MRI thorax. Also image the head for metastasis if neurological symptoms.
- Serum alpha fetoprotein and βHCG (elevated in germ cell tumours).
- Assess for evidence of tumour lysis (renal function, calcium, phosphate, uric acid).
- Biopsy:
  ○ Less invasive options include biopsy of enlarged peripheral lymph nodes, aspiration of pleural or pericardial effusions and sputum cytology.
  ○ If full blood count abnormalities (cytopenias or blast cells), consider peripheral blood flow cytometry and/or bone marrow biopsy.
  ○ Consider diagnostic bronchoscopy or mediastinoscopy/biopsy.

Management aims to relieve symptoms and treat the underlying disease:
- Sit upright and supplemental oxygen.
- Assess for immediately life-threatening features, i.e. cerebral oedema (confusion, coma), airway compromise (e.g. stridor) or haemodynamic instability (hypotension, syncope without precipitating factors such as bending).
- If life-threatening features:
  ○ Endovascular stenting (symptomatic relief in 24–48 h) [6] prior to diagnostic testing, followed by anticoagulation. Consider early radiotherapy for malignant obstruction, with steroids to prevent post-radiation swelling.
- If due to thrombosis, anticoagulate and remove the venous catheter if present. Local catheter-directed thrombolysis has been used, but care must be taken if brain metastases have not been excluded and thrombolysis is not recommended following stent insertion due to increased morbidity [5].
  ○ Intubation may be necessary to protect a threatened airway.
  ○ Steroids can be considered if lymphoma is suspected but may reduce diagnostic yield of subsequent tissue biopsy.
  ○ If no life-threatening features, proceed to tissue biopsy, staging and multidisciplinary review. External beam radiotherapy or chemotherapy may be used for malignant disease. For lymphoma patients, chemotherapy may be the only treatment required.

Median survival of patients presenting with malignant SVC syndrome is approximately 6 months, but prognosis depends on the underlying tumour [6].

Chemotherapy- or radiotherapy-induced lung injury

Chemotherapy-induced pulmonary toxicity can be acute, severe and life-threatening although subacute, often later-onset, pulmonary fibrosis also occurs. A significant number of chemotherapy agents used for haematological malignancy have been implicated and include bleomycin, methotrexate, procarbazine and carmustine (BCNU); all-*trans*-retinoic acid (ATRA); rituximab; imatinib; dasatinib; alkylating agents (busulphan, melphalan, cyclophosphamide, chlorambucil); and antimetabolites (methotrexate, cytosine arabinoside, 6-mercaptopurine, azathioprine, gemcitabine, fludarabine).

Acute (or hypersensitivity) pneumonitis can occur after the first dose of chemotherapy or several months after starting treatment. Presenting features are progressive dyspnoea and a non-productive cough. A low-grade fever is often present, and examination may reveal fine crackles. Radiological changes can include interstitial/reticular changes, ground-glass opacities, pleural effusions and/or a diffuse or focal alveolar pattern (consolidation) (Figure 35.1). Lung function tests show a reduced diffusing capacity for carbon monoxide. Histological findings from lung biopsy are variable and may show an inflammatory interstitial reaction, fibrin

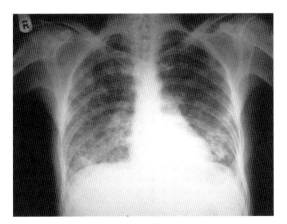

Figure 35.1 Chest XR of drug-induced pneumonitis resulting from 6 months of nitrofurantoin. Source: Reproduced with permission of Dr E. Paramasivam, Leeds, UK.

and collagen deposition in the septal walls or organizing pneumonia.

Other patterns of lung injury include allergic infusion reactions (e.g. rituximab), pleural effusions (e.g. bleomycin, imatinib, dasatinib), thromboembolic disease (e.g. thalidomide), alveolar haemorrhage or eosinophilic pneumonitis (e.g. gemcitabine). Non-cardiogenic pulmonary oedema can occur due to endothelial inflammation and vascular (capillary) leak. Non-cardiogenic pulmonary oedema has been reported with high-dose cytosine arabinoside, generally responding to discontinuation of therapy and oxygen and diuretic therapy [7]. Vascular leak has also been associated with a differentiation syndrome in patients treated with ATRA for acute promyelocytic leukaemia, and its management is discussed in Chapter 4. Later-onset pulmonary fibrosis has most often been associated with bleomycin, busulphan and carmustine.

No single test is diagnostic of chemotherapy-induced pneumonitis, and diagnosis rests on an appropriate clinical/radiological picture and exclusion of other causes. The major differential in an immunocompromised patient is infection, and typical symptoms and signs of infection may be absent due to a lack of inflammatory reaction. Other noninfective differentials include transfusion-associated reactions, pulmonary oedema, haemorrhage or progressive/relapsing disease.

Management:
- Careful investigation for infective causes. Bronchoalveolar lavage or lung biopsy may be appropriate when excluding infection or malignancy.
- Acutely, consider empirical antimicrobial therapy.
- Withhold suspected chemotherapy agent.
- Corticosteroids if severe or deteriorating pneumonitis.

With prompt management, changes are usually fully reversible although some patients require ventilatory support and not all survive. The decision to re-challenge with chemotherapy will depend on the implicated drug and the patient's individual circumstances.

Bleomycin
Pulmonary fibrosis can occur in up to 10% of patients and can be fatal. It typically presents subacutely in the first 6 months with a dry cough and breathlessness. Toxicity is associated with total doses greater than 450 U, increasing age, combination chemotherapy, thoracic radiotherapy, renal impairment and exposure to high doses of inspired oxygen. The latter may

potentiate bleomycin-induced lung injury, even if given several years later:

• Oxygen should be avoided in patients previously exposed to bleomycin unless hypoxic. For example, avoid high oxygen doses during clinical procedures and in the peri-operative period.

• High-dose oxygen should only be used for immediate life-saving indications, and the minimum dose used to maintain oxygen saturations at a lower target range of 88–92% [8].

If bleomycin lung injury is suspected, discontinue bleomycin, investigate to exclude infection, optimize fluid balance and consider steroid therapy.

Radiotherapy

Radiation involving lung tissue can cause a pneumonitis but is less likely with a smaller volume irradiated (rare if <10%), lower total dose (rare if total dose <20 Gy) and delivery in more fractions. Chemotherapy prior to radiotherapy is a risk factor for pneumonitis. Pneumonitis can also occur within the radiation field when chemotherapy is given to patients who received prior thoracic radiotherapy.

Acute pneumonitis usually presents with symptoms of breathlessness, cough, low-grade fever or pleuritic chest pain, typically 2–3 months after treatment. Diagnosis may be made clinically and from chest XR changes (early changes typically ground-glass or diffuse haziness confined to the radiation field), but the differential includes infection and relapse such that lung biopsy is sometimes required. More established fibrosis may evolve over 6–24 months. Steroids are usually given for acute radiation pneumonitis, for example prednisolone 1 mg/kg for several weeks and then tapered [7].

Malignant spinal cord compression

Myeloma and non-Hodgkin's lymphoma (NHL) cause 10–20% of all cases of MSCC. Other common causes are solid organ tumours of prostate, breast, lung and kidney. MSCC is usually extradural, arising from vertebral involvement extending into the epidural space, although paravertebral masses can also spread through intervertebral foramen. The earliest symptom of compression is progressive back pain, occurring in over 90% of patients, often for weeks or months prior to diagnosis. This provides an opportunity to intervene prior to the onset of permanent neurological injury. A focal weakness occurs

in 75%, and at diagnosis, approximately half have sensory symptoms and bowel or bladder disturbance. Cord compression is the first feature of the malignancy in approximately 20% of cases of MSCC, and this is more common in myeloma and lymphoma than solid organ tumours.

Management

• Have a low tolerance for investigating back pain in cancer patients.

• If MSCC is suspected, urgent MRI (or CT if this is not available) of the whole spine is required since multiple lesions may be present.

• See Chapter 22 for MSCC management of myeloma.

• The goals of treatment are to relieve pain, stabilize the spine, prevent paralysis and control local progression.

• Steroids are typically given as part of initial management, e.g. dexamethasone 10 mg IV bolus and then 16 mg daily orally in divided doses, followed by a taper.

• Definitive therapy for lymphoma patients may involve surgical decompression, radiotherapy, systemic chemotherapy or combinations of these. Surgical intervention is more likely if there is spinal instability, prior radiotherapy to the site or when diagnostic biopsy is required.

Renal failure following high-dose methotrexate

High-dose methotrexate describes doses typically $\geq 1\,g/m^2$ used to treat patients with lymphoma affecting the central nervous system (CNS) and as prophylaxis against CNS relapse in patients with acute ALL and high-risk NHL. Methotrexate is a folic acid antagonist mainly cleared in the urine. High concentrations can lead to acute renal dysfunction, elevated plasma concentrations and subsequent systemic toxicity including myelosuppression, mucositis, rash and less frequently pneumonitis or encephalopathy. As an approximate guide, toxicity risk is increased with methotrexate levels greater than 5–10 μmol/L at 24 h, greater than 1 μmol/L at 48 h and greater than 0.1 μmol/L at 72 h after administration [9].

Preventative measures include stopping drugs that can increase methotrexate toxicity (e.g. trimethoprim, trimethoprim–sulphamethoxazole, proton pump inhibitors, NSAIDS or penicillins), dose modification for pre-existing renal impairment, aggressive hydration to maintain urine output and urinary alkalinization with sodium bicarbonate (usually to maintain urine pH ≥7.0), which improves methotrexate solubility. Folinic acid (leucovorin) rescue counteracts methotrexate and is introduced 24–36h after methotrexate. Urinary pH, renal function, urine output and methotrexate plasma levels are then monitored, and treatment continues until plasma methotrexate levels are reduced (usually to <0.1 µmol/L). Severe renal toxicity can sometimes occur despite all these measures.

Management

• Patients with delayed methotrexate elimination have been managed successfully by increasing the dose and/or frequency of folinic acid rescue and with careful adjustment of fluid balance and alkalinization.

• If, despite these measures, there is a toxic plasma methotrexate level resulting from delayed clearance in a patient with deteriorating renal function (e.g. serum creatinine ≥1.5 times upper limit of normal (ULN) or oliguria), consider treatment with glucarpidase. Glucarpidase is a recombinant bacterial carboxypeptidase enzyme that converts methotrexate to inactive metabolites. In clinical studies, a median 97–99% reduction in plasma methotrexate is achieved within 15min. This response is often sustained, but this is less likely when pretreatment methotrexate levels are greater than 50 µmol/L. Methotrexate levels should be monitored, and further treatment may be required. Glucarpidase was licensed in the USA in 2012 but is currently an unlicensed orphan medicine in the UK. The recommended dose is 50 U/kg intravenous injection over 5min. Leucovorin is a substrate and should be avoided for 2h before or after glucarpidase. Methotrexate levels should only be measured by a chromogenic assay for 48h after administration of glucarpidase (metabolites can lead to an overestimate of methotrexate level when using immunoassays).

• In patients with renal failure, haemodialysis or haemofiltration can be used to reduce the plasma methotrexate concentration (haemodialysis with a high-flux dialyzer appears most effective). However, the plasma methotrexate level rebounds following dialysis, which limits its usefulness.

Inadvertent administration of intrathecal vincristine

Bolus intravenous vincristine is widely used as part of combination chemotherapy for lymphoma, leukaemia and solid organ malignancies. Over 60 cases of inadvertent administration of intrathecal vincristine have been reported and show that this is usually a fatal event. Vincristine binds tubulin, forming neurofilament aggregates and results in an ascending radiculomyeloencephalopathy. Initial neurological effects are in the lower limbs followed by autonomic dysfunction (e.g. constipation, abdominal pain or difficulty with micturition), progressing to respiratory failure and death within days or weeks [10]. Management recommendations are based on six surviving patients where treatment was immediately started. Surviving patients had paraparesis or tetraparesis, and all hospitals administering intrathecal chemotherapy must have a policy outlining the steps required to ensure safe practice and prevention of such a tragic error.

Management [11]

The following treatment should be initiated immediately after the injection:

1 Remove as much CSF as is safely possible through the lumbar access.

2 Insert an epidural catheter into the subarachnoid space via the intervertebral space above the initial lumbar access and commence CSF irrigation with lactated Ringer's solution. Fresh frozen plasma should be requested, and when available, 25 mL should be added to every 1 L of lactated Ringer's solution.

3 Urgent insertion of an intraventricular drain or catheter by a neurosurgeon (keep patient fasted for theatre and sat upright) and continuation of CSF irrigation with fluid removal through the lumbar access connected to a closed drainage system. Lactated Ringer's solution should be given by continuous infusion at 150 mL/h or at a rate of 75 mL/h after the fresh frozen plasma has been added.

The rate of infusion should be adjusted to maintain a spinal fluid protein level of 150 mg/dL. Supportive care should be provided in a high dependency environment.

The following measures have also been used in addition although their roles in the reduction of neurotoxicity are not clear:

• Folinic acid has been administered intravenously as a 100 mg bolus and then infused at a rate of 25 mg/h for 24 h and then bolus doses of 25 mg 6 hourly for 1 week.

• Intravenous administration of glutamic acid 10 g over 24 h, followed by 500 mg three times daily by mouth for 1 month.

• Pyridoxine has been given at a dose of 50 mg 8 hourly by intravenous infusion over 30 min.

Lymphoma involving the pericardium

Although primary cardiac lymphomas occur, involvement most commonly arises from direct extension of systemic disease such as high-grade B-cell lymphoma. The differential diagnosis of an effusion in patients with haematological malignancy would include:
• Infection (e.g. viral, bacterial including mycobacteria, fungus)
• Kaposi's sarcoma (in HIV patients)
• Uraemia (if renal failure)
• Radiation (if recent mediastinal radiotherapy)
• Drugs (e.g. imatinib)

Symptoms of pericardial effusion include dyspnoea and chest discomfort. Symptoms can be of abrupt onset when increased pericardial pressures lead to impaired ventricular filling and falling cardiac output (cardiac tamponade). Tachycardia is common; pulsus paradoxus is present in about 30% of patients, and Beck's triad of hypotension, raised jugular venous pressure and decreased heart sounds may be present in tamponade [6].

Investigation and management
Electrocardiography may show low-voltage waveforms and electrical alternans; chest XR may show an increased transverse cardiac diameter (water-bottle heart). Echocardiogram is the imaging method of choice to define its size, position and haemodynamic significance. The classical picture is of right ventricular collapse in early diastole. Patients with a large or symptomatic effusion will require echocardiogram-guided pericardiocentesis, which can be an emergency bedside intervention for tamponade. Insertion of an indwelling drainage catheter could be considered at pericardiocentesis to prevent re-accumulation.

When the pericardial effusion is the presenting feature of a suspected haematological malignancy, standard investigations would include a staging CT and consideration of a lymph node or bone marrow biopsy. Pericardial fluid can be sent for cytology, flow cytometry, microscopy and culture. Pericardial biopsy may be required.

Consider peripheral blood testing for HIV, troponin, inflammatory markers and blood cultures if pyrexial.

Patients with recurrent effusions may require surgical intervention, but post-operative paradoxical haemodynamic instability has been reported, requiring intensive care support for vasopressor-dependent hypotension. Definitive therapy for the underlying malignancy must also be considered to prevent progression or recurrence.

References

1 Howard SC, Jones DP, Pui CH. The tumor lysis syndrome. N Engl J Med 2011;364(19):1844–54.
2 Cairo MS, Bishop M. Tumour lysis syndrome: new therapeutic strategies and classification. Br J Haematol 2004;127(1):3–11.
3 Cairo MS, Coiffier B, Reiter A, Younes A. Recommendations for the evaluation of risk and prophylaxis of tumour lysis syndrome (TLS) in adults and children with malignant diseases: an expert TLS panel consensus. Br J Haematol 2010;149(4):578–86.
4 Coiffier B, Altman A, Pui CH, Younes A, Cairo MS. Guidelines for the management of pediatric and adult tumor lysis syndrome: an evidence-based review. J Clin Oncol 2008;26(16):2767–78.
5 Lepper PM, Ott SR, Hoppe H et al. Superior vena cava syndrome in thoracic malignancies. Respir Care 2011;56(5):653–66.
6 McCurdy MT, Shanholtz CB. Oncologic emergencies. Crit Care Med 2012;40(7):2212–22.
7 Abid SH, Malhotra V, Perry MC. Radiation-induced and chemotherapy-induced pulmonary injury. Curr Opin Oncol 2001;13(4):242–8.
8 O'Driscoll BR, Howard LS, Davison AG. BTS guideline for emergency oxygen use in adult patients. Thorax 2008;63(Suppl. 6):vi1–68.
9 Widemann BC, Adamson PC. Understanding and managing methotrexate nephrotoxicity. Oncologist 2006;11(6):694–703.
10 Reddy GK, Brown B, Nanda A. Fatal consequences of a simple mistake: how can a patient be saved from inadvertent intrathecal vincristine? Clin Neurol Neurosurg 2011;113(1):68–71.
11 Hospira UK Ltd. Summary of Product Characteristics. Summary of Product Characteristics May 7, 2009 [cited March 20, 2013]; http://www.medicines.org.uk/EMC/searchresults.aspx?term=Vincristine&searchtype=QuickSearch (accessed on November 21, 2013).

APPENDIX A

Adult, Paediatric and Neonatal Haematology Reference Intervals

Quentin A. Hill

Department of Haematology, Leeds Teaching Hospitals NHS Trust, Leeds, UK

In order to understand a laboratory value, the reference interval (previously *normal values* or *normal range*) for healthy individuals is required. Some haematological values in healthy individuals vary depending on age, gender and ethnicity. Further variation can occur at a local level due to differences in the analytical process as well as collection, transport and storage of specimens. For these reasons, local reference intervals should always be used where available. However, local reference intervals are sometimes difficult to achieve, for example, with neonates, where even published data has limited sample size, which can affect the precision of the reference limits.

The intervals provided in Tables A.1–9 are therefore only a guide to values expected in healthy individuals.

Reference intervals are typically based on the mean value ±2 standard deviations, thereby encompassing 95% of the reference (healthy) population. As well as recognizing that some healthy individuals will have values outside the reference interval, clinical context is essential to interpret results. For example, varying degrees of left shift on the blood film is a *normal* physiological response to severe sepsis, pregnancy or administration of growth factors but in a different context may be the presenting feature of a bone marrow disorder.

Haematology in Critical Care: A Practical Handbook, First Edition. Edited by Jecko Thachil and Quentin A. Hill.
© 2014 John Wiley & Sons, Ltd. Published 2014 by John Wiley & Sons, Ltd.

Adult reference intervals

Table A.1 Adult values for the full blood count, haematinics and common tests of coagulation.

	Male and female	Male	Female
Haemoglobin (g/L)		135–180	115–160
PCV (haematocrit)		0.40–0.52 (40–52%)	0.37–0.47 (37–47%)
MCV (fL)	78–100		
MCH (pg)	27–32		
White cells (×10^9/L)			
Total	4–11		
Neutrophils	2.0–7.5		
Lymphocytes	1.0–4.5		
Monocytes	0.2–0.8		
Eosinophils	0.04–0.4		
Basophils	<0.1		
Platelets (×10^9/L)	150–400		
Reticulocyte count (%)	0.8–1.8		
Ferritin (serum) (µg/L)	10–322		
Vitamin B12 (ng/L)	211–911		
Folate (serum) (µg/L)	5.4–24		
PT (s)	9–14		
APTT (s)	23.5–37.5		
APTT ratio	0.8–1.2		
Derived fibrinogen (g/L)	1.6–5.9		
Clauss fibrinogen (g/L)	1.3–5.0		
Thrombin time (s)	10–18		

Source: Local reference intervals at Leeds Teaching Hospitals NHS Trust, September 2013. Reproduced with permission of Dr Mike Bosomworth, Head of Blood Sciences. Copyright Leeds Teaching Hospitals NHS Trust.
MCV, mean corpuscular volume; MCH, mean corpuscular haemoglobin; PCV, packed cell volume; PT, prothrombin time; APTT, activated partial thromboplastin time.

Table A.2 Adult normal ranges for various haemostatic and anticoagulant factors.

Test	Method	Range	No. of subjects
Bleeding disorders			
FVIII:C	One stage assay	58–209 IU/dL	25–30
VWF:Ag	ELISA	46–146 IU/dL	25–30
VWF:Rco	Visual Agglutination	50–172 IU/dL	25–30
FIX	APTT based	62–144 IU/dL	25–30
FII	PT-based	84–132 IU/dL	25–30
FV	PT-based	66–126 U/dL	25–30
FVII	PT-based	61–157 IU/dL	25–30
FX	PT-based	74–149 IU/dL	25–30
FXI	APTT-based	60–150 U/dL	25–30
FXII	APTT-based	50–180 U/dL	25–30
FXIII	Pentapharm assay	59–163 U/dL	20
α_2-Antiplasmin	Chromogenic	67–103 U/dL	20
Thrombotic disorders			
Antithrombin activity	Chromogenic	85–131 IU/dL	80
Antithrombin antigen	ELISA	83–124 IU/dL	30
Protein C activity	Chromogenic	79–142 IU/dL	80
Protein C antigen	ELISA	75–131 IU/dL	25–30
Protein S total	ELISA	71–136 IU/dL	80
Protein S free	Latex	Males 74–143 IU/dL	40
		Females 67–125 IU/dL	40

Source: Local normal ranges from the Royal Hallamshire Hospital, Sheffield, Key et al. [1]. Reproduced with permission of John Wiley & Sons, Ltd.

Paediatric and neonatal reference intervals

Table A.3 Normal blood count values from birth to 18 years.

Age	Haemoglobin (g/dL)	RBC (×10^{12}/L)	Haematocrit	MCV (fL)	WBC (×10^9/L)	Neutrophils (×10^9/L)	Lymphocytes (×10^9/L)	Monocytes (×10^9/L)	Eosinophils (×10^9/L)	Basophils (×10^9/L)	Platelets (×10^9/L)
Birth (term Infants)	14.9–23.7	3.7–6.5	0.47–0.75	100–125	10–26	2.7–14.4	2.0–7.3	0–1.9	0–0.85	0–0.1	150–450
2 weeks	13.4–19.8	3.9–5.9	0.41–0.65	88–110	6–21	1.5–5.4	2.8–9.1	0.1–1.7	0–0.85	0–0.1	170–500
2 months	9.4–13.0	3.1–4.3	0.28–0.42	84–98	5–15	0.7–4.8	3.3–10.3	0.4–1.2	0.05–0.9	0.02–0.13	210–650
6 months	10.0–13.0	3.8–4.9	0.3–0.38	73–84	6–17	1–6	3.3–11.5	0.2–1.3	0.1–1.1	0.02–02	210–560
1 year	10.1–13.0	3.9–5.1	0.3–0.38	70–82	6–16	1–8	3.4–10.5	0.2–0.9	0.05–0.9	0.02–0.13	200–550
2–6 years	11.0–13.8	3.9–5.0	0.32–0.4	72–87	6–17	1.5–8.5	1.8–8.4	0.15–1.3	0.05–1.1	0.02–0.12	210–490
6–12 years	11.1–14.7	3.9–5.2	0.32–0.43	76–90	4.5–14.5	1.5–8.0	1.5–5.0	0.15–1.3	0.05–1.0	0.02–0.12	170–450
12–18 years											
Female	12.1–15.1	4.1–5.1	0.35–0.44	77–94							
Male	12.1–16.6	4.2–5.6	0.35–0.49	77–92	4.5–13	1.5–6	1.5–4.5	0.15–1.3	0.05–0.8	0.02–0.12	180–430

Source: Arceci et al. [2]. Reproduced with permission of John Wiley & Sons, Ltd.
Red cell values at birth derived from skin puncture blood; most other data from venous blood.
MCV, mean corpuscular volume; RBC, red blood cell; WBC, white blood cell.

Table A.4 Red blood cell (RBC) values (mean ± 1 SD) on the first postnatal day from 24 weeks' gestational age.

Gestational age (weeks)	24–25 (n=7)	26–27 (n=11)	28–29 (n=7)	30–31 (n=35)	32–33 (n=23)	34–35 (n=23)	36–37 (n=20)	Term (n=19)
RBC (×10^{12}/L)	4.65±0.43	4.73±0.45	4.62±0.75	4.79±0.74	5.0±0.76	5.09±0.5	5.27±0.68	5.14±0.7
Haemoglobin (g/dL)	19.4±1.5	19.0±2.5	19.3±1.8	19.1±2.2	18.5±2.0	19.6±2.1	19.2±11.7	19.3±2.2
Haematocrit	0.63±0.04	0.62±0.08	0.60±0.07	0.60±0.08	0.60±0.08	0.61±0.07	0.64±0.07	0.61±0.074
MCV (fL)	135±0.2	132±14.4	131±13.5	127±12.7	123±15.7	122±10.0	121±12.5	119±9.4
Reticulocytes	6.0±0.5	9.6±3.2	7.5±2.5	5.8±2.0	5.0±1.9	3.9±1.6	4.2±1.8	3.2±1.4
Weight (g)	725±185	993±194	1174±128	1450±232	1816±192	1957±291	2245±213	

Source: Zaizov and Matoth [3]. Reproduced with permission of John Wiley & Sons, Ltd.
Counts performed on heel-prick blood. MCV, mean corpuscular volume.

Table A.5 Haemoglobin values (g/dL, median and 95% range) in the first 6 months of life in iron-sufficient (serum ferritin ≥10 µg/L) preterm infants.

	Birthweight		Birthweight	
Age	1000–1500 g	Number tested	1501–2000 g	Number tested
2 weeks	16.3 (11.7–18.4)	17	14.8 (11.8–19.6)	39
1 month	10.9 (8.7–15.2)	15	11.5 (8.2–15.0)	42
2 months	8.8 (7.1–11.5)	17	9.4 (8.0–11.4)	47
3 months	9.8 (8.9–11.2)	16	10.2 (9.3–11.8)	41
4 months	11.3 (9.1–13.1)	13	11.3 (9.1–13.1)	37
5 months	11.6 (10.2–14.3)	8	11.8 (10.4–13.0)	21
6 months	12.0 (9.4–13.8)	9	11.8 (10.7–12.6)	21

Source: Lundström et al. [4]. Reproduced with permission of Elsevier.
All infants had an uncomplicated course in the first 2 weeks of life, and none received exchange transfusion.
Counts obtained from venous and skin puncture blood.

Table A.6 Values for mature and immature neutrophils and the ratio of immature to total neutrophils in 24 infants <33 weeks gestation.

	Mature neutrophils (×10⁹/L)		Immature neutrophils (×10⁹/L)		Immature : total ratio	
Age (h)	Median (range)	Mean	Median (range)	Mean	Median (range)	Mean
1 (n = 10)	4.64 (2.20–8.18)	4.57	0.11 (0–1.5)	0.30	0.04 (0–0.35)	0.09
12 (n = 17)	6.80 (4.0–22.48)	8.61	0.27 (0–1.6)	0.48	0.04 (0–0.21)	0.06
24 (n = 17)	5.60 (2.61–21.20)	7.64	0.14 (0–3.66)	0.47	0.03 (0–0.17)	0.05
48 (n = 20)	4.98 (1.02–14.43)	6.24	0.13 (0–2.15)	0.44	0.02 (0–0.17)	0.05
72 (n = 22)	3.19 (1.28–13.94)	4.63	0.16 (0–2.42)	0.38	0.3 (0–0.25)	0.05
96 (n = 21)	3.44 (1.37–16.56)	5.33	0.23 (0–3.95)	0.45	0.05 (0–0.37)	0.07
120 (n = 17)	3.46 (1.27–15.00)	4.98	0.25 (0–2.89)	0.44	0.05 (0–0.21)	0.07

Source: Adapted from Lloyd and Oto [5]. Reproduced with permission of BMJ Publishing Group.

Table A.7 Normal limits of the immature: total and immature: segmented granulocyte ratios in healthy neonates

	Day 1	Day 7	Day 28
Immature : total	0.16	0.12	0.12
Immature : total (African)	0.22	0.21	0.18
Immature : segmented	0.3 (neonatal period)		

Source: Arceci et al. [2]. Reproduced with permission of John Wiley & Sons, Ltd.

Table A.8 Mean and range of values for neutrophils, band forms and lymphocytes (×10⁹/L) in African neonates.

	Day 1	Day 7	Day 28
Neutrophils	5.67 (0.98–12.9)	2.01 (0.57–6.5)	1.67 (0.65–3.2)
Band forms	1.16 (0.16–2.3)	0.55 (0–1.5)	0.36 (0–0.39)
Lymphocytes	5.10 (1.4–8.0)	5.63 (2.2–15.5)	6.55 (3.2–9.9)

Source: Summarized from Scott-Emuakpor et al. [6]. Reproduced with permission of John Wiley & Sons, Ltd.
Data based on 100-cell differential count. Pooled data on preterm, term and post-term neonates as no statistical difference between the mean values of these groups.

Table A.9 Reticulocyte counts (×10⁹/L) in the first year of life in term infants

Age	Reticulocytes
1 day	110–450
7 days	10–80
1 month	10–65
2 months	45–210
5 months	30–120
12 months	40–140

Source: Arceci et al. [2]. Reproduced with permission of John Wiley & Sons, Ltd.

References

1 Key N, Roberts HR, Makris M, O'Shaughnessy D, Lillicrap D (eds.). Practical Hemostasis and Thrombosis second edition. Oxford: John Wiley & Sons, Ltd; 2009. Reproduced with permission of John Wiley & Sons, Ltd.

2 Arceci RJ, Hann IM, Smith OP (eds.). Pediatric Hematology. 3rd edition. Oxford: John Wiley & Sons, Ltd; 2006. Reproduced with permission of John Wiley & Sons, Ltd.

3 Zaizov R, Matoth Y. Red cell values on the first postnatal day during the last 16 weeks of gestation. Am J Hematol 1976;1(2):275–8.

4 Lundström U, Siimes MA, Dallman PR. At what age does iron supplementation become necessary in low-birth-weight infants? J Pediatr 1977;91(6):878–83.

5 Lloyd BW, Oto A. Normal values for mature and immature neutrophils in very preterm babies. Arch Dis Child 1982; 57(3):233–5. BMJ Publishing Group. http://adc.bmj.com/content/57/3/233.full.pdf+html (accessed on November 22, 2013).

6 Scott-Emuakpor AB, Okolo AA, Ukpe SI. Pattern of leukocytes in the blood of healthy African neonates. Acta Haemat. 1985;74:104–7.

Index

Haematology in Critical Care: A Practical Handbook, First Edition. Edited by Jecko Thachil and Quentin A. Hill.
© 2014 John Wiley & Sons, Ltd. Published 2014 by John Wiley & Sons, Ltd.